The Stored Tissue Issue

The Stored Tissue Issue

Biomedical Research, Ethics, and Law in the Era of Genomic Medicine

ROBERT F. WEIR
ROBERT S. OLICK

WITH JEFFREY C. MURRAY

UNIVERSITY PRESS

2004

OXFORD
UNIVERSITY PRESS

Oxford   New York
Auckland   Bangkok   Buenos Aires   Cape Town   Chennai
Dar es Salaam   Delhi   Hong Kong   Istanbul   Karachi   Kolkata
Kuala Lumpur   Madrid   Melbourne   Mexico City   Mumbai   Nairobi
São Paulo   Shanghai   Taipei   Tokyo   Toronto

Published by Oxford University Press, Inc.
198 Madison Avenue, New York, New York 10016
www.oup.com

Oxford is a registered trademark of Oxford University Press

Library of Congress Cataloging-in-Publication Data
Weir, Robert F., 1943-
The stored tissue issue : biomedical research, ethics, and law in
the era of genomic medicine/
by Robert F. Weir, Robert S., Robert S. Olick, with Jeffrey C. Murray.
p. cm.   Includes bibliographical references and index.
ISBN 0-19-512368-9
1. Preservation of organs, tissues, etc.–Moral and ethical aspects.
I. Olick, Robert S.
II. Murray, Jeffrey C.
III. Title.
RD127.W45 2004   174′.29–dc22   2003190051

9 8 7 6 5 4 3 2 1

Printed in the United States of America
on acid-free paper

To Brooke and Berkeley
RFW

To Sarah, Stephen, and Grant
RSO

Preface

A few years ago we agreed that the professional and scholarly literature on "the stored tissue issue" too frequently takes an adversarial, almost combative approach. Commonly, biomedical investigators are pitted against research participants, bioethicists, health-law attorneys, and anyone else who raises questions about traditional research practices.

We decided to follow a different path, in part because everyone has a stake in the conduct and achievements of biomedical research. Yet we did not want to minimize the competing interests that make this issue controversial or to underplay the important changes that need to take place in some research practices. Rather, we set out to write a multidisciplinary analysis of this complex subject that offers, we hope, a reasonably balanced approach to a highly charged issue and a set of recommendations that make good sense.

Premises

The approach we take in this book reflects five premises regarding biomedical research with human tissues. These premises are recurring themes of the book and are the foundation on which our substantive points, critiques, arguments, and recommendations are based.

Gift and Gratitude. All of us are beneficiaries of modern biomedical research, in terms of both past, present, and future scientific discoveries and medical advances and the voluntary participation in research studies by innumerable persons worldwide. Many of these studies, of course, use various human tissues obtained from individuals. Much of this collaborative research process depends on gifts and gift giving. On one side of this process, countless persons voluntarily give of themselves, literally, by permitting various tissues to be taken from their bodies for diagnostic, therapeutic, and research purposes, even though in research settings they often know that they will not benefit personally from the research done with the tissues. On the other side of this process, countless biomedical professionals also give of themselves by using their knowledge, skills, time, energy, and technological equipment to discover new knowledge about the human genome, the wonders and complexities of human existence, and effective medical interventions that will improve the health and lives of many persons in each passing human generation.

The appropriate response to this mutual gift giving is gratitude, even if some of the "gifts" for research are obtained under questionable conditions. That gratitude properly goes in two directions: gratitude to the persons in all countries who have voluntarily permitted tissues to be obtained from their bodies and used for scientific and medical purposes and gratitude to all the biomedical professionals who have worked and continue to work diligently to increase our knowledge about who we are, at least scientifically, and to improve our individual lives through better health and health care.

The theme of gift and gratitude has to be qualified in one important way. Participants in human tissue research studies—the individual sources of subsequently banked DNA samples—cannot all be correctly grouped together as gift-giving "donors" to biomedical research. Many of these participants—those who are patients—can form no donative intent because they are often unaware that their tissue samples may end up being used in research studies. Unlike individuals who make decisions to donate their usable solid organs and tissues to others at the time of death, and unlike persons who donate their bodies, if later usable as cadavers, to medical schools for anatomical teaching and research purposes, many patients are apparently unknowing gift givers because they are unaware that their tissues, obtained for diagnostic and therapeutic purposes, may subsequently also be used for research purposes. In addition, patients sometimes may have a vague idea that their tissues may later become research material (and they may have signed a general consent document to that effect), but they are not aware of any specific research plan, or even a range of possibilities for the research studies in which their samples may later be used.

Mutual Respect. The appropriate relationship between individuals who participate in collaborative research studies and biomedical professionals who conduct those research studies is one of mutual respect. For that reason, we do not use the language of "subjects" in this book to denote the individuals, families, and groups who participate, either voluntarily or involuntarily, in biomedical research studies, even though we know that this language is the language of the federal regulations and is widely used by scientific investigators. We believe that the use of this term—commonly intended by scientists and others to be merely descriptive—runs the risk of being subordinative, demeaning, and disrespectful toward other persons, especially since the same language is often used indiscriminately by scientific investigators to refer to all animals used in research studies, whether they are humans, chimpanzees, dogs, mice, or other animals. We will, instead, refer to human "participants" in research studies.[1]

Even as we raise many ethical questions about the way some human tissue research is done, we do not question the integrity of individual investigators or the collective motives of members of professional research-oriented societies. Yet we have no doubt that ethical mistakes have been made by some investigators, that some widely accepted research practices violate the moral and legal rights of research participants, and that the unprecedented commercial possibilities of some current research in genetics and other biomedical fields pose unprecedented ethical challenges to scientific investigators (and, indirectly, to the rest of us). We are also convinced that it is necessary to make some changes in the ways human tissue research is done, not only to protect the individuals and groups who participate via their stored tissues in these research studies but also to preserve the respect that vast numbers of persons still have for the biomedical research enterprise and the scientists who carry out the research.

The Need for Critique. We believe that research with human tissues is essential for the ongoing improvement of human health. We also believe that the international debate that emerged in the 1990s—and continues to this day—about common research practices with stored tissues and the risks these practices pose to some individuals, families, and groups has the possibility of producing positive change in the way that human tissue research is done worldwide. We have been participants in this debate, and we hope this book is a major contribution to it. For that reason, even as we affirm our ongoing support for biomedical research, we will devote much of this book to a critique of some tissue-based research practices, several ethically problematic cases, and some institutional and federal policies that support these practices. We will also make a number of recommendations for change and improvement along the way.

The Need for Choice and Protection. Unfortunately, the achievements and benefits gained through biomedical research sometimes come at a substantial price: ignoring the rights and needs of research participants to exercise informed choice, to avoid having personally objectionable research done with their tissue samples, and to take preventive steps to protect themselves, their families, and the ethnic, racial, or cultural groups with whom they identify from having genetic information about them get in the wrong hands. This problem takes many forms and occurs in many places. Sometimes the problem occurs because of inadequate disclosures about DNA banking practices in research consent documents, even with approval of the documents by Institutional Review Boards (IRBs). Sometimes the problem occurs in hospital and clinical settings because of inadequate disclosures in admissions forms and by physician-investigators regarding the possibilities of post-diagnostic research and secondary research. Sometimes the problem occurs in isolated parts of the globe when geneticists and other biomedical investigators provide inadequate disclosures to indigenous groups about planned research with their tissues and possible profits from that research. These failures of disclosure may be the result of carelessness, lack of knowledge or insight, or, occasionally, the misguided belief that "what they don't know won't hurt them."

We all want to benefit personally—and we want our children and succeeding generations to benefit—from the yet-to-be-discovered knowledge that is possible through scientific research. But achieving that success at the cost of ignoring or sacrificing basic rights is too great a price to pay. For that reason, much of this book will focus on informed consent, the right of persons to express choice and have that choice honored, concerns about possible genetic discrimination against individuals/families/groups, the rights of individuals and indigenous populations to protect their DNA and the genetic information imbedded in it, and related matters of concern that have been voiced in recent years by many people in many countries. In short, we agree with the statement made by a committee of the Health Council of the Netherlands: it is important for persons to "have a say in what happens" with tissues removed from their bodies for diagnostic, therapeutic, and research reasons.[2] Having a say is of critical importance even if, as is usually the case, genetics research poses no meaningful threat of physical harm to participants.

The Need for Greater Public Awareness and Support. Most multidisciplinary committees and commissions worldwide that have analyzed this issue have expressed the hope for greater public awareness and support of human tissue research. We agree, and we think that the best way to improve public support and secure better funding for biomedical research is by greater disclosure about the purposes, processes, and procedures of this research. It is time, given both the scientific possibilities and psychosocial risks in the era of genomic medicine, for scientists, physicians, and other health-care professionals to make substantial improvements in their research-related consent documents, brochures, videos, Web sites, and other methods of communicating with the people on whom their professional work depends. It is time for scientific investigators to provide more information about their common, everyday practices in working with human tissues—about which the general public knows very little. We will discuss several studies of public attitudes about research with stored tissues that support this view.

Greater disclosure should occur in multiple ways and should address how human tissues are obtained, the scientific purposes for which they are collected, why they are stored in laboratories for years, the reasons why they are sometimes coded and other times anonymized, the ways in which they are shared with other investigators around the globe, why some scientific studies need tissue samples from thousands of individuals, the possible psychosocial risks for participants in tissue-based research, and other concerns. This greater disclosure may be costly to scientific investigators and their research teams in terms of extra time, effort, and expended funds. But these costs will be outweighed by greater gains in public awareness and support, enhanced appreciation for human tissue research and the work done by investigators and their multidisciplinary teams, and, we hope, increased funding for biomedical research. The alternative is unacceptable: "A continued escalation of individual concerns surrounding the research use of human tissue could begin to erode the trust that is the foundation of the patient-physician and participant-researcher relationships."[3]

Organization of This Book

This book is divided into three parts. Part I focuses on the transition from decades of unquestioned research practices in the biomedical sciences to an ongoing, international controversy about research with stored tissue samples. In Chapter 1 we describe and analyze three paradigm and problematic cases we call John Moore, NHANES III, and DeCODE Genetics. Chapter 2 provides a description of the available information regarding stored tissues in the United States, several surveys of public opinion about genetics research, the multidisciplinary literature on genetic privacy and genetic discrimination, and some relevant concerns of research scientists. Chapter 3 contains a descriptive interpretation of the initial period of this controversy in the United States. We discuss several competing positions developed by some leading health-law attorneys, a number of biomedical organizations, and a multidisciplinary task force assembled by the National Institutes of Medicine. Chapter 4 indicates why the field of molecular genetics has a particularly significant role in this debate about research, rights, and rewards. We discuss a variety of topics relevant to the DNA banking practices common to genetics laboratories: biological sampling methods, the several types of stored human tissue, the types of information contained in tissue samples, techniques used for anonymizing samples, DNA sequence storage, and new technologies for DNA research.

Part II analyzes current laws and policies in the United States, as well as the recommendations made by multidisciplinary committees in several other countries. Chapter 5 focuses on recommendations made by distinguished panels of experts in the Netherlands, England, Canada, the Council of Europe, and the Human

Genome Organization. In Chapter 6 we give a summary and assessment of the federal policies governing human tissue research in the United States. Then in Chapter 7 we expand on our discussion of the John Moore case and also survey the current legal landscape in the United States concerning matters of ownership and control of body parts, patenting biological sequences, genetic privacy and discrimination, and other topics pertinent to an understanding of the larger legal framework for human tissue research. Chapter 8 discusses the National Bioethics Advisory Commission report on research with stored biological samples, the most comprehensive analysis of this topic yet provided to or by the federal government.

Part III deals with the ethical, professional, and legal implications of current research practices with stored tissues. Chapter 9 provides a comprehensive analysis of the need to update the process of informed consent so that research participants and patients will have more knowledge about research practices commonly used with stored tissues—and more opportunities to communicate their preferences and choices regarding how their tissue samples may be used in research. In Chapter 10 we move beyond informed consent to discuss a variety of other ethical and legal implications of human tissue research. The book concludes with Chapter 11, where we propose an agenda for the near future consisting of a number of recommendations that we believe will, if carried out in practice, improve public understanding of, participation in, and support for research done with banked DNA samples.

Notes

1. The authors of a recent Institute of Medicine (IOM) report on IRBs also use this more respectful terminology. The IOM report, "Responsible Research: A Systems Approach to Protecting Research Participants," is available at http://www.iom.edu.
2. Health Council of the Netherlands, Committee on Human Tissue for Special Purposes, *Proper Use of Human Tissue* (The Hague: Health Council of the Netherlands, 1994), p. 31.
3. Ted Ashburn, Sharon Wilson, and Barry Eisenstein, "Human Tissue Research in the Genomic Era," *Arch Intern Med* 160 (2000): 3381.

Acknowledgments

We are thankful for many types of support we received while working on this book. More than anyone else, Jeff Murray, a pediatrician and geneticist, has been invaluable to our research efforts. From the beginning of our research to the writing of the last draft, Jeff has provided numerous comments, suggestions, and practical words of advice. He has helped us gain a better understanding of the work done by genetics investigators and their research teams by providing written descriptions of laboratory practices with stored tissues, copies of relevant papers in scientific journals we do not usually read, insightful observations about research studies being done worldwide, critiques of chapters, and an experienced understanding of the ethical problems inherent to human tissue studies. We could not have written this book without his many contributions along the way.

We are also thankful for the two universities that supported us during the process of research, writing, and revision. At the University of Iowa (UI), Robert Weir received a grant from the Obermann Center for Advanced Studies to co-direct (with Jeff Murray) a national, interdisciplinary faculty research seminar on the topic of this book. Seminar participants who made especially important contributions to our thinking about this issue were Jon Merz, Ken Kipnis, Amy Sparks, Bill Freeman, and Dorothy Vawter. In addition, the university granted Robert Weir a developmental leave to write portions of the book.

Both of us benefited from conversations about the ethical and legal aspects of this complex issue with our colleagues at Iowa in biomedical ethics and medical humanities, especially Kirk Payne, Lauris Kaldjian, Susan Lawrence, Susan Zickmund, and Cheryl Erwin. Later at the State University of New York, Upstate Medical University (SUNY Upstate), Robert Olick also benefited from thoughtful comments from colleagues in the Center for Bioethics and Humanities: Kathy Faber-Langendoen, Sam Gorovitz, and other members of the works-in-progress group.

Others helped us in a variety of ways. Dana Turkel, Bill Woodbury, and Ben Sodey provided Rob Olick with invaluable research assistance. Several persons in the UI Department of Pediatrics contributed material for the book: Shiva Patil, Kathy Mathews, Brian Schutte, and Judy Miller. Four members of the UI Department of Pathology helped Robert Weir have a better understanding of how tissue samples are stored, processed, and used in pathology labs: Michael Cohen, Robert Robinson, John Kemp, and Robert Folberg. Susan Johnson and Roger Williamson in the Department of Obstetrics and Gynecology also made helpful contributions to portions of the book, as did Trish Wasek, the Director of the UI Human Subjects Office. The photograph on the front cover was obtained with the help of Jeff Murray and Alexandre Vieira.

In addition, Vicki Hudachek spent countless days typing and proofreading multiple drafts and raising important questions about some of the wording of the manuscript. At Oxford University Press (OUP) Jeff House, as always, was insightful in his comments, helpful with his advice, gentle but persuasive in his few critical remarks about the manuscript, and patient in his willingness to wait while we dealt with several unavoidable delays during the process of writing. An anonymous reviewer for OUP was also very helpful in making some suggestions that greatly strengthened the book. Further, the professional editing and design skills of Lynda Crawford, Margery Heffron, and Eve Siegel at OUP improved our book in countless ways.

Robert Weir is especially indebted to Richard Caplan, now retired from the UI faculty, for many years of friendship, collaboration, and lively intellectual dialogue.

Finally, our thanks go to Jerry and Sally, our wives, who have been supportive of us and this book project in ways too numerous to count. The book is dedicated, respectively, to our granddaughters (RFW) and children (RSO).

Contents

Part III   Ethical, Professional, and Legal Implications

I

FROM UNQUESTIONED TRADITIONAL PRACTICES TO A CONTROVERSY ABOUT RESEARCH, RIGHTS, AND REWARDS

1

Unprecedented Cases, Debatable Changes, and New Challenges

> The conjunction of remarkable advancements in electronic information technology and basic biomedical research, especially in molecular genetics and genomics ... augers profound changes in the way that society will deal with the fundamental issues of health and disease in coming years. The changes, on balance, offer great promise of enhancing understanding, diagnosis, treatment and prevention of human diseases.... At the same time, however, the changes are generating deep public concerns that arise in part from philosophical and ethical considerations of individual autonomy and privacy and, in part, from pragmatic concerns about the security and confidentiality of sensitive, personally identifiable medical information, which, in the hands of insurers, employers and others, could be harmful to individuals and their families.
> American Association of Medical Colleges, 1997[1]

> We are not just talking about creating a market for Iceland's DNA. This isn't fish or lamb's wool we are dealing with here. This particular product is the spirit of the human species, and before Iceland turns its DNA into a commodity—and one that they may not even earn their fair share of money from—I just hope they know what they are doing.
> Henry T. Greely, 1999, Stanford University School of Law[2]

The importance of biomedical research with human tissue samples can hardly be doubted. Research using human tissues is one of the three legs on which modern medical progress stands. Along with research done with nonhuman animals (e.g., mice, dogs) and research done in chemistry and pharmaceuticals, research with tissue samples obtained from patients and research participants is essential to the success of modern medicine.

The funding for biomedical research by governments, pharmaceutical companies, biotechnology companies, and private organizations has recently increased significantly in many countries. Public funding for research in the United States may double over a five-year period. In the United States, the National Institutes of Health (NIH) now receives over $27 billion a year, and that money is used to

3

fund more than 36,000 research awards. Whenever NIH administrators make appeals for even more funding, they present as notable examples some of the recent achievements by investigators in molecular genetics, cancer research, and other fields of research using human tissues.[3] As another example, Britain also plans to significantly increase funding for scientific research, with projections of an $8.2 billion budget for science over a three-year period (2001–2004). By a substantial margin, the largest increase in the U.K. science budget is for genomics research.[4]

Numerous examples can be given of the ways that collecting, storing, and doing research with human tissues has benefited nearly everyone alive today, especially those of us living in industrialized, urbanized societies. All of us are beneficiaries of previous research done with stored tissues. Much of this research has, in fact, become such a common contributor to modern life and good health that many of us take it for granted. Thus, rather than provide a long list of scientific and medical achievements that benefit us all, we give but one example—blood banking—to illustrate both the importance and commonness of collecting, banking, and carrying out research studies with tissue samples.

The practice of collecting blood, banking blood samples of various types, and doing research with those samples has been around since early in the twentieth century. Several scientific discoveries early in the century made the practice possible and useful: the discovery of blood groups (A, B, and O), the identification of the Rh positive and negative groups, the development of blood-storage techniques (by adding sodium citrate to prevent blood coagulation), and the subsequent development of longer-term blood storage methods. Later discoveries led to the now-common practices of freezing components of blood (red blood cells, platelets, and plasma fractions) for a year or longer. The result has been a dramatic increase in blood banking. Since the first blood bank in the United States was opened in 1937, the practice of banking blood has increased to the point that there are now more than 2,200 institutions (e.g., blood banks, hospital transfusion services, research laboratories) affiliated with the American Association of Blood Banks.[5]

Several practices common to blood banks are also relevant to various aspects of the issues we address in this book. Blood banks have traditionally depended on volunteer donors, kept track of individual donors as well as the type of blood identified with those donors, and recontacted donors as needed to meet the occasional critical need for rare blood types. The anonymity of donors has therefore not been preserved, nor have blood samples been "anonymized" as they often are in other research settings; rather, blood banks have steadily improved the logistics of keeping in contact with donors. In addition, the administrators of blood banks have traditionally affirmed the importance of the process of informed consent by disclosing appropriate information to donors, having them sign one or more consent documents (e.g., for plateletpheresis), and, at least in some research-related blood banks, giving donors one or more options regarding the use of their blood or blood components for research purposes.

By contrast, other examples from the United States and elsewhere indicate that some biomedical research has been and is being conducted with blood and other stored tissue samples with insufficient attention to the process of informed consent, the choices of potential participants in research studies, and other ethical and legal concerns pertinent to human tissue research. Three such case studies—John Moore, NHANES III, and DeCODE Genetics, Inc.—illustrate some of the reasons for the ongoing international controversy over biomedical research with banked DNA samples.

The John Moore Case

John Moore was a harbinger of things to come. A resident of Seattle, he was in Alaska working on the Trans-Alaska pipeline in 1976 when he was diagnosed with hairy cell leukemia, a rare and potentially fatal type of cancer. Later that year, on the advice of his father, a physician in Southern California, he traveled to the UCLA Medical Center to have additional diagnostic tests performed. While hospitalized, he was a patient of David Golde, M.D., who confirmed the diagnosis of hairy cell leukemia using blood samples and some bone marrow tissue. Golde recommended that Moore undergo a splenectomy to slow down the progress of his disease and save his life. Moore signed a surgical consent document, and surgeons subsequently removed his abnormally large spleen (a surgical procedure no longer used for patients with hairy cell leukemia). Before the surgery, however, and undisclosed to Moore, Golde and Shirley Quan, Ph.D., a research colleague, already knew that "certain blood products and blood components were of great value in a number of commercial and scientific efforts"; that access to blood with these components would be scientifically important and commercially advantageous; and that they had made arrangements, without Moore's knowledge or consent, to have portions of his spleen taken to a research lab following the surgery.[6]

Moore returned to the UCLA Medical Center many times over the next seven years, convinced that the visits were necessary for his medical care. Each time, additional tissue samples were taken, ostensibly for diagnostic and therapeutic purposes: more blood, blood serum, and bone marrow aspirate, plus some skin and sperm. Unknown to Moore, in 1979 Golde and Quan established an immortalized cell line using Moore's T-lymphocytes. They also produced scientific publications based on their work with an "anonymous" cell line, applied with the Regents of the University of California for a patent on the cell line in 1981, and began to negotiate agreements for the commercial development of the cell line and products (e.g., lymphokines) to be derived from it. Biotechnology firms predicted a potential market for these products of more than $3 billion within a decade.

In 1983 Moore signed a second consent document, this time as a participant in a research study. On the form he explicitly refused to agree with a statement that would have granted the University of California "any and all rights I, or my heirs, may have in any cell line or any other potential product" which might be developed from the tissue samples obtained from me."[7] He also hired a law firm to investigate the facts in his case and any violation of his legal rights that might have occurred. In 1984 a patent was issued on the cell line, naming Golde and Quan as the inventors and the Regents as the assignee of the patent. That same year Moore, whose attorneys had read a description of the cell line (the "Mo" cell line from a Seattle patient) in a scientific paper by the investigators, brought suit against Golde, Quan, the Regents, and others. The 1990 decision of the California Supreme Court recognizing Moore's rights of informed consent but denying his claim of property rights to the cell line was a landmark decision, raising many of the issues that we will discuss in this book. A closer analysis of *Moore v. Regents of the University of California* is included in Chapter 7.

The NHANES III Study

The NHANES longitudinal study was also a harbinger of things to come. NHANES, the National Health and Nutrition Examination Survey, was a three-part series of medical and epidemiologic studies carried out by the Centers for Disease Control and Prevention (CDC). Since 1966, more than 85,000 persons have participated in the studies, including NHANES II in 1976–80 and NHANES III in 1988–94. The Hispanic Health and Nutrition Examination Survey, conducted in 1982–84, was a related but more focused CDC study. Most pertinent of all the studies to the topic of this book, NHANES III had multiple purposes: to provide a natural history of diseases in the population, give an accurate description of the diseases in the country, monitor changes in the health of the population, study the etiology of diseases, and establish empirical data for recommended changes in health policy. In contrast to the first two surveys, NHANES III was the only national survey in which physician examinations were performed to measure individuals' health. NHANES III was also different from the other two studies in that it took place well into the era of molecular genetics, so that genetic investigators and epidemiologists at the CDC were able to use scientific techniques with stored tissue samples that had not been possible in the earlier NHANES studies.

The NHANES III methodology involved identifying 40,000 noninstitutionalized persons from 81 counties in 26 states, with high sample rates for children aged 1 and older, racial minority groups, and older adults. These individuals were interviewed by CDC personnel regarding their nutrition practices, reproductive health, physical activity, mental health, and health habits. Most of them (29,314 persons of all races) were given extensive physical examinations with multiple lab tests of blood and urine, and they were explicitly promised a long-term follow-up; the NHANES III consent document stated that "after several years, we will check back with you to note any changes in your health."[8] Participants were also given home-study examinations regarding their socioeconomic status, demographic information, and environmental influences. Numerous publications from CDC investigators followed.[9] All the medical and health data were linked to other personal information to facilitate the multiple purposes of the study and to make long-term follow-up more valuable. By the mid-1990s, CDC scientists had also produced an archive of approximately 19,500 blood samples stored in liquid nitrogen and immortalized cell lines from approximately 8,500 participants.

To meet the ethical and legal requirements for informed consent, the NHANES III administrators, working with the Institutional Review Board (IRB) at the CDC, initially prepared a very detailed and technical statement on consent to be given to prospective participants in the study. Later judged to be too technically difficult, that document was replaced by a simple six-page booklet with descriptive text and pictures about NHANES III. The only language in the booklet pertaining to informed consent for banked samples is a one-sentence, descriptive statement: "A small sample of your blood will be kept in long-term storage for future testing."[10]

Very few of the adults who voluntarily participated in NHANES III probably remember reading that sentence. Presumably, very few paused to wonder about the implications it might have for them or, possibly, for their families. Likewise, very few parents, if any, who granted permission for their young children or adolescents to participate in the study probably gave much thought to the possible benefits or harms that might come to their children from later scientific studies done with their stored blood samples. The language of "DNA banking" was hardly commonplace at the time of this study. Few participants would have had reason to ask the CDC physicians, nurses, and scientists about that sentence.

Yet some CDC investigators were subsequently bothered by an important ethical problem. On the one hand, they possessed what they described as an invaluable "national treasure chest" of health information on a cross-section of the U.S. population and an unmatched archive of nationally representative DNA samples for biomedical research. On the other hand, they became concerned about the paucity of information they had provided the NHANES III participants about the possible research uses of their stored blood samples. The consent document had seemed satisfactory when it was developed in the 1980s. But Karen Steinberg, Ph.D., chief of a molecular biology branch at CDC, later observed, "I didn't think it was all right" for molecular research with DNA samples in the 1990s.[11] In light of the professional literature in the 1990s on molecular genetics and ethics, Steinberg and some of her CDC colleagues wondered whether they had adequately informed the sample population regarding the planned storage and scientific uses of their blood samples. They also wondered whether the persons in the study population had understood themselves to be consenting to long-term research on their banked blood samples and whether the CDC would perhaps need to get additional, more specific consent from these persons (the cost of "re-consenting" the participants was estimated at $2 million) before carrying out the planned research with the stored samples.

The *Moore* decision and NHANES III study illustrate some of the developments that have come about over the past two decades in terms of research on stored tissue samples. During this period, new techniques in molecular biology have transformed not only the life sciences, biomedical research, and clinical medicine, but also the traditional, unquestioned practices of storing blood by freezing it and storing portions of surgery-derived tissue in formalin-fixed containers and paraffin blocks in pathology laboratories. These practices have now been supplemented by new ways of storing an almost endless variety of human tissues for diagnostic and research purposes. Physicians and biomedical investigators in pathology, genetics, internal medicine, obstetrics and gynecology, pediatrics, psychiatry, anatomy, epidemiology, and numerous other fields frequently store tissue samples from patients and research participants (and tissue supply companies) in freezers, on slides, in wet tissue cultures, and in cylinders of liquid nitrogen for long periods of time; many of them also store DNA that has been extracted from tissue samples.

In academic medical institutions, these stored tissues are regularly used for diagnostic purposes, multiple kinds of educational sessions, numerous types of research, and sometimes for other purposes, such as the calibration of scientific machines. In addition, biomedical investigators routinely transform some banked biological materials into immortalized cell lines that can be kept indefinitely and shared with other scientists throughout the world in multiple research protocols. Outside academia, stored tissue samples (and extracted DNA) are used by commercial labs for diagnostic and research purposes, by the Federal Bureau of Investigation (FBI) and state departments of forensic sciences for the purposes of crime prevention and improved criminal prosecutions, and by the Department of Defense for the purpose of more accurate identification of dead bodies.

As the *Moore* decision and NHANES study indicate, however, the extraordinary achievements of biomedical researchers in the era of molecular biology have been accompanied by numerous ethical and legal questions. What are the interests and rights of the patients and research participants from whom the stored tissue samples come? As scientists supplement traditional, unquestioned research practices with new scientific methods, how important is it to replace the traditionally uninformed or minimally informed participation in research by persons in clinical and research settings with more substantive, more rigorous requirements regarding informed consent? How important is it to provide patients and research participants with more information about planned or possible research with *their to-be-stored tissue samples* so that they can *exercise choice about participating in the research* via their DNA samples?

In one important way, *Moore* and NHANES are similar: they clearly indicate the unprecedented possibilities for scientific success in the era of molecular genetics. Both involved gifted biomedical investigators intent on achieving important scientific goals that could only be accomplished by seizing an unusual opportunity for successful research with human tissue samples, with Moore's tissue samples (especially the spleen) being highly unusual themselves and the tissue samples in the NHANES study being unusual only because of the nationally representative population pool from which they came.

In other ways, the cases are significantly different. Moore's experience involved a patient who involuntarily became a participant in a research protocol; the NHANES case had thousands of persons who willingly participated in this national research study. The Moore case had a physician-investigator who deceived his patient, violated the requirements of informed consent, and later (after Moore refused to grant permission on the research consent form) sent Moore another research consent form with an attached request to "Please circle 'I do.'"[12] With NHANES, some CDC scientists were willing to postpone further research until troubling questions about informed consent had been satisfactorily answered. *Moore* was aberrant in that it had several interested parties pursuing the possibility of a huge monetary gain, whereas the research carried out in NHANES was more conventional, and not motivated, as far as we know, by the thought of great personal or institutional profit. *Moore* centered on legally significant questions of ownership and commercial rights connected with a cell line; NHANES has not been challenged or tested in court. One other important difference: we do not know what any of the more than 29,000 persons who participated in NHANES III thought about matters pertaining to the control and ownership of tissue samples and cell lines, but we do know what John Moore thinks.

> To learn that their position was that they owned a part of me.... I think demeaned is a good word.... I mean, by God, they thought so little of me. To learn all of a sudden, I was just a piece of material.... There was a sense of betrayal.... I mean, why didn't he just tell me? Why didn't he just discuss it with me?... To me, it was a total invasion of a person's right to control the use of their own genetic code, their own flesh and blood.... I certainly have no objection to scientific research but ... it was like rape. In a sense, you've been violated ... for dollars.[13]

Moore's comments will seem hyperbolic to some readers. The case itself can be interpreted in three quite different ways: *(1)* as an extreme example of a physician-investigator willing to ignore a patient's interests and rights for the sake of professional advancement and personal financial gain, *(2)* as an extreme example of an individual patient-research participant willing to jeopardize biomedical progress for his own ego and financial gain, or *(3)* as a highly unusual, but very important, example of the competing interests and rights in the ongoing controversy over research with stored tissues. We choose the third perspective.

For us, whatever one may think of the individuals involved, *Moore* was grounded in a number of important questions that persist today. We will discuss all of them in this book. The most significant of these questions are: Do physicians have a responsibility to inform patients that their tissue samples collected for diagnostic and therapeutic purposes (in this case, portions of spleen, and samples of blood, blood serum, and bone marrow aspirate) may later also be used for research purposes? If a physician knows that he or she plans to use a patient's tissue sample in a research protocol, should the patient be given that information before the sample is taken? If a biomedical investigator anticipates the possibility or likelihood of a patent application and commercial profit (both being unusual events), should the research participant from whom the sample originates be informed about these possibilities before the sample is obtained? Moreover, should the research participant be rewarded with a share of the profits realized from research done with his or her unusual tissue sample, even if the tissue is transformed through laboratory techniques into a permanently living cell line (e.g., the creation of lymphoblastoid cell lines by Epstein-Barr virus)? Or did the court correctly conclude that Moore did not retain any ownership interest in the biological materials (either the stored tissue samples or the cell line) he contributed?[14]

Likewise, NHANES III, as it was discussed in subsequent meetings at the CDC and the NIH in 1994–95, brought into sharp focus a number of important questions. Are there important scientific and ethical differences between research done on "existing" stored tissues, and planned research on human tissues not yet collected or stored? Should research on archival samples (e.g., tissue stored in paraffin blocks in pathology labs for years or dried neonatal blood spots stored for months or years) conform to current policies and recommendations regarding informed consent? If so, does that mean that scientific investigators, interested in doing potentially significant research on existing stored tissues for which there was inadequate informed consent earlier, must now either (a) go to the expense, logistical difficulties, and hassle of "re-consenting" the patients or research participants, if that is even possible, or (b) forgo the research? Or if not, does such research on archival specimens possibly escape the current requirements of informed consent, and therefore IRB review, because the federal regulations on research permit (1) IRB exemptions for some research on previously existing, truly anonymous samples, and (2) IRB waivers for studies of identifiable samples under certain conditions?

In subsequent NHANES studies and other prospective studies involving long-term research on banked tissue specimens from numerous participants, how specific and technical will the information in the consent document(s) need to be? If a proposed study is longitudinal in nature (e.g., population-based genetics or epidemiologic studies), how should investigators adequately inform potential research participants about the kinds of research that might be done on their stored tissue samples in the future? If the planned research is going to involve transforming tissue samples into cell lines, should potential research participants be informed in advance about the multiple research studies planned for the cell line(s)?

DeCODE Genetics

A third research study continues to raise important questions about research with stored tissue samples and offers some new twists regarding the rights of the persons from whom the tissues come and the rewards that may accompany the research.

Kari Stefansson, M.D., Dr. Med., a neuropathologist at Harvard Medical School, returned to his native Iceland in 1996 to launch a for-profit venture that combines several ingredients: the DNA of that remarkably homogeneous population, the laboratory techniques of molecular genetics, the compliance of the Icelandic Parliament, the public trust of the Icelandic population, and the investments of international biotechnology firms and pharmaceutical companies. With venture capital of $12 million from investors in the United States, Stefansson established DeCODE Genetics, Inc., a population-based genomics company in Reykjavik (but incorporated in the United States), founded on the principle that only a homogeneous population can quickly yield the genetic clues to the medical mysteries of common diseases.[15]

Iceland has such a population: 270,000 citizens in a country that has been largely isolated from the rest of the world for 1,100 years. Moreover, this population offers several other unusual advantages to scientific investigators: extensive computerized genealogical records going back 10 centuries, population-wide clinical records beginning with the national health service in 1915, a large human tissue bank dating from the 1940s, and an educated, largely cooperative population.[16]

Stefansson's goals are (1) to index the heredity of the entire nation of Iceland using a combination of stored blood samples, new blood samples, genealogical records, family histories, and centralized clinical records, and (2) to use this unique database to study the genetic causes of dozens of common diseases. To accomplish these goals, he helped sponsor a bill in the Icelandic Parliament intended to prohibit the export of human DNA from Iceland and promote the development of biotechnology in Iceland. He also succeeded in getting Hoffmann-La Roche, a pharmaceutical company based in Basel, Switzerland, to invest $200 million over five years in DeCODE. A condition of this financial agreement was that Hoffmann-La Roche is obligated to donate to the Icelandic population samples of any pharmaceutical products resulting from its collaboration with DeCODE for the lifetime of the relevant product patents.[17]

The national database that DeCODE is developing, with assistance from the Icelandic government, was initially called the Genotypes, Genealogy, Phenotypes and Resource database.[18] Now it is simply called the Icelandic Healthcare Database (IHD).[19] To win public trust for this commercial enterprise, DeCODE indicated it would use North American-type consent forms in its solicitation of new blood samples, all genetic research would be done with anonymous samples only, stored samples and derivative DNA data would be kept confidential, no individual research results would be reported to research participants or third parties, any DeCODE-created diagnostic tests resulting from this research would be provided free to physicians and patients in Iceland, and any other international biotechnology and pharmaceutical companies signing on to collaborate with DeCODE would be required to follow the Hoffman-La Roche model of donating quantities of patented products in sufficient numbers for the Icelandic population. In addition, the company stated that no patient information from clinical records would be added to the IHD until all identifiers had been removed and replaced with encrypted identification numbers, with the computerized list that links names to coded IDs being kept inside a double-locked safe in a guarded room.

To date, Stefansson's efforts have produced mixed results. On the one hand, he and his scientific collaborators have initiated research studies on 25 common diseases and claim to have isolated 15 specific disease genes. For example, they needed only 10 weeks using blood samples from 16 affected families in the Icelandic database to map the locus of a familial essential tremor gene to chromosome 3q13.[20] They continue to solicit blood samples from individuals and families in Iceland, promote the genetic homogeneity of Iceland as the richest natural genetics laboratory in the world, and look for additional commercial partners in other countries. A law passed in 1998 enabled DeCODE to become a virtual monopoly in genetic studies in Iceland and an actual monopoly with exclusive rights to market the IHD database abroad for 12 years.[21] The database itself now contains the family histories of over 75% of the approximately 800,000 Icelanders who have ever lived.

As another indication of its powerful position in Iceland, DeCODE is now the funding center for Icelandic genetics; it annually outspends the Icelandic government's entire research budget of $65 million.[22] The genomics company has also succeeded in selling DeCODE stock to Icelanders and other investors, with a July 2001 initial public offering on NASDAQ raising $194 million.[23]

On the other hand, from the beginning, many Icelandic geneticists and other scientists have been critical of DeCODE's business practices. Many physicians continue to be concerned about the potential loss of their patients' privacy, some individuals and families remain unwilling to contribute blood for DeCODE research studies, and many persons are disturbed about some of the ethical implications of its scientific work.[24] The company's stock price has plummeted since it went public. Even some internationally prominent geneticists who recognize the scientific importance of the Icelandic population voice reservations about Stefansson's project. Mary-Claire King, the American geneticist credited with mapping the BRCA1 gene, acknowledges that the scientific information gained from the DeCODE studies "could become one of the treasures of modern medicine. . . . The population there is like a gift from heaven." Yet she counsels,

This is what colonial treasure hunters have done for hundreds of years. It is not that it wasn't important to find gold, diamonds, and minerals in Africa or Mexico. It was taking the treasures away and the absolute evisceration of the societies that were there which were wrong. This is the twenty-first-century version of that. It is an elegant approach. . . . But there is a price. And if the price is the destruction of the field of genetics in Iceland— or the loss of the trust patients put in their doctors—then perhaps elegance isn't all that matters.[25]

Stefansson seems not to be bothered by his critics. In fact, given the scientific achievements of DeCODE to date, his response to ongoing criticisms of his company and the national database is sometimes dismissive:

Our right to develop medicine does not come free. We have a moral obligation to do what we can to move forward. There are opposing needs: to protect privacy and push science forward. There are times when they clash. Medicine today would simply not exist if privacy was the only need, the only right that anyone ever considered important.[26]

Three particular ethical concerns about the situation in Iceland will also be recurring themes in this book. First, even in a country whose citizens have national identification numbers and access to a national health system, there appears to be substantial concern (at least by a vocal minority) about the threat that DeCODE and its database represent to personal *privacy*. This concern seems to be exacerbated by the realization that the database, though national and multigenerational in scale, is nevertheless built around a small population, smaller than many of the cities in the world. Even when it is possible to rule out the type of discriminatory use of personal genetic information that could result in the loss of health insurance in the United States, a significant number of Icelanders still seem to be uneasy about the prospect that an enormous amount of personal information about them, including genetic information about them and their families, will be contained in one national database.

Second, many Icelanders are concerned that the new law permits Stefansson and his colleagues to reverse the normal requirements of *informed consent*. Rather than requiring DeCODE-funded investigators to get individuals to consent voluntarily (to opt in) to participation in various research studies, the law uses an opt-out, or presumed-consent mechanism: it presumes that 270,000 people are willing research participants in DeCODE studies unless individuals specifically request exemption in writing. Individuals who do fill out the opt-out forms and send them to the Director of Public Health will still not be able to get DeCODE (or government health officials) to remove the personal and medical information about them that is already in the database.[27]

Third, the *commercial* aspects of the DeCODE project bother many people, for different reasons. For some, the sheer amount of money involved is disconcerting, especially when it may become a corrupting influence on individual scientists and lead to badly done science. For others, the problem with the commercialization of Icelandic genetics is the unprecedented creation of a monopolistic scientific company backed by national law. For still others, the problem is the disproportionality between the enormous profits anticipated by DeCODE and the limited identifiable benefits to be gained by the rest of the Icelandic population: several hundred high-tech jobs and some free pharmaceutical products.[28]

Like *Moore* and NHANES III, the DeCODE database project raises important questions with implications for biomedical research practices anywhere in the world. For example, should scientific investigators make good-faith efforts to contact living, identifiable persons (in this instance, most of them still living in Iceland) for consent before using archived tissue samples from the 50-year-old tissue bank for genetic research? Should research teams try to contact surviving family members for permission before carrying out research studies on archived tissue samples from individuals who are now dead? Given the small size of the population in Iceland, how might these genetics investigators (or an impartial review committee) determine whether it would be impracticable to try to make such contacts?

In terms of prospective sample collection, will the new blood samples to be used in genetics research really be anonymous (or, more likely, be anonymized after collection), or will they be linkable to actual people in a manner similar to the way that medical records added to the national database will be linkable to actual patients? Should Icelanders who passively consent to provide blood samples be given any information about possible secondary research uses of the samples (e.g., for research purposes other than the identification of genetic causes of common diseases)? Will they be given specific information about the conditions of ownership and control of stored DNA samples or transformed cell lines (namely, that the stored biological materials will become the property of DeCODE)? Should potential research participants in Iceland be given more information about the commercial aspects of this research enterprise? Other than the possibility of some free diagnostic tests and free medications that may be forthcoming from DeCODE's collaborative research arrangements—significant benefits in the view of DeCODE supporters—do the citizens of Iceland have any financial share in DeCODE's corporate profits if they provide the blood samples that are essential to this research project?

Regarding other implications of scientific research done, at least partially, for huge financial gain, will Icelanders who opt out and refuse to provide blood samples still be entitled to free diagnostic tests and medications produced by DeCODE and its commercial partners? Does the new law significantly limit the personal and commercial rights of Icelanders? Does the working arrangement between DeCODE and the Icelandic government give this genomics company an unfair, monopolistic advantage in genetics-related drug discovery, as Stefansson's critics claim? In trying to protect Iceland's unique genetic heritage from external, "bleed and run" researchers, does Stefansson open himself to some of the same criticisms because of his commercial arrangements with transnational corporations with headquarters outside the country? Or put another way, is DeCODE open to the criticism sometimes directed at international "genehunters," namely a willingness to disregard the interests and rights of the "natives" in the search for genes and financial gain?

Some other developments are worth noting. Within Iceland, DeCODE's questionable business practices have motivated some of its critics to establish an alternative company. A small group of Icelandic scientists and business leaders have started an alternative biotechnology firm that also plans to mine Iceland's genetic riches, but without a monopolistic use of Icelandic medical records. Instead, the company called UVS—the initials stand for three legendary Icelandic witches—has worked out agreements with the Icelandic Cancer Society and two hospitals to do genetics research with volunteer patients, specifically some of the adult patients who have refused to permit their medical data to be included in the national database.[29]

Moreover, some of the Icelandic geneticists and other scientists who oppose DeCODE have formed an organization called Mannvernd, a word meaning "protection of humans." The founders of Mannvernd maintain in their mission statement that the DeCODE database project "infringes on human rights." Their Web site quotes (with several translation options) virtually all of the critical comments made about the DeCODE project by scientists, ethicists, attorneys, and journalists any place on the planet.[30]

In addition, the Icelandic Medical Association (IMA) has become one of DeCODE's severest critics. The IMA has advised its members to protest the national database by refusing to submit patient records and by encouraging patients to fill out and mail in the opt-out forms. In 1999 the World Health Organization (WHO) officially backed these IMA resistance efforts, at least in part because the Icelandic law and database guidelines do not provide satisfactory protection of the privacy rights of children, of individuals or families with serious medical conditions, or of the deceased members of families.[31] Partially because of these IMA efforts, more than 18,000 Icelanders (over 10% of the adult population) have officially opted out of the research plan.[32] The IMA opposition to DeCODE will continue, it seems, as long as the genomics company insists on gaining access to patients' medical records on the basis of presumed consent, rather than the voluntary, informed consent of individual patients.[33]

Outside Iceland, DeCODE's scientific success with its DNA bank (linked with the genealogical database and the medical records database) has motivated some geneticists in other countries to develop national gene-hunting projects based on the unusual genomic "gold mines" in their countries. In Sweden, for example, a biotechnology firm called UmanGenomics has been given exclusive rights by the Swedish Medical Research Council to produce and sell genetic information gained from blood samples stored in a 15-year-old "Medical Bank," or DNA bank, in a geographically isolated part of Sweden.[34]

In Estonia, some geneticists have established a not-for-profit organization called the Genome Center Foundation. They have also been given the rights by the Estonian government to catalog information on the health status and genetic makeup of 75% of the nation's population of 1.4 million people by using health questionnaires and blood samples. At a projected cost of $90–$150 million over the next 10 years, they plan to identify prominent disease genes in the Estonian population and hope to establish a national database that might, perhaps, later be used in collaboration with DeCODE's Icelandic database. The Estonian Genome Project is expected to begin in 2004.[35]

In Denmark, serious proposals have been made by scientists to turn the entire country into a cohort for study. This tantalizing prospect for investigators is made possible by the government-controlled system of approximately 200 databases (80 medical databases, 120 demographic databases) containing large amounts of information on each of the country's five million people. Although access to the databases is tightly restricted at the present, some scientists hope that they will soon be permitted to link all of the national databases (some of which are connected with tissue collections) by gaining access to the personal identification number that follows each Dane from cradle to grave.[36]

Britain's Medical Research Council and Wellcome Trust have agreed jointly to fund the U.K. Biobank project, a molecular genetics and epidemiologic study that will involve collecting genetic, health, and lifestyle data over 10 years from 500,000 volunteers, a cohort twice the size of the population of Iceland. Although participation in the $120 million study will be voluntary, some physicians, ethicists, and opposition groups have raised questions regarding the use of "blanket" or general informed consent, the limits that will be placed on access to the database, and whether this study might later become a DeCODE type of government-backed, genetics study of the entire British population. Three features, however, distinguish this study, scheduled to begin in 2004, from the DeCODE project: a diverse population, the scientific goal of trying to quantify the roles of genes and environmental influences on common diseases, and public funding and ownership of the project.[37]

The Challenges Presented in Writing This Book

The questions raised by the Moore, NHANES, and DeCODE cases indicate some of the terrain to be covered in this book. The terrain will be rugged and filled with obstacles, because the multiple issues involved in discussing the subject of research with stored tissue samples are complex, diverse, and difficult. Some of the terrain will consist of scientific territory, as we describe the multitude of ways that biomedical investigators in various fields use stored specimens for a variety of scientific purposes, as we interpret the particular contributions and challenges presented by molecular genetics, and as we address questions that spark disagreement among scientific investigators (e.g., Are anonymized samples really anonymous?). Some of the terrain will involve territory that is more analytical and ethical, as we address issues pertaining to individual rights, disclosure and informed consent, confidentiality and privacy, "anonymous" samples, the role of "community" in consenting to research protocols, discrimination and other harms that can result from genetic research, secondary research use of samples, and so on. Some of the terrain will be legal in nature, as we interpret relevant federal and state laws and major court cases, assess current federal regulations, discuss international codes and legal guidelines, and address legal issues such as the ownership and control of biological samples, patents connected with human biological materials, and the commercialization of research done with biological materials.

We also face other challenges. In contrast to most issues in bioethics and research ethics, the subject of this book has in recent years become a highly emotional area that has brought about an unprecedented number of related developments: policy statements from professional medical societies in the United States, international policy statements, guidelines from national genetics organizations, debates between biomedical investigators and privacy advocates, proposed model laws, disagreements between geneticists and pathologists, published documents from consumers of genetic services, published concerns about stigmatization by some minority groups in the United States (e.g., Ashkenazi Jews, Native Americans), a model consent document by the National Action Plan on Breast Cancer, several NIH-sponsored meetings, and many reports by national commissions (e.g., in the Netherlands, England, Canada, and the United States) and international organizations.

The issue is emotional, the stakes are high, and the efforts to shape professional and public opinion have been intense because, at its core, the subject of research on stored tissue samples presents a fundamental dilemma to those of us who try to be informed, thinking persons. On the one hand, we place great importance on biomedical research, realize in varying degrees that we have personally benefited from research done in earlier years with stored tissues, and ardently hope that we and our families will benefit from future discoveries and achievements by biomedical investigators using stored specimens. On the other hand, we also place great importance on personal privacy and autonomy, realize in varying degrees that the success of some biomedical investigators using banked samples has been achieved without adequate regard for the interests and rights of research participants and patients, and fervently hope that future research done with stored DNA samples will avoid the harms of insufficient disclosure, financial greed, discrimination, and group stigmatization that have, unfortunately, characterized some research in the past.

We face a formidable challenge in our plan to develop a reasonable, defensible position on this divisive, global topic. We know that the task will not be easy and that we will not persuade all readers of this book. But that should come as no surprise. As Larry Gostin, a law professor at Georgetown University, has observed, "The legal and ethical issues about the use of stored tissue are probably the most profound, complex, and troubling of any ethical issue we have in science today. . . . It pits two fundamental values against each other, and there's no easy resolution."[38] Two molecular pathologists agree. Wayne Grody, a pathology professor at UCLA, and Mark Sobel, a pathologist at the National Cancer Institute, have commented on "the intrinsic thorniness of the issue," pointing out that "the unprecedented power of modern molecular genetic technology brings opportunities for both spectacular scientific advances and sober philosophic reflection."[39]

Given these challenges, our goals can be stated concisely. We intend this book to be comprehensive in its data and resources, interdisciplinary in its analysis, fair and persuasive in its arguments, and realistic in its proposed solutions. We know that our call for significant changes to enable patients and research participants *to exercise meaningful choice* in the ways their tissue samples are used in biomedical research (choices they frequently do not have at the present time) will be controversial. By the end of the book, readers will be able to assess whether we have met these goals.

Cases and Vignettes

Each chapter, with the exception of the concluding chapter, ends with brief descriptions of several real cases. Some of the cases, both here and in other chapters, are intended to illustrate why many persons and professional groups interpret human tissue research almost entirely in terms of the enormous societal benefit such research has produced and will continue to produce. Others are intended to show why other persons and several nonprofessional groups tend also to focus on the possible harms that such research can do. Still other cases are like vignettes, in that they are intended to illustrate the expansive scientific purposes for which DNA can be studied and some of the ethical and legal problems that may be involved in some of these tissue studies. We hope that reading these cases, individually and collectively, encourages serious thinking about the complex issue of biomedical research with DNA samples in the era of genomic medicine.

In 1959, a 25-year-old man died of unexplained causes in the Manchester Royal Infirmary. The unusual symptoms included weight loss, fever, night sweats, ulcers, and multiple infections. After the autopsy, tissue samples were routinely stored. The case was reported in the *Lancet*. Many years later, when AIDS had been defined, the physicians who had seen the mysterious earlier case realized that the patient's symptoms had been consistent with human immunodeficiency virus (HIV) infection. In 1987, aided by polymerase chain reaction (PCR) technology, pathologists and geneticists in Manchester used the tissue samples stored in the pathology archive to prove that the patient's cells had indeed been infected with HIV, thus making the 1959 case the earliest documented case of HIV infection in Britain. They also compared the HIV strain from the late 1950s with strains prevalent today and with related chimpanzee viruses and demonstrated that the human form of the HIV arose about 100 years ago when it diverged from the chimpanzee virus.[40]

Tutankhamen ("King Tut") was the enigmatic boy pharaoh of the eighteenth dynasty, perhaps the most interesting of the Egyptian dynasties. Before he died and his body was mummified and entombed in the fourteenth century B.C.E., he had no reason to think that centuries later his body would become the object of scientific study. He might have expected Anubis, the Egyptian god of the realm of the dead, to decide his future in the life to come, and he may have feared future grave robbers who might steal the valuable objects entombed with him. But he could not have imagined that in the future the DNA in the remaining portion of his body would be analyzed by scientists from Egypt, Japan, and other countries, along with the residual DNA of other members of his dynasty. Yet that has happened, with his remains having been studied by professionals in human genetics, medicine, anthropology, and evolutionary biology.[41]

For over 50 years the Framingham Heart Study has been a traditional epidemiologic study funded by the National Heart, Lung, and Blood Institute. The original research participants in Framingham, Massachusetts, have been undergoing medical examinations and blood tests since 1948 in order to help investigators find the causes of cardiovascular disease; many of their children have participated in the Offspring Study since 1971. Since the early 1990s, however, the heart study has been transformed by molecular genetics. Biomedical investigators have been collecting blood samples for the purposes of DNA extraction and the creation of immortalized cell lines. They now have over 5,000 samples from both cohorts—the original participants and their children—and plan to create a renewable DNA resource for the ongoing study. In addition, they now collaborate with the Mammalian Genotyping Service at the Marshfield Clinic (in Marshfield, Wisconsin) that scans the DNA samples to study genetic markers for hypertension, osteoarthritis, osteoporosis, and diabetes.[42]

A leading law/medicine journal published a hypothetical case based on the Icelandic Health-care Database that is comprised of data from various health institutions in the country. The case assumes that the health institutions are fairly small (given the small national population), as is the size of the population in their respective parts of the country. According to the case, "Jon" has Huntington disease and lives in a town with 2,000 residents. Jon receives some treatment at his local hospital, which later transfers his medical information to the national database. The author writes, "The small population in Jon's region, and the even smaller number of people with Huntington's disease in that area, would make it relatively easy to identify Jon as one of the few people living in the hospital's service area who have that particular disease. Moreover, due to the extensive genealogical data that are available, it would be easy to map Jon's family tree, assuming that Jon was identified, and thereby identify all of his family members who are predisposed to Huntington's disease."[43]

The Kingdom of Tonga, in the South Pacific, has a population of 108,000; its people are geographically isolated, homogeneous, and have easily traceable family pedigrees. The government of Tonga planned to give exclusive rights to the genetic makeup of its citizens to Autogen Ltd., an Australian biotechnology company. Autogen hoped to get all of the adults in Tonga's chain of 170 islands to provide DNA samples for research purposes. Unlike DeCODE's presumed consent process with an opt-out provision, individuals who took part in the Tongan DNA collection would have been required to give express, informed consent. Yet the project was terminated because the Tonga Human Rights and Democracy Movement convinced many citizens that there had been inadequate public discussion of the plan, the research study failed to incorporate the traditional Tongan role of the extended family in decision making, and the commercialism in the project represented exploitation of Tongans.[44]

As these cases illustrate, the subject matter of this book is complex and controversial, the stakes are high, and reasonable people disagree about what should be done to protect the interests of biomedical researchers *and* the interests of the persons from whom tissue samples come. Stated another way, reasonable people disagree about how to foster an environment in which important, ethically responsible biomedical research can be conducted in the era of genomic medicine. This book recommends a series of changes that would foster such an environment.

Notes

1. American Association of Medical Colleges, "Patient Privacy and the Use of Archival Patient Material and Information in Research," unpublished paper, April 1997, p. 1.
2. Quoted by Michael Specter, "Decoding Iceland," *The New Yorker,* January 18, 1999, pp. 49–50.
3. The National Institutes of Health provides substantial information on its Web site: www.nih.gov. Also see David Malakoff, "Biomedicine Gets Record Raise As Congress Sets 2002 Spending," *Science* 295 (2002): 24–25; and William Frist, "Federal Funding for Biomedical Research: Commitment and Benefits," *JAMA* 287 (2002): 1722–4.
4. John Pickrell, "Gene Jocks, Data Crunchers Hit Jackpot," *Science* 290 (2000): 1669–70.
5. Elisa Eiseman and Susanna B. Haga, *Handbook of Human Tissue Sources: A National Resource of Human Tissue Samples,* (Rockville, Md.: RAND, 1999), p. 128. Also see Mike Mitka, "FDA Wants More Restrictions on Donated Blood," *JAMA* 286 (2001): 408.
6. *Moore v. Regents of the University of California,* 51 Cal. 3d 120, 271 Cal. Rptr. 146, 793 P.2d 479, (1990).
7. UCLA School of Medicine consent document, "Informed Consent for Use of Blood and Bone Marrow Tissue for Medical Research Concerned with 'Growth of Human Hematopoietic Cells in Vitro,'" September 20, 1983, on file with the authors.
8. Centers for Disease Control and Prevention, U.S. Department of Health and Human Services, "National Health and Nutrition Examination Survey III," January, 1994, p. 3.
9. Some examples: Ronette Briefel et al., "Total Energy Intake of the US Population: The Third National Health and Nutrition Examination Survey, 1988–1991," *Am J Clin Nutr* 26 (1995): 1072S–80S; Carlos Crespo et al., "Leisure-Time Physical Activity Among US Adults," *Arch Intern Med* 156 (1996): 93–98; Ross Anderson et al., "Relationship of Physical Activity and Television Watching with Body Weight and Level of Fatness Among Children," *JAMA* 279 (1998): 938–42; and Amanda Sue Niskar et al., "Prevalence of Hearing Loss Among Children 6 to 19 Years of Age," *JAMA* 279 (1998): 1071–75.
10. CDC, p. 3.
11. Eliot Marshall, "Policy on DNA Research Troubles Tissue Bankers," *Science* 271 (1996): 440.
12. Beth Burrows, "Second Thoughts about U.S. Patent #4,438,032," *Genewatch* 10 (October 1996): 5.
13. *Ibid.,* pp. 6, 8.
14. *Moore.*
15. Bernhard Palsson and Snorri Thorgeirsson, "Decoding Developments in Iceland," *Nat Biotechnol* 17 (1999): 407.
16. Eliot Marshall, "Tapping Iceland's DNA," *Science* 278 (1997): 566.
17. Vicki Brower, "Mining the Genetic Riches of Human Populations," *Nat Biotechnol* 16 (1998): 337–40.
18. This information is available on DeCODE Genetics' Web site: http://www.decode.com.
19. Jeffrey R. Gulcher and Kari Stefansson, "The Icelandic Healthcare Database and Informed Consent," *N Engl J Med* 342 (2000): 1827–30.
20. Jeffrey R. Gulcher et al., "Mapping of a familial essential tremor gene, FET1, to chromosome 3q13," *Nat Genet* 17 (1997): 84–87. Among DeCODE's achievements is the discovery of the first gene that underlies common forms of stroke. See Nicholas

Wade, "Scientists in Iceland Discover First Gene Tied to Stroke Risk," *New York Times,* September 22, 2003, pp. A1, A23.

21. *Act on a Health Sector Database.* No. 139/1998 (123d sess., 1998–99).

22. Specter, p. 46.

23. Michael Fortun, "Open Reading Frames: The Genome and the Media," *Genewatch* 14 (September 2001): 11.

24. Marshall, p. 566.

25. Specter, p. 44.

26. Specter, p. 49.

27. Gulcher and Stefansson, p. 1827. Also see David Winickoff and Einar Arnason, "The Icelandic Healthcare Database" (two letters), *N Engl J Med* 343 (2000): 1734.

28. Henry T. Greely, "Iceland's Plan for Genomics Research: Facts and Implications," *Jurimetrics* 40 (2000): 153–91.

29. Martin Enserink, "Start-Up Claims Piece of Iceland's Gene Pie," *Science* 287 (2000): 951.

30. Mannvernd: Association of Icelanders for Ethics in Science and Medicine. Reykjavik, Iceland. (See www.mannvernd.is/english/index.html.)

31. Ricki Lewis, "Iceland's Public Supports Database, But Scientists Object," *The Scientist* 13 (1999): 33.

32. George J. Annas, "Rules for Research on Human Genetic Variation—Lessons from Iceland," *N Engl J Med* 342 (2000): 1831.

33. Alison Abbott, "Iceland's Doctors Rebuffed in Health Data Row," *Nature* 406 (2000): 819.

34. Allison Abbott, "Sweden Sets Ethical Standards for Use of Genetic 'Biobanks,' " *Nature* 400 (1999): 3; and Annika Nilsson and Joanna Rose, "Sweden Takes Steps to Protect Tissue Banks," *Science* 286 (1999): 894.

35. Lone Frank, "Storm Brews Over Gene Bank of Estonian Population," *Science* 286 (1999): 1262–63; and Gwen Kinkead, "To Study Disease, Britain Plans a Genetic Census," *New York Times,* December 31, 2002, pp. D5, D8.

36. Lone Frank, "When an Entire Country Is a Cohort," *Science* 287 (2000): 2398–99.

37. David Dickson, "Partial UK Genetic Database Planned," *Nat Med* 6 (2000): 359–60; Kinkead, pp. D5, D8; and Melissa Austin, Sarah Harding, and Courtney McElroy, "Genebanks: A Comparison of Eight Proposed International Genetic Databases," *Community Genetics* 6 (2003): 41–42.

38. Evelyn Strauss, "The Tissue Issue: Losing Oneself to Science?" *Sci News* 152 (1997): 190.

39. Wayne W. Grody and Mark E. Sobel, "Update on Informed Consent for Stored Tissue Research," *Diagn Mol Pathol* 5 (1996): 80.

40. The Nuffield Council on Bioethics, *Human Tissue: Ethical and Legal Issues* (London: Nuffield Council on Bioethics, 1995), p. 37.

41. Soren Holm, "The Privacy of Tutankhamen—Utilizing the Genetic Information in Stored Tissue Samples," *Theor Med Bioeth* 22 (2001): 437–49.

42. Rebecca Voelker, "Two Generations of Data Aid Framingham's Focus on Genes," *JAMA* 279 (1998): 1245–46.

43. Hrobjartur Jonhantsson, "Iceland's Health Sector Database: A Significant Head Start in the Search for the Biological Grail or an Irreversible Error?," *Am J Law Med* 26 (2000): 50.

44. Heidi Forster, "Legal Trends in Bioethics," *J Clin Ethics* 12 (2001): 84; and Austin, Harding, and McElroy, pp. 41–42.

2

Concerns About Some Common Research Practices

> In the United States, ... [s]ome institutions ... have archived specimens of human tissues that are more than 100 years old. Historically, these stored tissue samples have been used by the biomedical community for educational and research purposes. More recently, stored tissues have played a major role in the understanding and treatment of such diseases as cancer, HIV/AIDS, and heart disease. However, the use and storage of human tissues raises several legal, ethical, and societal issues.
>
> Elisa Eiseman and Susanne Haga, 1999
> *Handbook of Human Tissue Sources*[1]

> The concern is that, while such potentially sensitive information [about individuals] is becoming increasingly easier to obtain, adequate safeguards and procedures for handling this information are not yet in place. Therefore, the current system for protecting tissue donors, which has worked well in the past, is becoming and will continue to become increasingly obsolete.
>
> Ted Ashburn, Sharon Wilson, and Barry Eisenstein, 2000,
> Pfizer, Inc.; Beth Israel; and Harvard Medical School[2]

Storing human tissues for biomedical research purposes has been a common practice for decades, yet until a few years ago there were no reliable data in the United States or elsewhere on the approximate numbers or types of tissues in storage at government laboratories, universities, or commercial tissue banks. Likewise, the two statements quoted above remind us that expressions of concern about the multiple uses and possible abuses of our continually expanding knowledge in human genetics have been common for many years—long before and, we predict, long after the Human Genome Project (HGP)—yet there has been little information compiled about these concerns or how they may play influential roles in the current controversy over research with stored tissues.

We provide both kinds of information in this chapter, beginning with an overview of the available data about human tissues in storage in the United States to highlight both the magnitude and variability of this very common scientific practice. We then discuss concerns about biomedical research with stored tissues that seem to be held by many potential research participants and by geneticists and other scientists who do human tissue studies, including a shared concern about the difficulty of protecting genetic privacy and preventing genetic discrimination. The chapter concludes with an overview of additional ethical issues that will be discussed later, an explanation of the terminology that we use throughout the book, and some illustrative cases.

The Available Data About Tissues in Storage

When the National Bioethics Advisory Commission (NBAC) decided in 1997 to do a report on research with stored tissue samples, its members realized that there was no national database on the types of human biological materials currently being stored, the diversity of ways by which tissue samples were stored for diagnostic and research purposes, or even a "ballpark" number of the total tissue samples stored. They therefore commissioned Elisa Eiseman of the Science and Technology Policy Institute at RAND to develop an inventory of stored tissue samples in the United States. Part of the national data that Eiseman and her colleagues collected was included in the 1999 NBAC report on stored biological materials.[3]

Gathering reliable data about stored tissue samples is difficult because of the various types of human biological materials being stored, the variety of forms in which they are stored, the diverse places (ranging from national repositories to private companies to pathology departments to the freezers in numerous researchers' labs) in which they are stored, and the sheer number of stored tissues and other biological materials in this country. Nevertheless, Eiseman, Susanne Haga, and other RAND colleagues succeeded in gathering some preliminary national data for the NBAC report, and later published a much more complete inventory of stored human tissue samples.[4]

Based on data collected from many institutions and mathematical models used for estimating numbers over time, Eiseman and Haga's updated national inventory indicates that there are *more than 307 million tissue specimens* currently being stored by the military, academic medical centers (especially pathology departments), federally funded research institutes and tumor registries, academic and commercial DNA banks, sperm/ovum/embryo banks, nonprofit tissue banks, and departments of forensic sciences. Most of these stored tissues were originally collected for diagnostic and therapeutic purposes. In addition, there are innumerable tissue samples stored by biomedical investigators outside repositories.

Eiseman and Haga estimate that the more than 307 million tissues now in storage came from approximately 178 million clinical cases, with additional human tissue samples being accumulated at a rate of more than 20 million samples per year. The difference between the estimated number of stored specimens and the estimated number of cases is due to the fact that a single case (e.g., a biopsy) can produce tissue samples stored in several forms: a formalin-fixed section, a paraffin block,

Table 2.1 Overall summary of stored tissue samples in the United States[5]

TYPE OF REPOSITORY	NUMBER OF CASES	NUMBER OF SPECIMENS	CASES/YEAR
Large Tissue Banks, Repositories, and Core Facilities	>2.8 million	>119.6 million	390,790
Longitudinal Studies	>340,088	>508,088	
Pathology Specimens	>160 million	>160 million	>8 million
Newborn Screening Laboratories	>13.5 million	>13.5 million	<10,000 to >500,000
Forensic DNA Banks	1.4 million	1.4 million	
Sperm, Ovum, and Embryo Banks	>200	>9,900	>2,300
Umbilical Cord Blood Banks	>18,300	>18,300	
Organ Banks		>75,500	>75,500
Blood Banks		~12 million	~12 million
Grand Total	**>178.0 million**	**>307.1 million**	**>20.5 million**

From Elisa Eiseman and Susanne B. Haga, *Handbook of Human Tissue Sources,* p. 141. Reproduced by permission of the RAND Corporation.

one or more frozen samples, a number of histologic slides, several extracted DNA samples for genetic analysis, and so on. Table 2.1 summarizes the national data.

Some of the data provided in the RAND national inventory indicate both the magnitude and the complexity of the problem. In general terms, the vast majority of stored tissues (an estimated 265.5 million diagnostic and therapeutic samples from more than 176 million cases) are in three types of settings: the National Pathology Repository at the Armed Forces Institute of Pathology (AFIP), pathology departments in Graduate Medical Education (GME) teaching institutions, and newborn screening laboratories in the 50 states.[6] More specific examples from Eiseman and Haga:

• Approximately 120 million tissue samples are stored in *large tissue banks, repositories, and core facilities* in almost every sector of the scientific and medical communities: the *military* (the AFIP has more than 92 million specimens at the National Pathology Repository and more than 2 million DNA samples at the Department of Defense's DNA Specimen Repository for Remains Identification); *tissue banks funded by NIH* (e.g., the National Cancer Institute funds the Cooperative Human Tissue Network for multiple kinds of cancer research and the 14 breast tissue banks of the National Action Plan on Breast Cancer Specimen and Data Information System; the National Heart, Lung, and Blood Institute maintains 1.5 million samples of serum, plasma, and cells in its Blood Specimen Repository; the National Institute of Mental Health has 1,200 brains in its brain collection; National Institute on Aging funds several Alzheimer Disease centers that store human brains, brain slices, cerebrospinal fluid, and blood samples); *research universities and academic medical centers* (e.g., the AIDS Specimen Bank at the University of California at San Francisco, the Human Brain Bank at the University of Pittsburgh, the Breast Cancer Tissue Bank at the University of Washington); *commercial enterprises* (e.g., PathServe, Clontech, and LifeSpan BioSciences, which stores 175 different types of human tissues and has over one million normal and diseased human samples); and *nonprofit/noneducational organizations* (e.g., the American Type Culture Collection, the Biologic Specimen Bank, the Biomedical Research Institute, and the Coriell Institute for Medical Research, which has 35,000 cell lines in storage from 1,000 genetic diseases).

- Many samples (e.g., blood, slides of tumors) are stored in state-based and national *tumor registries* (e.g., the federal Surveillance, Epidemiology, and End Results [SEER] Program has tissue samples and database information on 2.3 million cancer cases, with approximately 125,000 cases being added each year).
- Over 508,000 samples are stored as diagnostic and research parts of *longitudinal health studies* funded by the federal government, as best illustrated by the CDC's NHANES projects (blood and urine samples from more than 85,000 participants), the NIH Women's Health Initiative (blood samples from 336,000 participants), the Harvard Physicians' Health Study (more than 22,000 participants), the Framingham Heart Study, and the Bogalusa Heart Study.
- The largest (other than the AFIP) and oldest collections of stored human biological materials are *pathology specimens,* with more than 8 million cases being accessed each year and more than 160 million specimens currently in storage in four diverse kinds of settings: *pathology departments at GME teaching institutions* (there were 1,687 accredited GME teaching institutions in 1997), *clinical service and diagnostic laboratories* not associated with GME teaching institutions (there are approximately 640,000 such labs that perform tests on human specimens), *DNA diagnostic laboratories* (GeneTests, a national directory of DNA diagnostic labs, lists 148 such labs, with 90% of the labs regularly banking DNA samples as a service to referring physicians, genetic investigators, and families at risk for specific genetic disorders), and the *CDC* (e.g., the National Center for Infectious Diseases has stored blood samples from 100,000 Alaskan natives).
- Another large source of banked DNA exists in the form of dried blood spots that have been collected for years by *newborn screening laboratories* in all 50 states, the District of Columbia, Puerto Rico, and the Virgin Islands, with a current total of more than 13.5 million newborn screening cards in storage and new cards being stored at a rate of 10,000–500,000 cards a year, depending on state populations.
- Approximately 12 million blood samples are stored each year by *blood banks.* The American Red Cross collects and stores a three-day supply of fresh blood, 20,000 units of frozen blood, and the world's largest registry of frozen rare blood (fresh red blood cells can be stored for up to 42 days, fresh platelets for up to 5 days, frozen plasma for one to five years, and frozen whole blood for more than 10 years. "Old" platelets and red blood cells are sold to scientific researchers, and "old" plasma is used for making Factor VIII and other blood derivatives).

- Numerous types of *specialized tissue collections* exist, as illustrated by *brain and brain tissue banks* (e.g., Harvard has more than 5,000 brains stored in its Brain Bank; Duke has more than 1,000), *cryopreserved embryos* in the 280 fertility programs in the United States (e.g., the Genetics & IVF Institute freezes more than 2,300 embryos annually), and private and public *umbilical cord blood banks* that collectively have more than 18,000 units of umbilical cord blood cryopreserved in liquid nitrogen for the long-term purpose of providing autologous or allogeneic umbilical cord blood transplants to patients with blood diseases, cancer, or certain genetic disorders.

- Other types of biological materials are collected by *organ and tissue banks* affiliated with the American Association of Tissue Banks; these banks work with organ and tissue transplant programs to recover, process, store (in freezers), and distribute over 75,000 specimen samples for transplantation each year (donated organs and tissues not suitable for transplantation are available for education and research purposes).

- Other types of DNA samples are stored in *forensic DNA banks* by the FBI and state departments of forensic sciences for the purposes of improved criminal identification and prosecution; nationwide, approximately 1.4 million blood samples and other DNA samples (e.g., saliva, cheek smears) have been taken from convicted sex offenders, violent felons, and various other criminals either at sentencing or before release from prison.[7]

Segments of Public Opinion

We currently *stand at a crossroads* regarding human tissue research. Biomedical investigators have succeeded in collecting and storing the massive numbers of human tissue samples described above, but many of us are unaware of the extent to which this has been accomplished, or even that it has occurred. Tissue has frequently been collected without appropriate disclosure to patients and research participants about why tissues are needed for research purposes and what investigators plan or hope to do with them. Perhaps as a result, there is a growing body of evidence suggesting that a significant portion of the American public is not convinced they want their tissues to be used for scientific studies. Persons surveyed usually support biomedical research and value the achievements gained through research, but many remain unconvinced that research studies on banked tissue samples is a trustworthy enterprise that they should personally support with samples of their own blood, cheek cells, urine, skin, and other tissues.

To document this increasing problem, we present the findings of six studies of public opinion. Each indicates that segments of the U.S. general public want more information disclosed about research that may be done with their tissues. In addition, many people seek a more active role in making decisions about how their tissues will be used in research studies, and they have significant concerns about the virtual absence of information currently being provided about human tissue research, especially in clinical settings.

A University of Iowa Pilot Study. Carried out at the University of Iowa in 1996, this first survey was a pilot study of 93 patients in a family medicine outpatient clinic (response rate, 94.9%). For that reason its findings are of limited value, but nevertheless are important. We found substantial support for human tissue research, with 52% of the persons indicating that it is "very important" and 54% declaring support for the general idea of participating in research studies. We also found substantial concern about the ways that human tissue research occasionally uses samples collected in routine patient care. For example, 69% of the respondents agreed "it is necessary" for physicians to inform patients "if research might be conducted on their tissue sample," although only 3% of them reported that they had ever been informed that such research was a possibility. A large majority (73%) stated that they would be "very" or "somewhat bothered" if post-diagnostic research were done on their tissue samples without their consent.[8]

A National Action Plan on Breast Cancer Study. In 1996–97 the leaders of the National Action Plan on Breast Cancer developed a Model Consent Form for Biological Tissue Banking. Wanting a final version of the consent document that would be usable and effective in clinical settings, they hired Prospect Associates in Rockville, Maryland, to carry out a qualitative study of reactions to the proposed consent form. That company recruited a diverse representation of the population in Baltimore, Houston, Los Angeles, and Minneapolis as participants in 26 focus groups. Each group had 10 to 15 participants. Sixteen focus groups were conducted with general consumers (divided among African Americans, Hispanic Americans, Asian Americans, and white Americans), four groups contained breast cancer patients, four had family members of cancer patients, two were comprised of physicians, and two were limited to nurses. Each participant was identified by demographic data: gender, age, race/ethnicity, income level, and educational level.

Each group was led by a moderator and met for 90 minutes. The participants were first asked to read a draft version of the Model Consent Form, written in simple English. It contained information about tissue banking research in surgery (including information about "extra tissue" that might be removed during surgery) and three statements to which projected future patients were to respond with yes or no: permission for surgeons to keep some tissue for cancer-related research, permission for tissue to be kept for research about "other medical questions," and permission to be contacted again in the future to take part in more research. Participants were then asked to fill out a questionnaire describing their reactions to the form, followed by a group discussion about the form and, more generally, about tissue banking.[9]

The qualitative summary report about the focus groups is instructive, even though lacking in statistics, because of what it says regarding public support for human tissue research. The report describes several recurring concerns in all the meetings: (*1*) the meaning, implications, and limits of "extra tissue"; (*2*) the limitations of confidentiality with this research (e.g., cancer patients and family members expressed fear about health insurance implications); (*3*) widespread mistrust of the medical profession (recurring reasons included the profit motive in research, the inability to guarantee confidentiality, vagueness about the kinds of research being done, silence about how long tissue would be kept for research, and the refusal to report results to research participants); and (*4*) the problematic procedures that may used in administering the consent form (the "overwhelming" majority view was that surgeons should discuss the form with patients several days prior to surgery to permit time for reflection and a possible change of mind).[10]

An NBAC Study. A third study was commissioned by the National Bioethics Advisory Commission in 1998–99. Carried out by the Center for Health Policy Studies (CHPS), this qualitative study took the form of structured mini-hearings held with specific population subgroups in seven cities: Richmond (educated baby boomers); Honolulu (urban neighbors); Mililani, Hawaii (suburban neighbors); San Francisco (young adults); Cleveland (African Americans); Boston (senior citizens); and Miami (Jewish women). Not intended to be representative of the national population or even an entire subgroup population, the mini-hearings represented an effort by NBAC to get a variety of perspectives on human tissue research from nonexperts.[11]

The mini-hearings were open to the public, but only 7 to 14 individuals were invited to be active participants in the recorded discussions. Sessions were led by a moderator, attended by a member of NBAC, and assessed by several persons from CHPS who made cross-group comparisons. The participants answered questions regarding their knowledge about human tissue research, listened to several hypothetical scenarios, discussed a variety of issues raised by the moderator, and completed a pre- and post-discussion questionnaire.

If the planners of these meetings expected a diversity of opinions, they got it. In fact, the opinions expressed on tissue ownership, informed consent, privacy and confidentiality, stigmatization, third-party concerns, sponsorship of research, and safeguards for tissue-based research were so diverse that common themes and majority views were elusive, if not impossible to document accurately. At least one point, however, was clear: "many people *are not aware that tissue may be stored and later used for research.*"[12] CHPS had three recommendations for NBAC: a nationally representative survey of public opinion about human tissue research is needed, the consent process for tissue-based research needs to be improved, and public education materials about tissue-based research and privacy concerns need to be developed.[13]

A Georgetown University/University of Maryland Study. Two important studies of public opinion about genetics research with stored tissues were published in 2001. A multidisciplinary group at Georgetown University and the University of Maryland published the results of a survey among Ashkenazi Jews. The investigators were interested in examining the attitudes of this group toward genetics research with anonymized samples and in seeing if there were significant concerns, even when research was done with individually anonymized samples, about the possibility of stigmatization and discrimination based on the group identity of the participants. Moreover, the survey provided data about the perceived importance of informed consent for human tissue research in clinical and research settings and about attitudes toward personal participation in a variety of research studies.[14]

The sample size was 273 persons, with an age range of 18–90. The central feature of the survey was the presentation of two hypothetical scenarios, one in which a patient provides a blood sample as part of routine care in a clinical setting and the other involving a voluntary research participant who provides a blood sample for a research study of a specific genetic mutation common in the Ashkenazi Jewish population. Later, in both scenarios, a group of researchers wants to use the now-anonymized blood sample for a secondary research study of another genetic mutation found in the Jewish community. After each scenario, survey participants were presented with eight hypothetical research studies, each of which could have been the secondary research study in the two scenarios, and were asked (*a*) if written informed consent should have been required for the reuse of their DNA, and (*b*) if they would be willing to participate via their anonymized DNA samples in each of the eight hypothetical studies.[15]

The results of the survey were clear. The majority of the persons surveyed believed that written consent should be required for the reuse of stored samples regardless of whether the DNA was collected in a clinical or research setting. For all eight hypothetical studies, 70%–75% of the survey participants thought that written consent for post-diagnostic studies with samples initially obtained in clinical settings was more important than it was for secondary research following an initial research study (60%–65% opted for written consent for secondary research). As to willingness to participate in the eight hypothetical studies, a high percentage of the survey participants (85%–90%) were willing to participate via their DNA samples in genetics studies focusing on physical illnesses (both treatable illnesses if discovered early and untreatable illnesses) and psychiatric illnesses (mental illnesses or alcoholism). By contrast, only 72%–75% were willing to participate in genetics studies focusing on behavioral traits (such as intelligence or creativity), and even fewer (60%–70%) were willing to participate in studies examining potentially stigmatizing or stereotype-confirming traits (such as frugality or homosexuality).

Most respondents who believed that written informed consent should be required in clinical and research settings also indicated that they would usually be willing to provide consent if asked by genetics investigators, and said, to the surveyors' surprise, that they would not be reluctant to give their DNA samples for genetics studies of mental illness or behavioral traits. The authors concluded: "The present study . . . suggests that some individuals feel strongly that additional written consent should be required for re-use of samples."[16]

A Study by the CDC. The largest, most representative, and perhaps most important public opinion study, also published in 2001, was done by a CDC multidisciplinary group. The rationale for this quantitative study of public attitudes toward the donation and storage of blood samples for genetics research was twofold: there is a need for population-based research to assess the frequencies of genetic variants and their associations with human diseases, and this research depends on public attitudes toward the donation and long-term storage of blood samples. Simply put, the "assessment of the public's attitudes is crucial; the generalizability of and implications from population-based genetic studies will depend on the willingness of the public to participate."[17]

The CDC study was based on data from the 1998 American Healthstyles survey of health attitudes and behavior, an annual population-based market research survey. The 1998 version of the survey included seven statements about genetics, with four statements pertaining to blood donation and storage for genetics research. Of the 3,130 Healthstyles survey participants, 2,621 (84%) responded to the genetics statements, to which they indicated agreement/disagreement on a 1–5 scale. The statements about blood donation and storage were worded as follows:

1. I would be willing to donate blood for research to find genes that affect people's health.
2. If I donated blood for a specific health research project, I would not mind if the blood was stored and used later for health research in genetics.
3. I would donate my blood for health research in genetics but want a guarantee that researchers would not provide the test results to anybody except me.
4. I would anonymously donate my blood for health research in genetics, even though researchers would not be able to notify me if they discovered that I have a genetic condition.[18]

A substantial minority of persons participating in the survey (42%) indicated that they were in favor of both blood donation and long-term storage of their blood samples for genetics research. By contrast, 10% of respondents stated they would be willing to donate blood but not have it stored for long-term studies; 27% indicated they would not be willing to donate blood for genetics research, even with assurance of confidentiality and anonymity; and 21% would not be willing to donate blood or have it stored for genetics research under any circumstances.[19] The results of this study understandably concerned the CDC investigators because they were convinced that "genetic and epidemiologic research will rely equally on the increasing use of biological specimens and the willingness of individuals to participate in such studies by donating and allowing storage of their biological specimens."[20]

If truly reflective of the American public's attitudes about genetics research, the results of the CDC analysis clearly indicate that considerable work needs to be done to increase public support for and willingness to participate in long-term genetics research studies. The study's authors conclude: "Future studies in this area ... will need to include specific definitions for the donation and storage of blood specimens and *further define the intended use of these specimens* for study participants. ... Understanding [the public's attitudes toward genetic research] has far-reaching implications for future population-based studies."[21]

A Study by the Department of Clinical Bioethics, NIH. A study of 504 older adults published in 2002 provides additional data regarding the preferences and concerns of a selected group of the general public. This study seems to demonstrate that most sample sources are likely to think that it is important to give consent for human tissue research (with the importance given to consent declining as a respondent's age increases), to have some control over whether one's samples are used for research purposes, and to receive the results of possibly significant clinical findings.[22]

Unfortunately, the study has a number of flaws, including the use of a study population that would seem to be the least knowledgeable, and least representative of all adult age groups for a telephone-interview study about attitudes toward current human tissue research: older adults with a mean age of 65 (24% of persons surveyed were over 75), half of them being participants in ongoing Alzheimer studies, and all of them selected, in part, on the basis of a minimal standard of decision-making capacity (they could "remember the survey questions").

In addition, respondents were given no information about human tissue research, either with clinically derived samples or with samples obtained in research settings; provided with no information about the potential benefits and possible risks of research with stored samples; given incomplete options regarding the identity status of samples; and asked to respond to simplistic, vague scenarios. Thus, though the results are generally consistent with other survey findings, they should be interpreted cautiously.

Genetic Privacy and Genetic Discrimination

As indicated by these studies of public opinion, a significant portion of the U.S. population is concerned about human tissue research, especially when this work involves genetics studies of stored DNA samples. The nature of this concern, thus far, is fairly general. It will remain somewhat vague and diffuse until additional research studies by social scientists enable us to be more specific about its foci. At present the dominant concern expressed in these surveys seems to pertain to two related fears: (*1*) genetics investigators (and the "system" of biomedical research) will not adequately protect the privacy and confidentiality of our personal and familial genetic information, and (*2*) persons who participate, knowingly or not, in genetics studies via their stored DNA samples are at increased risk of becoming victims of genetic discrimination. Are these fears reasonable? Or are they largely based on anecdotal cases, inaccurate information, or misleading interpretations of scientific practices and the law?

Initially, we point out that though extant law may be more protective than some believe it to be, the current legal landscape in the United States provides a porous patchwork of protections for genetic information. As we discuss more completely in Chapter 7, the law does not guarantee that genetic information about individuals will be kept private and confidential or that it will be disclosed only with the individual's consent. The law also fails to establish uniform and strong protections against the use of genetic information to deny or restrict access to health insurance or employment (or other social goods).

We believe, as do many others, that law and policy must do more on both fronts and must move beyond the incrementalism of the past. This view is grounded in the belief that genetic privacy (indeed health information privacy generally) is an intrinsically important and personal value and that access to a person's genetic material and information about a person's genetic characteristics ought to be within the individual's control, to the greatest extent reasonable. Further, when third parties, in particular employers and health insurance companies, use information about a person's genetic predisposition to illness or disease to deny or limit important social goods when that person is asymptomatic (based on predicted future disability), this action can be an invidious form of status-based discrimination, akin to differential treatment based on race, gender, and ethnicity.

That said, the task of crafting the best, most comprehensive approach to these problems looms large, evidenced in part by the substantial variations among extant laws and policies and the range of challenging issues addressed—or left unaddressed. As Mark Rothstein notes, the tension between commitments to privacy and nondiscrimination and third-party claims of access implicates larger concerns about rights to health insurance and health care, and the information employers may justifiably claim is essential to have a safe and effective workforce and workplace, protect the public from harm, or serve other legitimate business needs. Moreover, relying on largely procedural rules (individual consent, restricted third-party access) may merely sidestep still more fundamental clashes with matters of equality of opportunity and allocation of resources.[23]

Our focus here is far more narrow—to elaborate on the prudential argument that doing more in this area is of critical importance to the research enterprise, and that investigators and IRBs should routinely assess and craft the informed consent process to include attention to concerns about privacy and the risks of genetic discrimination. The essential point is that there is good reason to believe that potential research participants would find the risks of disclosure of personal genetic information *material* to their decision whether or not to provide a tissue sample or allow information derived from that sample or already existing information to be used by an investigator. Hence, these concerns need to be addressed. In addition, greater assurances against these risks (with appropriate changes in law and policy) are likely to affirm and increase the public's desire to participate in genetics research.

Review of the data concerning attitudes toward and perceptions of the risks of "wrongful" use of genetic information strongly support this premise. Extensive empirical data comes from a national, random survey commissioned in 1996 by the National Center for Genome Resources. Using a combination of mailed questionnaires and telephone interviews, this study examined attitudes and perceptions among a wide range of stakeholders, including the adult population, physicians in primary care specialties, leaders of national patient-based organizations, scientists, and medical directors of health and life insurers. Among these groups, a majority believed that genetic information should be kept more confidential than other information in a person's medical record. Eighty-five percent (85%) of respondents felt that employers should be prohibited from gaining access to genetic information, while 69% felt that the same prohibitions should apply to health insurers and life insurers. A majority of respondents said that if health insurers or employers could get access to genetic test results, they would probably (36%) or definitely (27%) not take the tests. Physicians and industry leaders believed more strongly than the public "that patients would avoid testing unless confidentiality could be maintained." The authors concluded, "confidentiality of [genetic] testing and test results is a major concern for the public."[24]

These findings echo those of a 1995 Harris public opinion poll, in which over 85% of those surveyed were "very concerned" or "somewhat concerned" about the potential uses of genetic information by employers or insurance companies.[25] They are also consistent with findings that within populations at risk for Huntington disease, many would forgo testing to avoid the risks associated with disclosure,[26] and with several studies that have found evidence and fear of genetic discrimination. For example, in a frequently cited article, Paul Billings and colleagues report 41 separate incidents of possible discrimination, all but two involving either insurance (32) or employment (7).[27] Virginia Lapham and colleagues found that 22% of 332 members of genetic support groups nationwide believed they had been refused health insurance and 13% believed they had been denied employment or let go from a job.[28] And Lisa Geller and colleagues found that among individuals at risk to develop one of four selected genetic conditions (hemochromatosis, phenylketonuria, mucopolysaccharidoses, and Huntington disease) and parents of children with one of these conditions, nearly half of respondents (N = 917) reported experiencing discrimination by a variety of institutions, including health and life insurers and employers (other instances of reported discrimination involved educational institutions, adoption services, and blood banks).[29]

In sum, there is substantial collective evidence that people are widely concerned about genetic privacy and discrimination. Although data specifically probing comparable attitudes toward research participation are limited—one study suggests that similar apprehensions led some to decline to participate in clinical research protocols[30]—it follows that most of us would have similar concerns whether being asked for tissue samples or for release of genetic information in the course of clinical care or for research, perhaps especially so when research originates in the clinical setting. It also follows that reasonable research participants would want to know whether third parties would have access to genetic information about themselves and their families, and might base their decision to participate on an assessment of whether this possible third-party access might pose unacceptable risks of discrimination. IRBs and investigators need to be properly attentive to privacy and discrimination issues in the development and review of research studies. We return to some of these concerns later.

The primary challenge to the position we develop in later chapters can be pieced together from several sources and proceeds along the following lines: The available data tell us something about public attitudes and perceptions, but the message is generally suspect. In fact, genetic discrimination is a rare occurrence, and the contention that the threat is imminent is greatly exaggerated. Both within and outside the research community, there is concern that "hype" about genetic discrimination sends the wrong message about genetics studies and the uses of data about genetic risk and variation. Pointing to these concerns, researchers sometimes complain that there is no need to insert these issues into the informed-consent process until more substantial proof of genetic discrimination emerges. Rather, they maintain that we should focus our attention elsewhere unless genetic discrimination becomes a more widespread and realistic worry.

Supporters of this "wait and see" position can point to critiques of some of these studies that identify a number of limitations (some of which are noted by the authors themselves), including that the sample population was self-selected and highly sensitized (e.g., the Lapham and Geller studies), and that self-reports and anecdotal evidence may well overstate the extent of actual discrimination.[31] Further, there is some contrary empirical evidence suggesting genetic discrimination is not very prevalent. For example, studies conducted by Dorothy Wertz and colleagues in 1994–95 found a small number of reports of genetic discrimination among 1,084 genetic counselors, and 499 primary care physicians reported "only a few instances of refusals of employment or life or health insurance based on genetic information."[32]

In addition, a 1998 study of the impact of state laws against insurance discrimination, conducted by Mark Hall and Stephen Rich, concludes that actual discrimination in health insurance on the basis of genes is extremely rare. Their cross-sectional study of genetic counselors, insurance regulators, and insurance company representatives found "almost no well-documented cases of health insurers either asking for or using presymptomatic genetic test results in their underwriting decisions." Regulators reported so few complaints about genetic discrimination in health insurance that it "simply is not on their 'radar screen.'"[33] (On the other hand, genetic counselors reported that genetic discrimination is a prevalent concern, a finding consistent with the studies noted earlier.)[34] Relying in part on a review of some of this cumulative data, as well as an assessment of health insurance industry practices, one industry representative asserts that the rationale for enactment of nongenetic discrimination laws is based on "the erroneous belief that the threat of genetic discrimination by health insurers represents a clear and present danger."[35]

Whether or not one believes genetic discrimination to be a serious and current problem, several federal agency reports spanning a 10-year period provide additional reasons for widespread apprehension about the future. A 1989 study conducted by the Congressional Office of Technology Assessment (OTA), found that among Fortune 500 companies, 42% of the 330 respondents believed an applicant's health insurance risks to be a relevant factor in employment decisions. Thirty-six percent (36%) made a practice of conducting health assessments at some stage in the screening of job applicants. The OTA concluded that "growing concern among employers over the rising costs of employee health insurance, and the increased efforts to reduce those costs for the employer, are likely to increase the scope of health insurance screening in the workplace."[36] In 1993, a multidisciplinary NIH/Department of Energy task force on Genetic Information in Insurance reached a similar conclusion, warning that "[n]ew genetic tests in the context of risk underwriting by health insurers are likely to exacerbate an already severely troubled health care system."[37] In 1997, a U.S. Department of Health and Human Services report concluded that "as knowledge grows about the genetic basis of disease, so too does the potential for discrimination."[38] And in 1998, eight years after enactment of the Americans with Disabilities Act, the Equal Employment Opportunity Commission concluded that "[b]ased on genetic information, employers may try to avoid hiring workers who they believe are likely to take sick leave, resign, or retire early for health reasons (creating extra costs in recruiting and training new staff), file for workers' compensation, or use health care benefits excessively."[39] Various other sources further counsel that though the present-day reality of genetic discrimination is not accurately known, there is good reason to believe that if it is cost-effective—and legal—to use genetic information in the corporate personnel office and the insurance services office, it will be increasingly desirable to do so.[40]

The "wait and see" argument also misses several important reasons to maintain focus on strengthening privacy and nondiscrimination laws. Beyond commitment to the importance of these values and goals, other reasons that so many states have enacted genetic privacy and nondiscrimination laws and that Congress continues to debate the issue (taking some action in this area with HIPAA, the Health Insurance

Portability and Accountability Act and, once again, currently debating a federal genetic privacy and nondiscrimination law), are that the law serves important expressive functions and can shape, solidify, and change societal norms. Though they found few instances of actual genetic discrimination and could not conclude that state laws against discrimination in health insurance had prevented discrimination from occurring, Hall and Rich argue that these laws have shaped industry behavior, not through the heavy hand of legal threat, but by promoting and reinforcing social values and the industry's "more socially constructive instincts."[41] Through more effective and comprehensive efforts to shield privacy and protect against discrimination, the law's expressive and educative functions can be tapped to alleviate apprehensions and to "ensure public confidence in genetics research and use of genetic information."[42]

Relevant Concerns of Scientists

We are not aware of any surveys of geneticists, pathologists, epidemiologists, or other biomedical scientists who conduct human tissue research comparable to the studies of potential research participants discussed earlier. Similarly, we know of no literature that analyzes the specific concerns biomedical investigators may have about research with stored DNA samples comparable to the multidisciplinary literature on genetic privacy and discrimination. But we do have some knowledge, based on our interactions with scientific investigators and some of the professional literature that will be discussed in the next chapter, regarding relevant concerns of scientists about their work with stored tissues as well as some of their concerns about frequent efforts, often by research policy makers and nonscientists, to change some of their common research practices.

We therefore suggest that many, perhaps most, scientific investigators share, though from a different perspective, the general concerns of many potential research participants about threats to genetic privacy and the harms that could be done through acts of genetic discrimination against individuals and groups. For that reason, pathologists, geneticists, and other scientists working with stored tissues usually take multiple steps in their laboratories, research protocols, computer use, and electronic communications to protect the stored samples in their possession, the identification of sample sources, and any derivative information from the samples that is stored in their databases. Because of the nature of their work, many of these scientists seem to have a heightened awareness of the psychosocial harms that could come to research participants if their personal and familial genetic information came into the possession of individuals, companies, or governments that might use that information for discriminatory reasons.

Scientists who carry out human tissue studies also have concerns that differ substantially from those of potential research participants. While both groups place great importance on the benefits of biomedical research and are concerned about the possibility that research using the techniques of DNA banking could, by negligence or intention, contribute to the loss of genetic privacy and the increased likelihood of genetic discrimination, scientists are concerned about (*1*) obtaining sufficient numbers of specific types of tissues from research participants, patients, clinicians and other investigators, and tissue supply companies to do their specialized, condition-specific or disease-focused research studies; (*2*) receiving grants to enable them to do the research that must be done to prevent disease, treat illness, and improve physical and mental health; (*3*) being slowed down by government regulations and IRB requirements from doing the timely, state-of-the-art research that is likely to get funded; (*4*) being distracted from doing good science by unfounded reports and anecdotal cases about genetic discrimination and other psychosocial harms occurring when genetic information about an individual or family is used for the wrong reasons; and (*5*) losing out to scientific competitors who move ahead to get major grants, notable scientific awards, patents for their discoveries, and, in a few cases, significant personal wealth. All of these concerns may influence investigators' views of proposals to change traditional, common research practices.

Other Ethical and Legal Concerns

In addition to genetic privacy and genetic discrimination, we also discuss in later chapters a number of other ethical and legal concerns related to research with stored tissues. We give substantial attention to the process of informed consent—how it can be improved, how it can be more relevant to the practice of DNA banking, and how appropriate informed consent is sometimes replaced by other versions of "consent" that do not provide patients and research participants with opportunities to express meaningful choice about whether and how their tissues will be used for research purposes.

We also address ownership and control of the body and its parts, post-diagnostic research with clinical samples, anonymized tissues, human embryonic stem cell research, research on cadaveric tissues, vulnerable research participants, the increasing commercialism of human tissue research, the use of databases in human tissue research, and some special issues in forensic settings. In addition, we subsequently "unpack" the concept of psychosocial harm by delineating multiple harms that are possible in genetic studies and thus may be unintended consequences of research done with identified or coded samples, or alternatively, with anonymous or anonymized samples.

On Terminology

We want to be as clear in this book as the subject matter permits us to be. To that end, we point out that the language used by biomedical professionals and in the professional literature in reference to stored tissue samples is almost as diverse as the tissue samples. For decades pathologists have referred to the clinically derived materials they work with as "specimens," "archived specimens," and "patient material." More recently, some geneticists have tended to refer to the human biological materials they analyze in their labs (when they are making global references) as "tissues," "tissue samples," "blood samples," or "DNA samples." More commonly, of course, molecular geneticists refer to the specific molecular portions of the tissues they are studying (e.g., portions of chromosomes, polymorphic fragments of base-pair sequences) or to the techniques they use in their analytical work, rather than to the "larger" tissues themselves.

Recent multidisciplinary professional literature regarding the controversy over research with stored tissue samples has also used a variety of terms for the materials being studied: "body tissues," "research samples," "biological samples," "materials of human origin," "human tissue specimens," "stored specimens," "biosamples," "biomaterials," "banked genetic materials," "human biological materials," and so on. A multidisciplinary paper from an NIH workshop on this issue illustrates the terminological and definitional challenges we face: "In this article, the term *tissue sample* will include all samples that can serve as DNA sources, including not only solid tissues, but also blood, saliva, and any other tissues or body fluids containing nucleated cells."[43]

As far as we can determine, this variation in terminology occurs for a number of reasons:

1. Traditional, discipline-specific terms of reference are hard to give up.
2. Different writers or groups of writers use different terminology, either by choice or as a result of carelessness or inconsistency.
3. Some professional groups and individuals use generic, inclusive terminology that can include (*a*) tissues that already are being stored *and* (*b*) tissues that have not yet been collected.
4. Some writers distinguish (*a*) all human DNA-containing tissues from (*b*) the derivatives of such tissues, such as extracted DNA and transformed cell lines.
5. Some persons fail to distinguish between (*a*) human DNA-containing biological *materials* and (*b*) the DNA-related *data* that can be derived from a tissue sample or cell line.
6. Some researchers use terminology that enables them to make distinctions that are important to them: between "tissue specimens" and "tissue samples," or between blood and other tissues, or between tissues and organs, or between tissues and subtissue units such as cells and DNA.
7. Others use terminology that suggests a distinction between (*a*) "valuable" human tissues that can be used for important clinical and research purposes and (*b*) hair, nail clippings, saliva, sweat, and other "waste" tissues that seem to have importance only for forensic scientists.

8. Still others try to distinguish between (*a*) all nongametic human tissues, and (*b*) human sperm, ova, and, for obvious reasons, embryos.

As an example of the importance placed on terminology, we observe that NBAC originally announced plans to produce a report on research with "stored tissue samples." They also commissioned several papers concerning the appropriate research use of stored tissue samples. In their published report, however, NBAC members changed terminology and stipulated that they would be using the language of "human biological materials," which they define to include the following:

[T]he full range of specimens, from subcellular structures such as DNA, to cells, tissues (e.g., blood, bone, muscle, connective tissue, and skin), organs (e.g., liver, bladder, heart, kidney, and placenta), gametes (i.e., sperm and ova), embryos, fetal tissues, and waste (e.g., hair, nail clippings, urine, feces, and sweat, which often contains shed skin cells).[44]

In our view, some of the terminological distinctions used in the literature are important, while others are inaccurate or unpersuasive. Accordingly, for the purposes of greater clarity and increased understanding, we now (*1*) make some definitional points about the components of stored tissues and (*2*) explain some of the terminology that we use in this book.

It is important to understand that a human cell contains DNA, the information-containing macromolecule, which itself is converted into a messenger RNA, and that this messenger RNA is eventually translated into a protein composed of amino acids. Although DNA contains the information in the cell, proteins do most of the actual work in the cell. Tissue samples from human beings may contain one or more of these parts depending on how they are processed.

For example, whole blood contains within it white blood cells, which have within them DNA, messenger RNA, and protein. These cells can be stored *frozen*, in which case all of the components are preserved. Alternatively, the cells can be transformed into *a permanently living cell line*, a lymphoblastoid cell line, in which all of the components are retained, but with the possibility that some of the messenger RNA and protein may not be exactly representative of a normal white blood cell contained within a living human. As still another alternative, all of the components of *white blood cells can be extracted* using various chemical means so that isolated collections of DNA or RNA or protein can also exist.

Each of these different materials requires different types of processing and contains, in some cases, slightly different or complementary information. For example, the protein and messenger RNA materials do not contain all of the information contained within the DNA, since much of the DNA is comprised of regulatory regions or other stretches of DNA of unknown function that do not appear to be transcribed to RNA or translated into protein. Alternatively, since the protein and messenger RNA do the bulk of the work in the cell, these materials can sometimes take on specific forms that give a direct indication of how a particular cell is functioning that may not be apparent from inspection of the DNA alone.

With these definitional points in mind, we point out that the terminology we use in this book is based on six guidelines:

1. We most commonly use "stored tissue samples" as the form of reference for the practices and issues we analyze in the book.
2. We restrict "stored tissue samples" to tissues obtained from humans.
3. We use "biological materials," "human biological materials," "specimens," "specimen samples," and "DNA samples" as general, inclusive synonyms for "stored tissue samples," even though we have just pointed out that the scientific techniques used in labs sometimes extract DNA from tissue samples and thereby separate DNA from the messenger RNA and protein in the original samples.
4. We mean by "stored tissue samples" and its synonyms: (*a*) *samples of human tissue* wherever found, however obtained, and however stored, as well as (*b*) *cellular and molecular fractions* (especially DNA) of human tissue and (*c*) *derivatives* of human tissue, such as extracted DNA and transformed cell lines.
5. We make four distinctions regarding the identity status of stored samples by referring to "identified" samples (the glass tube, slide, or cup containing a tissue sample retains the name of the person from whom the tissue came); "linked" or "coded" samples (the container for a sample has a numerical code that disguises the identity of the sample source, but is linked, most often by computer, to the name of that individual patient or research participant); "anonymous" samples (samples that were originally collected without any identifiers of the sample sources; no person, or computer, on the research team can identify a specific sample source with certainty, even if a legitimate need to know arises); and "anonymized" samples (samples that were originally identified, but the identifiers have been irreversibly stripped or disguised; these samples cannot be linked to the persons from whom they came even if a legitimate need to do so arises, although the samples may be linkable to previously obtained clinical and/or demographic information about those individuals).
6. We use "DNA banking" to mean two kinds of storage of DNA-related information for possible future use: (*a*) the *stored biological material,* including tissue samples, extracted DNA, and/or immortalized cell lines, and (*b*) the *stored genetic data* derived from a tissue sample, extracted DNA, and/or a cell line, including stored DNA sequence data and other relevant information about the human being from whom the stored sample came.

In the next chapter we discuss a number of important documents and policy statements that were distributed and published during the mid-1990s in the United

States. All received considerable discussion and criticism, but a proposed model law and an NIH/CDC workshop statement on informed consent in genetics studies drew the most attention.

Cases and Vignettes

A leader of Native American IRBs attended a national conference in which members from numerous local IRBs discussed the possibly ethnocentric nature of federal regulations designed to protect participants in research studies. The views expressed during the discussion ranged widely. Some physicians referred to human tissues left over from medical procedures as being "garbage." Other conference participants disagreed, noting that members of some Native American groups place great value on respectfully handling and keeping certain body parts that have been surgically removed. Others described a local IRB study showing that most post-partum women in a survey had expressed a preference for giving consent before research was done on their placentas, even though they were told that their placentas would be anonymized before the research began.[45]

In 1999 the news media in England disclosed a startling fact to their readers and viewers: pathologists at Europe's busiest children's hospital, the Alder Hey Royal Liverpool Children's Hospital, had 2,500 pots in the pathology laboratory that contained the organs of dead children. The organs had been removed from the bodies post-mortem, but the children's parents, who had consented to the autopsies, had neither known about nor consented to the removal and storage of the organs. Similar disturbing news was subsequently disclosed about the Royal Infirmary in Bristol. There, too, organs removed during post-mortem examinations of children's bodies were stored for research purposes without parental knowledge or consent. The response from groups of parents was immediate, loud, and angry. The news media was filled with denunciations of physicians, objections to the practices of secrecy, expressions of betrayal, and accusations of immoral conduct in the hospitals. The public furor did not begin to subside until March 2000 when the Royal College of Pathologists published new guidelines for post-mortem examinations in all National Health Service hospitals. The guidelines included detailed instructions for obtaining written, appropriately informed, parental consent, including new disclosures about where any retained organs would be stored, for how long, and for what purposes.[46]

Susan Lawrence, a medical historian at the University of Iowa, was expecting to receive proofs of an article on autopsy that she had written for a book, scheduled to be published in England in 2001. In November 2000 she received an astonishing e-mail from the book's editor: Because of the controversy surrounding the Alder Hey and Bristol hospital discoveries, which Lawrence had not heard about, there were some "incendiary" parts of the article's text that would have to undergo "some diplomatic changes." Simply put, two passages describing certain autopsy procedures would be deleted. One allegedly offending passage in the text was a descriptive sentence stating that "the remains of the dissected organs may or may not be replaced in the body; if not, they are disposed of as biohazardous waste." The other concerned medical autopsies requiring the consent of the immediate family, with this to-be-deleted portion: "which includes, either explicitly or implicitly, permission for the pathologists to take and to preserve organs and specimens of use to medical science." The book was, in fact, published in 2001 with these passages deleted in spite of the author's protests to the contrary.[47]

The advisory council to the director of the National Heart, Lung, and Blood Institute (NHLBI) has had to deal with a significant problem. The NHLBI has approximately 1.5 million blood samples, including samples from the Framingham Heart Study and multiple other studies. Yet the samples are stored elsewhere and are under the control of individual investigators and their universities—and some of the investigators do not want to share their data with other researchers. The result is that these blood samples could "remain on the shelf" forever unless the NHLBI decides to establish a policy mandating that investigators share all their genetics data gathered at NHLBI expense after a 12- to 18-month proprietary period. The advisory council has had to wrestle with one key question: How long should an investigator be allowed to retain exclusive control of data he or she has collected before turning it over to a central repository?[48]

Howard University plans to create a specialized DNA databank with samples provided by African Americans. Physicians and investigators will obtain blood samples or cheek swabs from 25,000 persons, most of them patients at teaching hospitals affiliated with Howard. Patients will be asked to sign consent forms permitting their samples to be used for research and any identifying data to be protected by an affiliated genomics company. Floyd Malveaux, M.D., dean of the medical school, has given several reasons for establishing the GRAD (Genomic Research in the African Diaspora) Biobank: (*1*) African Americans are often concerned that participating in genetics studies will result in genetic discrimination; (*2*) many African Americans trust Howard faculty members; (*3*) African Americans have higher incidences of certain medical conditions (e.g., high blood pressure, asthma, diabetes, renal failure) than other Americans; (*4*) investigators with existing DNA databanks often tend neither to obtain tissues from African Americans nor do research on the causes of high-frequency conditions in this racial group; and (*5*) Howard expects to make millions of dollars per disease studied. The GRAD Biobank will be managed by First Genetic Trust, a Chicago company that specializes in organizing genetic information while concealing individuals' identities.[49]

Notes

1. Elisa Eiseman and Susanne B. Haga, *Handbook of Human Tissue Sources: A National Resource of Human Tissue Samples* (Rockville, Md.: RAND, 1999), p. xvii.
2. Ted Ashburn, Sharon Wilson, and Barry Eisenstein, "Human Tissue Research in the Genomic Era," *Arch Intern Med* 160 (2000): 3378.
3. National Bioethics Advisory Commission, *Research Involving Human Biological Materials: Ethical Issues and Policy Guidance,* Vol. I (NBAC: Rockville, Md., 1999), pp. 13–15; also see Chapter 8 in this book.
4. Eiseman and Haga, *Handbook of Human Tissue Sources,* 1999.
5. *Ibid.,* p. 141.
6. *Ibid.,* p. xviii.
7. *Ibid.,* selected data from throughout the book.
8. Robert Weir and Robert Olick, "Pilot Study of Family Medicine Patients," part of an unfunded NIH grant proposal entitled "Informed Consent for Research on Stored Tissue Samples," Iowa City, Iowa, 1998, p. 34.
9. Prospect Associates, *National Action Plan on Breast Cancer: Model Consent Form for Biological Tissue Banking Focus Group Report* (Rockville, Md.: Prospect Associates, 1997), Appendix D.
10. *Ibid.,* pp. 5–6, 24–47.

11. James Wells and Dana Karr, "Mini-Hearings on Issues in Human Tissue Storage," in National Bioethics Advisory Commission, *Research Involving Human Biological Materials,* Vol. II: *Commissioned Papers* (NBAC: Rockville, Md., 2000), pp. G-1–G-53.
12. *Ibid.,* p. G-21, emphasis added.
13. *Ibid.,* p. G-22.
14. Marc Schwartz, Karen Rothenberg, Linda Joseph, Judith Benkendorf, and Caryn Lerman, "Consent to the Use of Stored DNA for Genetics Research: A Survey of Attitudes in the Jewish Population," *Am J Med Genet* 98 (2001): 336–42.
15. *Ibid.,* p. 337.
16. *Ibid.,* p. 342.
17. Sophia Wang, Fred Fridinger, Kris Sheedy, and Muin Khoury, "Public Attitudes Regarding the Donation and Storage of Blood Specimens for Genetic Research," *Community Genetics* 4 (2001): 19.
18. *Ibid.,* pp. 19–20.
19. *Ibid.,* pp. 18, 20.
20. *Ibid.,* p. 19.
21. *Ibid.,* p. 25, emphasis added.
22. Dave Wendler and Ezekiel Emanuel, "The Debate Over Research on Stored Biological Samples: What Do Sources Think?" *Arch Intern Med* 162 (2002): 1457–62.
23. Mark A. Rothstein, "Genetic Privacy and Confidentiality: Why They Are So Hard to Protect," *J Law Med Ethics* 26 (1998): 198–204. For an argument why health and life insurers should be permitted to use genetic information in underwriting just as they have used family history, smoking, and other health information for decades, see Robert J. Pokorski, "Use of Genetic Information by Private Insurers," in Timothy Murphy and Marc Lappe, eds., *Justice and the Human Genome Project* (Berkeley: University of California Press, 1994), pp. 91–109. For a critical response contending that this would lead to injustice in access to health care, see Norman Daniels, "The Genome Project, Individual Differences, and Just Health Care," in the same volume, pp. 110–32.
24. National Center for Genome Resources, "National Survey of Public and Stakeholders' Attitudes and Awareness of Genetic Issues" (Washington, D.C.: Schulman, Ronca and Bucuvalas, 1996).
25. U.S. Department of Health and Human Services, Report of the Secretary to the President, "Health Insurance in the Age of Genetics" (Washington, D.C.: July 1997), p. 4 (HHS Report).
26. Kimberly A. Quaid and Michael Morris, "Reluctance to Undergo Predictive Testing: The Case of Huntington's Disease," *Am J Med Genet* 45 (1993): 41–45.
27. Paul R. Billings et al., "Discrimination as a Consequence of Genetic Testing," *Am J Hum Genet* 50 (1992): 476–82.
28. Virginia Lapham, Chahira Kozma, and Joan O. Weiss, "Genetic Discrimination: Perspectives of Consumers," *Science* 274 (1996): 621–24.
29. Lisa N. Geller et al., "Individual, Family, and Societal Dimensions of Genetic Discrimination: A Case Study Analysis," *Sci Eng Ethics* 2 (1996): 71–88; also see Joseph S. Alper et al., "Genetic Discrimination and Screening for Hemochromatosis," *J Public Health Policy* 15 (1994): 345–58.
30. Karen Rothenberg and Sharon Terry, "Before It's Too Late—Addressing Fear of Genetic Information," *Science* 297 (2002): 196 (citing an unpublished paper).
31. Lapham, pp. 622–23; Geller, pp. 82–83. See Mark A. Hall and Stephen S. Rich, "Laws Restricting Health Insurers' Use of Genetic Information: Impact on Genetic Discrimination," *Am J Hum Genet* 66 (2000): 302; William Nowlan, "A Rational View of

Insurance and Genetic Discrimination," *Science* 297 (2002): 195–6; and Dorothy Wertz, "Society and the Not-So-New Genetics," *J Contemp Health Law Policy* 13 (1997): 310, all critiquing these studies.

32. Wertz, pp. 308–09.
33. Hall and Rich, p. 296.
34. *Ibid.*
35. Nowlan, p. 195.
36. U.S. Congress, Office of Technology Assessment, *Medical Monitoring and Screening in the Workplace: Results of a Survey—Background Paper,* OTA-BP-BA-67 (Washington, D.C.: USGPO., Oct. 1991), p. 45.
37. Task Force on Genetic Information and Insurance, NIH-DOE Working Group on Ethical, Legal and Social Implications of Human Genome Research, *Genetic Information and Health Insurance* (NIH Publication No. 93-3686, May 10, 1993), p. 5.
38. HHS Report, p. 3.
39. Equal Employment Opportunity Commission, "Genetic Information and the Workplace," January 20, 1998, available online: http://www.dol.gov/dol/_sec/public/media/reports/genetics.htm.
40. For example, other findings by Hall and Rich attest to these conclusions. "[F]our of six insurers said that, in the future, it is likely so much more genetic information will exist and predictive data will be so much more precise that genetic test results probably will be much more relevant to medical underwriting than now. . . . [W]hether this information will be used is largely a cost/benefit business decision, in response to market forces." Hall and Rich, p. 299.
41. *Ibid.*, p. 304.
42. Rothenberg and Terry, p. 197.
43. Ellen Wright Clayton et al., "Informed Consent for Genetic Research on Stored Tissue Samples," *JAMA* 274 (1995): 1786.
44. National Bioethics Advisory Commission, pp. 1–2.
45. William L. Freeman, "The Role of Community in Research with Stored Tissue Samples," in Robert F. Weir, ed., *Stored Tissue Samples,* pp. 275–76.
46. T.M. Wilkinson, "Parental Consent and the Use of Dead Children's Bodies," *Kennedy Inst Ethics J* 11 (2001): 337–58. Information about the new guidelines is provided on the Web. See Sarah Boseley, "Tougher rules on organ disposal" on this Web site: www.guardianunlimited.co.uk/nhs/story/0,2763,184356,00.html. Also see the British Department of Health's publication of the new guidelines on organ retention from post-mortem examinations at this Web site: http://www.doh.gov.uk/pm1.htm.
47. These e-mail comments were forwarded to us by our colleague Susan Lawrence.
48. Eliot Marshall, "Whose DNA Is It?" *Science* 278 (1997): 564–65.
49. Andrew Pollack, "Big DNA Files To Help Blacks Fight Diseases," *New York Times,* May 27, 2003, pp. A1, A20.

3

The Controversy over Stored Tissues, Research Practices, and Informed Consent

> Patients may expect that tissue samples will be used only for tests
> to provide information for their medical care. They may believe
> that samples will be discarded after testing, although the law often
> requires that samples be retained. When samples are obtained
> as part of medical care, patients may not be told [but should be
> told] about the possibility that these samples will be stored and
> used for research.
> NIH/CDC Workshop Statement, 1995[1]

> To give a description of each and every research protocol which
> might be performed on a patient's tissue is an unreasonable burden
> for the patient and the researcher. The current informed consent
> doctrine . . . is not well suited to research that does not involve
> patient therapy. General consent for use of the tissue should be
> sufficient. Society has a strong interest in research involving
> the use of human tissue which may be hampered by well-intended
> but intrusive regulations.
> College of American Pathologists, 1996[2]

As discussed in Chapter 1, the CDC had an ethical problem in 1994. Their investigators had completed NHANES III in 1991, some of the geneticists at CDC had approximately 19,500 blood samples and 8,500 cell lines in storage, and several publications based on these stored tissue samples had already appeared in leading medical journals. Yet some of the CDC scientists doing molecular genetic research were sufficiently concerned about the inadequacy of the informed consent process used in NHANES III that they were reluctant to continue this research. They turned to the CDC's Institutional Review Board for guidance.[3]

After considerable deliberation about the treasure chest of nationally representative DNA samples in the CDC's possession, the NHANES III consent process, and the federal regulations for research with human participants, the IRB sought advice from the National Center for Human Genome Research at the NIH (the NCHGR was renamed the National Human Genome Research Institute, or NHGRI, in 1997). The NCHGR, in turn, proposed that they enlist the participation of a multidisciplinary group of professionals and other interested persons to discuss the problem. The result was a national, invitational meeting in July 1994 on "Informed Consent for Genetic Studies: Using Stored Tissue Samples." The meeting was co-sponsored by the NCHGR and the CDC and held on the NIH campus.

The goal of this working meeting, from the perspectives of the NCHGR and the CDC investigators, was to produce a conference document that, when published, would not only help the CDC make a decision about the stored NHANES III blood samples and cell lines but also, they hoped, be a document with the status of an NIH "consensus statement" about the ways in which federal regulations on the informed consent process would be applied in various research settings involving genetics research with stored tissue samples. Ellen Wright Clayton, M.D., J.D., was selected as the meeting chairperson. The two-day meeting included presentations on the importance of population-based tissue samples to genetics research, the challenges of obtaining informed consent in a large, national, population-based DNA repository, state newborn screening programs, state cancer tissue repositories, the University of Utah tissue repository, the uniqueness of genetics studies, a University of Iowa study of DNA banking and informed consent, lessons from HIV seroprevalence studies, federal regulations governing informed consent and the use of stored tissue samples, the expectations of research participants about genetics research with their tissue samples, genetics studies with archival tissue collections, and the commercialization of products from genetics research. Discussions were lively and sometimes passionate, and a variety of positions were expressed about a range of subtopics related to the general theme of the meeting.

By the end of the meeting, the desired consensus on informed consent and genetics research with stored tissue samples had proved illusory. Instead, group discussions had exposed a "fault line" that repeatedly seemed to run between (*1*) some genetics investigators and other participants and (*2*) some bioethicists, health-law attorneys, and consumer advocates. The former group favored the retention of traditional research practices involving stored tissue samples without increasing investigators' responsibilities to inform sources of the samples about the planned research. The latter favored strengthening the informed consent process relating to the interests and preferences of research participants on genetics research with stored samples. In particular, participants in the meeting expressed important differences over traditional research uses of stored tissues, ownership and control of DNA samples, the impracticability of recontacting persons for consent to anonymize stored tissues, and the limits to be placed on the use of anonymized samples.

Consequently, the small group of participants assigned the task of drafting a paper reflecting the meeting's conclusions had a significant challenge: how to draft a paper that would call for increased attention to informed-consent matters by genetics investigators without accentuating the serious differences that had surfaced at the meeting. That challenge proved virtually impossible to meet; when the paper was finally published in *JAMA* more than a year later, the "consensus statement" (a designation given to the paper by the journal) was anything but a consensus.[4] Most participants at the meeting, including one of us (RFW), were willing to be listed as essentially agreeing with the paper's recommendations, but other participants at the meeting refused to do so.

In retrospect, it seems clear that no one who participated in this workshop guessed the importance it would have in the post-*Moore* controversy about biomedical research with stored tissues. After all, the common practices of collecting and storing human tissues for research purposes had gone largely unquestioned for decades, and these practices had become even more common in the era of molecular genetics.

Nevertheless, the NIH/CDC-sponsored meeting proved to be a watershed event in a number of ways. First, the meeting highlighted the unprecedented research possibilities provided by the techniques common to molecular genetics. Second, it demonstrated that a diverse combination of persons and groups had serious concerns about some of the research methods used with banked DNA samples. Third, it brought a number of differences of opinion between scientists and nonscientists into the open, especially regarding the appropriate role of informed consent in various genetics studies. Fourth, it showed that some concerns about research with banked tissues extended beyond geneticists to include some common research practices of pathologists, epidemiologists, and other biomedical investigators. Finally, the meeting and its resulting publication—by no means the starting point for this international controversy—served as a catalyst to motivate many professional societies to develop professional guidelines for human tissue research.

This chapter describes the controversy over research with stored tissues that surfaced at that meeting and continues to this day. We begin by raising many questions that characterize this controversy, not only because they are important for an understanding of the controversy itself but also because we will address many of them in later chapters.

Questions in the Ongoing Controversy

A number of questions asked before, during, and after the NIH/CDC meeting pertain to the role of informed consent and related ethical and legal considerations in scientific studies. Some focus on the role of informed consent in *prospective research studies*. For example, should patients and potential research participants be told about the possibilities of long-term storage of their tissue sample(s) and subsequent biomedical research on the sample(s)? What information, if any, should they be given about the likely nature of the planned storage of their tissue samples, including, perhaps, freezing the samples or biologically transforming them into immortalized cell lines, or computerized storage of their personal (and familial) genetic information in a DNA database? Should they be informed about the ways in which the confidentiality and privacy of their personal genetic information (derived from a DNA sample) will be protected, or about the possibilities of future secondary use of the stored sample for scientific purposes other than the purposes for which it was obtained? Should they be given information about the planned identity status of their stored sample in terms of whether it will be (*1*) identified as their sample, (*2*) linked to them (by using an identifying code) as the source of the sample, (*3*) completely anonymous as to individual origination, or (*4*) anonymized after collection? (For more complete descriptions of these terms, see Chapter 2.)

If identified or linkable genetic information about them is likely to be entered into a DNA database, should individuals be given written assurances that this information will not be disclosed to government officials who might request it for forensic purposes? What information, if any, should they be given by biomedical investigators about planned scientific uses of the tissue samples so that they can *communicate personal choices* about the control and ownership of the biological materials, future personal access to the information derived from the banked materials, access of third parties (including employers and health insurance companies) to the same information, the remote possibility that a particular DNA sample might become commercially valuable, and the possibility that they might subsequently want to withdraw their tissue sample (and/or derivative DNA data) from scientific storage?

The questions related to *retrospective studies* on stored tissue samples are different, but equally important to many participants in this ongoing controversy. Should archival tissue samples (e.g., paraffin blocks in pathology departments, neonatal blood spots in newborn screening laboratories) have a planned, limited "life span" in terms of a specified number of years for storage? Or should they be retained essentially forever for long-term clinical follow-up possibilities, epidemiological studies, or medico-legal purposes? How broadly or narrowly should *genetics studies* be defined in order to establish guidelines for the appropriate use of various molecular research methods with archival samples?

In terms of the *identity status* of the stored samples, should all such tissue samples be anonymized as a condition for long-term storage? Should some or all of the samples be retained as identified? Should they be linked or coded to allow disclosure to individual sample sources of potentially relevant clinical information that might be discovered? If some identified or linked samples are stored, should the persons from whom those samples came be recontacted (assuming they are still alive) for consent in the event that new diagnostic tests become possible, are promising in terms of possible benefit, and are wanted by physicians or scientific investigators? In the same kind of situation, should individuals be recontacted for consent in the event that promising new research possibilities come into being that did not exist when the samples were originally collected and stored?

If the residual stored samples are anonymous, does that status give investigators license to use them in whatever ways they regard as appropriate (e.g., as positive or negative controls, as biopsy specimens, as materials for virtually any kind of biomedical research) without ongoing IRB review? Does anonymity mean that such samples, including cell lines, are accessible to virtually any biomedical investigator (in any university, commercial firm, or country) who gets them in collaboration with other scientists and that the samples can then be used for any scientific purpose, without regard to whether such a purpose might be offensive or harmful in some way to the (now unknown) sample source? Can any samples be made truly anonymous, preventing even genetics investigators from tracing a tissue sample to the person from whom it came, even if there were a potentially beneficial clinical reason for that person to be identified?

Additional questions pertain to *post-diagnostic research* done with stored samples that were originally provided by patients in clinical settings. Do patients have any expectations as to what may be done with their blood draws, biopsy samples, or other tissue samples taken by nurses, phlebotomists, or physicians in a clinical setting after diagnostic tests have been completed? Does it matter, ethically, if the post-diagnostic research is subsequently done by *the same physician* who made the clinical request for a diagnostic sample, other biomedical researchers in the same academic or hospital department, researchers in other departments within the same university or hospital, or even biomedical researchers who finally end up with the tissue sample (or a portion of the tissue sample) in a commercial lab? Does it matter in terms of informed consent if the post-diagnostic research is done two weeks after a patient provides the tissue sample, or two or twenty years later under significantly different research circumstances (e.g., using investigative methods and technologies not available earlier)? The possibility of such post-diagnostic research is currently often undisclosed to patients or disclosed only in a vaguely worded sentence (e.g., as part of a hospital admissions form or a surgical consent document). Should this traditional practice be changed in the era of genomic medicine? Should physicians (including primary care physicians) and hospitals provide more information to patients about the possibility of post-diagnostic research, with the goal of obtaining adequately informed consent to this research practice?

We address many of these questions in this book. We also make some recommendations that we hope will take us beyond this seemingly endless list of controversial questions. At this juncture, however, we suggest that the controversy itself largely centers around three core questions pertaining to informed consent and related scientific, ethical, and legal concerns: (*1*) How specific do consent documents used in *research settings* need to be about the intended purpose(s) of a research study in order for research participants to give adequately informed consent? (*2*) How much information about the possibility of post-diagnostic research on stored samples needs to be given to patients in *clinical settings* in order for them to give adequately informed consent? (*3*) How much can the ethical and legal requirement of informed consent be expanded and strengthened before the *socially beneficial research* done by geneticists, pathologists, epidemiologists, and other investigators is seriously impeded?

Precursors to the NIH/CDC Workshop Statement

The Genetic Privacy Act. In early 1995 law professors George Annas, Leonard Glantz, and Patricia Roche began distributing a model piece of legislation called "The Genetic Privacy Act" (GPA). Drafted with ELSI funding (Ethical, Legal, and Social Implications of genetics), the model Act was intended as a proposal for federal legislation; it has also been discussed as a model by several state legislatures.[5]

The GPA is based on four premises: (*1*) genetic information is different from other types of personal information; (*2*) genetic information contained in DNA is like a "coded probabilistic future diary"; (*3*) this information can be accessible to many parties in the era of molecular biology; and, (*4*) because of the highly personal nature of the information and its accessibility, individually identifiable DNA samples need to be protected by law. Consequently, the overarching premise of the GPA

is that no stranger should have or control *identifiable* DNA samples or genetic information about an individual unless that individual specifically authorizes the collection of DNA samples for the purpose of genetic analysis, authorizes the creation of that private information, and has access to and control over the dissemination of that information.[6]

The proposed GPA addresses several of the concerns mentioned earlier, with most of the proposed legislation depending on the identity status of stored DNA samples. The central claim is that individually identifiable DNA samples are the property of the person ("sample source") from whom they come. If samples will be individually identifiable, the Act states that the sample source must grant advance authorization in writing to the collection, storage, and proposed use(s) of the samples, as well as to the possible disclosure of private genetic information gained from genetics analysis. The sample source (or that person's representative in the event of incompetency or death) also has other rights: to revoke consent to genetics analysis at "any time prior to the completion of the analysis," to inspect records that contain information derived from a genetics analysis, to prohibit the use of the DNA sample for research or commercial purposes "even if the sample is not in an individually identifiable form," to consent to the transfer of a DNA sample to other scientists for secondary research purposes, and to order the destruction of the sample upon the research study's completion or the withdrawal of the sample source from the study.

By contrast, the GPA would permit anonymous tissue samples to be used for research purposes if such use were not previously prohibited by the sample source. The authors emphasize: "Nothing in this Act shall be construed as prohibiting or limiting research on a DNA sample that cannot be linked to any individual identifier."[7] Moreover, research by pathologists, geneticists, and other scientists can be done on archival tissue samples, even if the stored samples are individually identifiable, as long as the samples were stored "prior to the effective date of this Act." However, no individually identifiable genetic information may be disclosed without the authorization of the sample source's representative.

That is a brief description of a model law written early in the debate over research with stored tissue samples. This document, even in unpublished form, turned out to be so controversial itself that it further fueled the fire of the larger controversy over research with stored samples, especially when the research involves molecular genetics.

American College of Medical Genetics. In late 1995 the American College of Medical Genetics (ACMG), the professional society of board-certified medical geneticists, contributed to the developing controversy by publishing a position paper on the storage and use of genetics materials in clinical and research settings. Written by John Phillips, M.D., and other members of the ACMG Storage of Genetics Materials Committee, the position paper emphasizes the importance of informed consent by patients and by participants in research studies.[8] Regarding the storage and use of genetics materials obtained for clinical tests, the authors recommend that patients be informed about the purpose and possible outcomes of the genetics test, the anticipated use of the blood or other tissue samples (including whether the sample will be stored for additional scientific purposes), and their options regarding future access to their genetic information and the possibility of subsequently requesting that the samples be destroyed. The ACMG committee also recommends that if samples are going to be stored, patients should be asked for permission to use the samples and the derivative genetics information in counseling and testing their relatives and for permission to anonymize the samples for the purposes of additional scientific research.

In terms of tissue samples obtained for investigational purposes, the ACMG committee recommends that potential participants in research be informed about the purpose and possible outcomes of the current research study, the investigator(s)' policy regarding the duration of sample storage and subsequent sample destruction, and the possibility that the research may lead to the development of diagnostic tests that, in turn, would raise several related issues (e.g., the need to disclose personal genetic information in a family setting and the remote chance that diagnostic tests will be commercially profitable). They also recommend that research participants be asked for permission to anonymize their samples for other types of research, and to be recontacted for additional consent for (currently unknown) future research efforts with their stored samples. As to research on archival samples, the committee points out the inherent conflict between the desirability (in terms of ethics and law) of recontacting individuals to secure their informed consent for ongoing research studies and the impracticability (in many research settings) of recontacting persons from whom samples were previously collected, but makes no specific recommendations regarding how this conflict can or should be resolved.

The NIH/CDC Workshop Statement

As indicated earlier, the report that came out of the writing group for the 1994 NCHGR/CDC meeting was controversial before and after its publication. Written by a multidisciplinary committee, the paper, "Informed Consent for Genetic Research on Stored Tissue Samples," was a generally accurate reflection of discussions during the meeting.[9] It understated some of the contentious points of the meeting, however, by saying simply that several important issues related to genetics research with stored samples needed further discussion.

The NIH/CDC workshop statement emphasizes the importance of conducting research with stored samples within the ethical and legal framework provided by federal regulations for the protection of research participants, and by local IRB review. The document addresses a range of situations and questions pertaining to genetics research on stored samples: whether (1) research with anonymous samples is exempt from federal regulations regarding informed consent and IRB review, (2) removing identifiers from existing samples can be done without the consent of the individual sample source, (3) limits (related to the preferences of sources, or the psychosocial risks of the research) need to be placed on the use of identified or coded samples, (4) genetics research can be done on samples (in pathology or elsewhere) previously obtained from now-deceased persons, (5) tissue samples from children can be used in genetics research, and (6) public health investigations involving genetics studies can be done without consent of the tissue sources.

The document makes several specific recommendations. Regarding previously collected samples, the paper emphasizes the distinction between anonymous samples and samples that are identifiable or linkable at the time a research project is proposed. Samples that are already anonymous (e.g., anonymous pathology samples that might be used for a genetics study) do not require informed consent for the obvious reason that it is impossible to identify the individual source. For this reason, research on existing, anonymous tissue samples is usually exempt from federal regulations. Even genetics studies with anonymous samples, however, should be reviewed by IRBs, at least in part to determine if the desired scientific information could be obtained in a protocol that allows individuals to consent. By contrast, research with stored, currently identified or linkable samples (e.g., samples originally obtained for diagnostic purposes, numerous kinds of pathological samples) requires informed consent if investigators plan to do genetics studies without anonymizing the samples.

What about the fairly common practice whereby investigators take existing identified or linked samples and make them anonymous for use in research by removing all identifiers or linking codes? Current federal regulations permit this practice of anonymizing samples without the consent of the individual source. But for the writers of this document, this practice is problematic, disingenuous, and occasionally deceptive when, for example, clinician investigators obtain a tissue sample for diagnostic purposes, know that they plan later to anonymize the sample for research purposes, do not convey that information to the source of the sample, and subsequently remove the identifiers without consent. Consequently, the statement's authors recommend that this practice be curtailed by changing the federal regulations and by having IRBs weigh the benefits of any such proposed research with to-be-anonymized tissues against the difficulty of requiring the investigators to recontact individual sources for their consent.

Regarding collecting samples in the future, the document is quite clear: "People should have the opportunity to decide whether their samples will be used for research."[10] In research and in clinical settings, information about possible research studies with tissue samples should be provided to individuals when their samples are collected. Whenever individuals agree to such research use of their tissues, the writers of this document recommend that they be given the following options: (1) are they willing to have their samples used in identified or linked research (with appropriate information about confidentiality, psychosocial risks, and possible withdrawal from the study), and (2) do they prefer or are they willing to have their samples stripped of identifiers and linking codes for use in research (again, with appropriate information about the investigators' personal interests, possible commercial benefit, and so on)? Additional recommendations involve giving research participants other choices about the research use of their tissue samples: are they willing to have their tissues shared with other scientists for secondary research purposes, to limit their tissue samples to certain kinds of research studies, and/or to restrict their tissue samples from being used in scientific studies they do not want to support?

This document, depending on one's views, represented either a major step in the direction of improving the process of informed consent for research with stored human tissues—or a major mistake that threatened many of the traditional, common ways of doing human tissue studies. How the core proposals about informed consent advocated in the document compare with the earlier proposals is illustrated in Table 3.1.

Table 3.1 Differing views about the applicability of informed consent to various human
tissue studies (a preliminary comparison)

Genetic Privacy Act:	Informed consent for research should include written authorization for genetics research on *identifiable* samples, but *not* on *anonymous* samples.
American College of Medical Genetics:	Patients have the right to consent to *post-diagnostic* genetics research on clinical samples, even if anonymized; research participants have the legal right to consent to *prospective* genetics tissue studies and, morally, to *retrospective* genetics studies on personal samples.
NIH/CDC Workshop Statement:	Research participants have the right to give specific, informed consent (with several options) to *prospective* or *retrospective* genetics research on *identified* or *linked* samples, including samples to be anonymized.

Critical Responses to the NIH/CDC Workshop Statement

Initial Response. Critical responses to the NIH/CDC "consensus statement" began even before the paper was published. Wayne Grody, M.D., Ph.D., wrote a sharply critical editorial in *Diagnostic Molecular Pathology* about the workshop statement when the paper was still in final draft form, arguing that traditional pathology practices were threatened by an undue emphasis on informed consent. He cautioned that the recommendations of the consensus document "would severely restrict access to archival clinical specimens for molecular genetic research and other purposes." The recommended choices to be given patients about the uses of their tissue samples would require "a multitiered consent form with more options and permutations than an airline frequent-flyer program." Moreover, the same lengthy consent form would have to be administered to patients in all sorts of settings: "every phlebotomy, urinalysis, sputum collection, and even haircut." If actually put into practice, "these restrictive and burdensome policies... would seriously impede, or completely block, a major proportion of molecular research on human disease, especially impacting those research questions that can be addressed in no other way" than through retrospective study of large numbers of archival specimens.[11]

Rapid Action Task Force. Soon thereafter, a so-called "Rapid Action Task Force" (RATF) of the American Society of Human Genetics (ASHG) circulated a draft proposal regarding "Informed Consent for Genetic Research."[12] Written by a committee chaired by Edward McCabe, M.D., the RATF draft criticizes the NIH/CDC workshop statement by affirming the "traditional research practices in human genetics" and calling for the development of consent forms that are "as clear and brief as possible." Accepting virtually all of the NIH/CDC document's recommendations regarding *prospective* genetic research, the RATF agreed that investigators needed to obtain informed consent for research on (*1*) anonymous samples and (*2*) anonymized samples, unless a particular research protocol qualified for a waiver under the federal regulations (e.g., the research could be classified as involving no more than minimal risk to the participants). The RATF's important differences with the earlier document pertained to *archival samples,* such as those contained in pathology labs and newborn screening labs.

American Society of Human Genetics. The RATF draft was subsequently revised by the board of directors of the ASHG, the premier society for professionals in genetics in this country, and published as a policy statement in the *American Journal of Human Genetics.* The published version differs significantly from the NIH/CDC document and the RATF draft, most notably by stating, in specific contrast to the RATF draft, that *informed consent is not necessary in prospective* genetics studies using (*1*) anonymous samples ("biological materials [that] were originally collected without identifiers and are impossible to link to their sources") or (*2*) anonymized samples ("biological materials that were initially identified, but have been irreversibly stripped of all identifiers and are impossible to link to their sources [but may be linkable] with clinical, pathological and demographic information [gained] before the subject identifiers are removed").[13] The ASHG policy statement also affirms the practice of anonymizing samples without consent in retrospective studies because the practice has two important benefits for investigators: it reduces the "chance of introducing bias" in a study by means of an incomplete study sample (some persons may refuse to consent, and others may be impossible to contact for additional consent); and "importantly, making samples anonymous will eliminate the need for [investigators to] recontact [sources] to obtain informed consent."[14]

Some Pathologists and Epidemiologists. In January 1996, additional concerns were expressed by some geneticists and pathologists attending a meeting convened by the NCHGR on "Genetics Research on Human Tissues: Conflicting Implications for Scientific Discovery, Informed Consent, and Privacy." As Richard Lynch, M.D., observed at the meeting, the role of pathologists as legal custodians of stored diagnostic tissue samples largely involves noncontroversial investigations of anonymous, anonymized, and coded samples, with biomedical benefits arising from each kind of research. He commented that "99 percent of what pathologists do with stored tissues is just aimed at better characterizing a lesion that already exists and has been excised by the surgeon."[15] But, as pointed out by privacy advocates at the meeting, problems arise when the tissue samples are subjected to genetics tests that may reveal personal genetic information that was neither known nor anticipated by the patient, the surgeon, or the pathologist, and that may now involve substantial risks of psychosocial harm for the source of the tissue sample and relatives of that person.

In April *JAMA* published letters responding to the NIH/CDC "consensus" paper that appeared four months earlier. One of the letters was especially critical of the document because of its implications for epidemiologic research. Written by Karl Kelsey, M.D., the letter stated that the requirement of "specific informed consent" for all genetics research "could greatly hamper epidemiologic study of gene-environment interaction." Moreover, such a requirement would be impossible to carry out in prospective studies that "necessarily involve testing hypotheses that did not exist at the time of specimen collection." Simply put, the letter stated that "requiring informed consent in every case is unreasonable and will impede research."[16]

College of American Pathologists. Later that year the College of American Pathologists (CAP) drafted a position paper, "Uses of Human Tissue," that was approved by 17 pathology societies. Stating that "the distinction between use of tissue for diagnosis and research is often unclear," the initially unpublished CAP paper points out that tissues used for research purposes can be collected in three different ways: (*1*) *prospective* collection for research requiring informed consent as part of a research protocol where "a patient's identity is clearly known to the researchers," (*2*) *concurrent* collection involving research done on preserved, "anonymized or linkable" portions of "therapeutic or diagnostic specimens left over after all the work necessary for the patient's care has been completed," and (*3*) *retrospective* collection involving the research use of "material already archived from specimens originally obtained for diagnostic and therapeutic purposes."[17]

Since any "left over" tissues from concurrent collection and the "already archived" tissues from earlier collection "can be made free of patient direct identifiers," the CAP paper contends that *general consent* for research (not "separate patient consent for each research study on archived or remnant tissues") is sufficient to protect the rights of patients. Written in response to the papers on genetics research and informed consent by the ACMG, the NIH/CDC committee, and the ASHG, this paper calls for general consent forms that are "worded broadly and include statements that tissues may be used in research approved by IRBs and for educational purposes." Such general consent forms would be simple and very general: "I __ CONSENT __ DECLINE TO CONSENT to the use of my tissues for research."[18]

Council of Regional Networks for Genetic Services. In December 1996, the Council of Regional Networks for Genetic Services (CORN) issued an unpublished position paper, "Issues in the Use of Archived Specimens for Genetics Research," that largely *went against the tide of criticism* directed at the NIH/CDC workshop document. The CORN paper points out that existing collections of tissues come in several forms, including: (*1*) newborn screening blood spots, (*2*) research samples in various labs, and (*3*) archived clinical specimens. Regarding post-diagnostic research on these samples, the paper states that "tissue specimens obtained for diagnostic and therapeutic purposes may reasonably be used for the continuing further advance of medical science."[19] As to new and future collections, the CORN paper emphasizes that increasing use of genetics studies in medicine means "the most forthright approach to the possibility of *multiple uses of new collections* would be an acknowledgement of the *assumption* that such specimens will be used in genetics research."[20]

In terms of anonymized samples, the CORN paper rebuts the frequent claim by genetics investigators that "use of anonymous samples is ethically justifiable, regardless of the purpose for which the samples were collected." Instead, it emphasizes the importance of (*1*) "the fiduciary relationship between medical professionals and their patients/subjects," (*2*) "the *right* of source persons to disclosure of possible future uses of their tissues," and (*3*) informed consent to *prospective* genetics studies, including, depending on relevant regulations and IRB requirements, research studies done on newborn screening blood spots and research carried out with surgical and other clinical specimens.

The paper then calls for the use of consent forms whenever a specimen is collected for "genetic study (either diagnostic or research)," and concludes with a proposed model consent document that is much more detailed and specific than the earlier NIH/CDC document published in *JAMA*. The model consent form would give the source of a tissue sample the options of (*1*) consenting to have an *identifiable* sample placed in storage (with 10 yes/no choices as to the types of research that could be done), (*2*) consenting to have an *anonymized* tissue sample stored for research (with 3 yes/no choices), or (*3*) refusing to consent to have "any excess specimen" stored in any form after the initial "genetic study and/or research purpose" for which the tissue sample was taken has been completed.[21]

Association of American Medical Colleges. A very different type of position paper was subsequently circulated by the Association of American Medical Colleges (AAMC). Titled "Patient Privacy and the Use of Archival Patient Material and Information in Research," the AAMC paper acknowledges the intense concerns over "genetic privacy" and the various technologies that "enable precise genetic information to be extracted from any human tissue sample that contains DNA." The initially unpublished paper points out that several legislative bills in Congress "threaten to burden, or even imperil, a large body of . . . research that is absolutely dependent on ready access to patient records and tissue samples, most often in coded, but linkable, form."[22]

The document emphasizes the importance of researchers having "ready accessibility of personally identifiable, i.e., linkable, archival patient materials, such as medical records and tissue specimens removed in the course of routine medical care." However, neither "the general public or legislators" recognizes the benefits that can be gained from "sophisticated genetic analyses on archival human tissue samples that may be decades old," or the clinical reasons why "all archival patient materials to be used in research cannot be made anonymous, that is, totally and irrevocably unidentifiable, or "the crushing financial, administrative and logistical burdens" that would accompany recent proposals for explicit informed consent for research on archival patient specimens.[23]

The AAMC document proposes several principles for research on stored samples, most of which are consistent with the earlier CAP position paper: the medical necessity of research on *archival* tissue samples, the medical benefits that can be gained from research on *linked* samples, the importance of protecting the confidentiality and privacy of *identified* patient information, the need for institutional confidentiality policies with severe penalties for violators, and the adequacy of permitting research on archival patient materials ("whether linkable or not") under "a general informed consent mechanism." The paper emphasizes the distinction between (*1*) "the forms of stringent informed consent appropriate for research in the typical clinical setting" and (*2*) the general informed consent that is sufficient for research on archived materials.

The paper concludes with a policy proposal for all clinical and research organizations: "[G]ive each patient at his/her first encounter with the health care system *two unique identifiers,* one for clinical use, the other for research." This proposal suggests that both numbers would be "permanently associated with the specific individual," and the linkage between the two numbers "securely maintained in a protected location [a databank] with controlled access," thereby protecting the confidentiality of the stored information.[24]

The debate about the meaning and applicability of informed consent for various human tissue studies continues, of course.[25] But the most contentious period of the controversy, at least in the United States to date, occurred in 1994–97, with numerous professional societies producing position papers and notable publications being done by academic professionals in several fields. Some of the views advocated during that period are further illustrated in Table 3.2.

Alternative Solutions

As should be clear by now, this controversy has numerous players: genetics investigators, pathologists, epidemiologists, federal regulatory agencies, the NIH, the CDC, several professional medical organizations, bioethicists, health-law attorneys, local IRBs, and interested groups of consumer advocates. The controversy in the United States has sometimes seemed in an oversimplistic way to be a debate between the authors and signers of the NIH/CDC "consensus" document, and the individuals and professional groups critical of it. Put in global perspective,

Table 3.2 Differing views about the applicability of informed consent to various human tissue studies

Genetic Privacy Act:	Informed consent for research should include written authorization for genetics research on *identifiable* samples, but *not* on *anonymous* samples.
American College of Medical Genetics:	Patients have the right to consent to *post-diagnostic* genetics research on clinical samples, even if anonymized; research participants have the legal right to consent to *prospective* genetics tissue studies and, morally, to *retrospective* genetics studies on personal samples.
NIH/CDC Workshop Statement:	Research participants have the right to give specific, informed consent (with several options) to *prospective* or *retrospective* genetics research on *identified* or *linked* samples, including samples to be anonymized.
Rapid Action Task Force (ASHG):	Research participants have the right to consent to *prospective* genetics research on any stored personal samples, unless this right is waived in a given study, but do *not* have the right to consent to *retrospective* genetics research on archival samples.
American Society of Human Genetics:	Research participants do *not* have the right to consent to either *prospective* or *retrospective* genetics studies whenever the samples are *anonymous* or *anonymized*.
College of American Pathologists:	Patients and research participants have the right to give informed consent to *prospective* research on *identified* or *coded* samples; otherwise, general consent is sufficient for all retrospective research and any prospective research on coded or anonymized samples.
Council of Regional Networks for Genetic Services:	Patients and research participants have the right to give specific, informed consent (with numerous options) to *prospective* genetics research, including research on samples to be anonymized, but *not* for *retrospective* genetics research or *post-diagnostic* genetics research.
Association of American Medical Colleges:	Patients have the right to give informed consent to *prospective* research on *identified* samples; otherwise, general consent is sufficient for all retrospective research and any prospective research on coded or anonymized samples.

however, this controversy represents an ongoing, international debate between (*1*) some multidisciplinary task forces, indigenous communities, and individuals in several countries who think that in the era of molecular genetics, increased emphasis needs to be placed on the distinctive importance of personal and familial genetic information, the right of personal choice about the use of one's body and the tissues taken from it, and the necessity of being able to exercise a measure of control over the research that can be done with one's tissues; and (*2*) some professional groups of biomedical scientists, pharmaceutical and biotechnology companies, and individuals in various countries who think that in an era of ever-increasing professional and legal regulations, renewed emphasis needs to be placed on the invaluable and often irreplaceable research resource represented by stored tissue samples, the inestimable societal and individual benefits that have been gained by means of biomedical research done with stored samples, and the serious threat posed to the continuation of these research efforts by unnecessarily restrictive policy proposals and laws aimed at strengthening the ethical and legal requirements of informed consent.

We conclude this chapter by taking a comparative look at the alternative solutions put forward by U.S. participants in this controversy over stored tissue samples, research practices, and informed consent. What do the various proposed solutions suggest be done to address the competing interests and values at stake with stored tissues? What recommended changes need to take place in current research practices to address concerns about informed consent that have been raised about research with existing collections of specimens, research with not-yet-collected samples, and any kind of research with stored samples that involves the possibility of psychosocial harm to individuals, families, and identifiable groups? Comparisons among the differing proposals advocated by various groups are summarized in Table 3.3.

Six possible solutions have been suggested and/or tried. One idea is to retain as many traditional research practices as possible, especially regarding retrospective research on archival samples. As illustrated by the CAP policy statement, the ASHG policy statement, and the AAMC policy statement, there are some

Table 3.3 What should be done now: comparisons of the differing proposals in the debate

1. *Retain Traditional Research Practices*	College of American Pathologists; American Society of Human Genetics; Association of American Medical Colleges
2. *Develop New Professional Guidelines*	American College of Medical Genetics
3. *Have More Consensus Meetings*	National Human Genome Research Institute (NIH)
4. *Recommend Changes in the Federal Regulations and IRB Practices*	Authors and signers of the NIH/CDC Workshop Statement
5. *Create Improved Consent Documents*	American College of Medical Genetics; NIH/CDC Workshop Statement; Rapid Action Task Force (ASHG); Council of Regional Networks for Genetic Services
6. *Mandate Changes by Statute*	Authors of the Genetic Privacy Act

pathologists, geneticists, and other biomedical investigators who downplay the importance of informed consent with stored tissues and want to continue traditional research practices, especially the practice of anonymizing samples without consent in pathology laboratories, newborn screening laboratories, and other locations for archived specimens.

The ASHG policy statement, while emphasizing the importance of informed consent in prospective studies using identifiable or identified samples, clearly favors placing greater weight on traditional research practices than on considerations of informed consent when the stored samples in question are samples that have been or could be anonymized without the consent of the sample sources or their relatives or surrogates. No mention is made of possible ways of anonymizing samples in an expanded context of informed consent, either by (1) recontacting the still-identifiable adult sources before anonymizing the samples (as had been discussed in the NCHGR/CDC meeting and NIH/CDC paper) or (2) initiating a request to an adult sample source (or the parent(s) of a neonatal sample source) for consent to anonymize samples for research purposes *before* the samples gain the status of "existing" or archival samples. The CAP and AAMC documents even raise questions about the importance of informed consent with identified or linked samples. Both policy statements emphasize the adequacy of a general consent statement that, whenever granted by an individual, would give researchers blanket permission to carry out virtually any kind of studies they choose with the tissue samples they secure from that person, including secondary research studies having significantly different purposes than those for which the sample was originally given.

Another possible solution is to recommend new professional society guidelines that can update professional practices in the light of new technological developments and new ethical and legal concerns about stored samples. This proposal's strongest feature is the importance it places on self-governance and change from within professional ranks, with the hope that choosing to adopt peer-influenced change will preclude imposed change from outside the profession (e.g., by law or federal regulations).

Thus the Storage of Genetics Materials Committee produced a position statement for the ACMG that briefly interpreted the concept of informed consent in the context of stored tissues, and then gave recommendations regarding the collection of tissue samples for prospective genetics tests in clinical and research settings as well as the currently acceptable uses of stored DNA or genetic materials. Similarly, the RATF made a proposal to the ASHG regarding the application of informed-consent considerations to prospective and retrospective studies that could have been helpful in modest ways in changing the practices of genetics investigators. The ACMG document, however, failed to make several needed recommendations pertaining to DNA banking and informed consent, and the RATF document, already primarily protective of the research interests of some of its authors, became even more protective of the research interests of investigators who use anonymized samples without consent in the revised form published by the ASHG.

A third solution is to try to arrive at consensus about acceptable research practices through special meetings of interested parties who have conflicting interests and concerns about stored DNA samples. This solution has been favored by the NCHGR at the NIH, as illustrated by the multidisciplinary meetings it planned and hosted in July 1994 and January 1996. In the first of these meetings, representatives from the CDC and NCHGR (now the NHGRI) met with invited genetics investigators, bioethicists, attorneys, and patient advocates in the hope of reaching agreement on whether the CDC could proceed to do research on its archived NHANES III tissue samples, or whether investigators at the CDC and elsewhere needed to gain more specific consent of individual sources before carrying out research on identifiable and/or anonymized tissue samples. In the 1996 meeting, several leading pathologists were invited to meet with NCHGR representatives, ELSI representatives, advocates for physicians and biomedical investigators, and patient advocates in order to enable the pathologists to express professional concerns over the issue of informed consent and research with stored tissues. Neither meeting resulted in unanimous agreement, but both meetings seem to have been beneficial. It appeared that compromise was possible on at least some of the issues in question, with several participants voicing hope for achieving a reasonable balance (e.g., in improved consent forms) in the near future between (1) the rights and preferences of individual patients and research participants and (2) the practices and interests of physicians and biomedical investigators. How much compromise is actually achieved remains to be seen, given the vested interests and high stakes involved in the debate.

A fourth solution is to recommend changes in the federal regulations and IRB review practices. The clearest example of this approach is the NIH/CDC workshop paper published in *JAMA*, which places considerable weight on the federal regulations (and related publications by the former federal Office for Protection from Research Risks, now named the Office for Human Research Protections) because they "are legally enforceable and because they are the embodiment of an attempt to strike a balance between the desire to increase knowledge and the protection of individual interests."[26] The document frequently quotes the regulations and sometimes goes to considerable lengths to show how the regulations can and should apply to some important research issues that have developed since the regulations were written, namely emerging questions about the collection and use of stored tissue samples.

Nevertheless, this proposed solution depends not merely on professionals in multiple fields being able to know, interpret, and apply the federal regulations to state-of-the-art concerns about the collection and use of stored DNA samples, but more importantly, their being able to bring about changes in the regulations (and their use by IRBs) so that they will continue to balance the competing interests of scientific investigators and individuals (and families) who participate in research studies. The NIH/CDC paper indicates several ways in which the regulations need to be updated, clarified, and changed to provide needed guidance for investigators and the IRB members who review their research proposals: appropriate limits to be placed on genetics studies with anonymous samples, IRB review of studies using anonymous samples, the practice of anonymizing existing samples, the limits of impracticability in securing consent, and the degree of deference to be given to individuals' preferences not to have their tissue samples used for specific types of genetics research.

A fifth possible solution is to produce updated consent forms in clinical and research settings that more accurately describe current research practices with stored samples and more adequately enable individuals to make informed choices about how their DNA samples (and the personal/familial genetic information contained therein) are to be used. The ACMG committee, the NIH/CDC workshop group, the RATF group, and the CORN position paper all maintain that many of the conflicts over stored tissues can be addressed by means of (1) more appropriately worded consent documents and (2) improved IRB review of research protocols using identified, linked, anonymous, or anonymized tissue samples. The catch, of course, is whether updated consent forms will be more protective of the rights of individual sources to make informed-consent choices about their banked tissues, or of the professional interests of biomedical investigators who frequently write the documents. The challenge will be to see if multidisciplinary interests can be reflected in updated consent documents that contain workable compromises, such as including modest amounts of information for patients about pathological research practices before any biological samples are collected as part of the surgery.

The CORN position paper, in fact, proposes the use of a model consent form that goes well beyond the general consent limit that the CAP and AAMC position papers find sufficient. In an effort to be "explicit and intentional about further uses" of tissue samples initially obtained for genetic diagnostic study or genetics research, the CORN Committee on Ethical and Legal Issues proposes that patients and research participants be given a consent document that contains "a menu of options, each to be marked affirmatively or negatively by the patient" or research participant. If an individual chooses to permit research on coded or *identifiable* samples, he or she can indicate specific preferences regarding secondary research, the requirement of additional consent in the future, the destruction of the specimen after this person dies, and the possibility of research having commercial implications. If the individual consents to research on *anonymized* samples, he or she can indicate preferences regarding secondary research, including whether that research is done by the same investigator(s) or by investigators in other facilities or institutions. If the individual does not consent to any research "after completion of the original testing for which the specimen was taken," that choice can also be expressed on the document.[27]

The sixth proposed solution is to mandate by statute the changes needed to protect individuals from unauthorized analysis of their DNA samples, disclosure of personal genetic information resulting from genetic studies, and transfer of their stored biological materials to other investigators. The most comprehensive attempt to work on this solution is the proposed Genetic Privacy Act written by George Annas, Leonard Glantz, and Patricia Roche. According to this model piece of legislation, an individual sample source has the right to determine who may collect and analyze a blood or other tissue sample, limit the purposes for which a DNA sample can be analyzed, know what information can reasonably be expected from the genetic tests, order the destruction of stored DNA samples, delegate authority to a surrogate to order the destruction of stored DNA samples, prohibit even the anonymous use of their samples in research, refuse to permit the use of the DNA sample(s) for research or commercial activities, and inspect (and obtain) copies of records containing information derived from genetic analysis of the DNA sample(s).[28]

This approach is, of course, quite different from the other strategies. Rather than relying on peer-influenced change, consensus-driven change, updated changes in the federal regulations, and research-oriented consent forms, this approach would force change through the power of law and the threat of legal penalties. Thus the proposed GPA has a section on civil remedies according to which a person (e.g., a clinician, a biomedical investigator, a professional in a biomedical lab) who violates the provisions of the GPA through negligence would be liable for a $25,000 fine plus other monetary damages, and a person who willfully violates the GPA would be liable for a $50,000 fine plus other monetary damages.

It remains to be seen whether this or any other proposal will actually work. At present, the GPA remains a controversial proposal for a model law that has been frequently discussed and often praised by advocates of change and informed consent. It has also been frequently rejected by scientific investigators, biomedical research societies, biotechnology companies, and some state legislatures as unnecessary and counterproductive to biomedical progress.[29]

In the next chapter, we describe some of the research practices common to molecular genetics. We also indicate why the complex field of genetics research has such a central role in the debate over research with banked DNA samples.

Cases and Vignettes

Geneticists working on the federally funded Human Genome Project became concerned in 1997 that geneticists in the private sector would win the race to establish an invaluable research database comprised of thousands of single nucleotide polymorphisms (SNPs) representative of the human genome. The specific concern was that a scientific consortium including Affymetrix, a biochipmaker, or another scientific consortium including Genset, a

French biotechnology company, would use biochip technology to identify 100,000 SNPs, gain patents, and then commercialize the process of searching for genetic anomalies through the use of a mutation-sensing "DNA chip." In response, the HGP-sponsored geneticists decided to develop a public database comprised of at least 100,000 single-base variations in human DNA obtained from blood samples from 100–500 people in four major population categories: African, Asian, European, and Native American. The SNPs project was projected to cost $20–$30 million. To kick-start the project, some investigators suggested beginning it by using cell lines in existing DNA collections, such as NHANES III, even though doing that would raise serious ethical questions about the informed consent originally given by the NHANES III participants.[30]

The physical remains of Christopher Columbus are well traveled, given the number of post-mortem trips they are claimed to have made over the centuries. Columbus died as an illustrious admiral in Valladolid, Spain, in 1506, having issued instructions that he should be buried in the Americas. Three years later his remains were moved to a family chapel on the island of La Cartuja in Seville. Years later a daughter-in-law received royal permission to move the explorer's corpse to Santo Domingo in the Dominican Republic. In 1795 the bones were moved, according to the Spanish version of the story, to Havana, where they remained until 1898. During the Spanish-American war, the bones were repatriated to Seville. According to the Dominican version of the story, the bones that were moved were those of someone else. Now, two Spanish teachers have asked the forensic specialists at the Laboratory of Genetic Identification at the University of Grenada to settle the historic dispute. Their plan is to have these DNA specialists test the skeleton of Hernando, an illegitimate son of Columbus' love affair with a woman from Cordoba, and compare the DNA results with the DNA found in the bones in the rival "Columbus" tombs in Seville and Santo Domingo.[31]

DNA Sciences, a biotechnology company in California, started using a Web site (see www.DNA.com) in 2000 in an attempt to recruit 50,000–100,000 altruistic persons willing to donate a sample of their DNA to help find disease-causing genes. The Web site's original invitation to participate in the Gene Trust Project declared, "The knowledge we gain from the gene trust has the potential to change medicine forever, but we can't do it without your help." Two years later the Web site's welcome stated, "We have had a tremendous and positive response to the Gene Trust Project and have begun several different studies with our Gene Trust Volunteer samples. At this time, we are not accepting any new registrations until we move to the next phase of our work." The Web page ended with a profile and photograph of one of the volunteers, who wanted to be a participant, via her blood sample, in the effort to find a cure for multiple sclerosis.[32]

A for-profit company—the First Genetic Trust, Inc. in Illinois—has a plan that will aid research efforts in pharmacogenomics, the interdisciplinary field that hopes to provide medicines tailor-made to an individual's genetic profile. Their plan, if it works, will also protect the confidentiality of individual's genetic information. Working with the Memorial Sloan-Kettering Cancer Center in New York, First Genetic Trust, serving as a third-party broker of genetic information, will invite individuals to store their DNA information in its confidential database, with each person having provided informed consent via the Internet. The company will then communicate that information in coded form to scientific investigators. Critics doubt that the plan will pass ethical and scientific muster [but administrators at Howard University in Washington, D.C., disagree, as indicated by a case in Chapter 2].[33]

Notes

1. Ellen Wright Clayton, Karen Steinberg, Muin Khoury, Elizabeth Thomson, Lori Andrews, Mary Jo Kahn, Loretta Kopelman, and Joan Weiss, "Informed Consent for Genetic Research on Stored Tissue Samples," *JAMA* 274 (1995): 1786.
2. College of American Pathologists, "Uses of Human Tissue," unpublished policy statement, August 1996, pp. 6–7.
3. Portions of this chapter are revised versions of two earlier papers: Robert F. Weir, "Advanced Directives for the Use of Stored Tissue Samples," in Robert F. Weir, ed., *Stored Tissue Samples: Ethical, Legal, and Public Policy Implications* (Iowa City: University of Iowa Press, 1998): 236–66; and Robert F. Weir, "The Ongoing Debate about Stored Tissue Samples, Research, and Informed Consent," in the National Bioethics Advisory Commission, *Research Involving Human Biological Materials: Ethical Issues and Policy Guidance,* Vol. II: *Commissioned Papers* (Rockville, Md.: NBAC, 2000): F-1 to F-21.
4. Clayton et al., pp. 1786–92.
5. George J. Annas, Leonard Glantz, and Patricia Roche, "The Genetic Privacy Act and Commentary," unpublished model law, February 1995.
6. *Ibid.*, p. 6, emphasis added.
7. *Ibid.*, p. 24.
8. American College of Medical Genetics, Storage of Genetics Materials Committee, "Statement on Storage and Use of Genetic Materials," *Am J Hum Genet* 57 (1995): 1499–1500.
9. Clayton et al., pp. 1786–92.
10. *Ibid.*, p. 1791.
11. Wayne W. Grody, "Molecular Pathology, Informed Consent, and the Paraffin Block," *Diagn Mol Pathol* 4 (1995): 156.
12. Edward R. B. McCabe et al., American Society of Human Genetics Rapid Action Task Force, "Report on Informed Consent for Genetic Research," unpublished document, pp. 1–10.
13. American Society of Human Genetics (ASHG), "Statement on Informed Consent for Genetic Research," *Am J Hum Genet* 59 (1996): 471–74.
14. *Ibid.*, p. 474.
15. Joan Stephenson, "Pathologists Enter Debate on Consent for Genetic Research on Stored Tissue," *JAMA* 275 (1996): 504.
16. Karl T. Kelsey, "Informed Consent for Genetic Research" (letter), *JAMA* 275 (1996): 1085.
17. College of American Pathologists, "Uses of Human Tissue," August 1996, pp. 7–8. For a related paper, see William Grizzle, Kay Woodruff, and Thomas Trainer, "The Pathologist's Role in the Use of Human Tissues in Research—Legal, Ethical, and Other Issues," *Arch Pathol Lab Med* 120 (1996): 909–12.
18. College of American Pathologists, "Uses of Human Tissue," p. 8. Three years later CAP published another version of this paper that had been revised by the Ad Hoc Committee on Stored Tissue. See William Grizzle et al., "Recommended Policies for Uses of Human Tissue in Research, Education, and Quality Control," *Arch Pathol Lab Med* 123 (1999): 296–300. The authors explained the publication of a revised paper in this manner: "Authors of the consensus statement recognized that there were portions of the statement that were being misinterpreted. The revision presented here clarifies points that have been misinterpreted." Among the revisions is a new concluding

sentence: "In the future, we recommend that all institutions put into place procedures to obtain simple [meaning "general or unspecified"] consent for the use of diagnostic specimens for research, education, and quality control studies."

19. Committee on Ethical and Legal Issues, Council of Regional Networks for Genetic Services (CORN), "Issues in the Use of Archived Specimens for Genetics Research: 'Points to Consider,'" unpublished manuscript, December 1996, p. 3.

20. *Ibid.*, p. 4.

21. *Ibid.*, pp. 7–8.

22. Association of American Medical Colleges (AAMC), "Patient Privacy and the Use of Archival Patient Material and Information in Research," unpublished paper, April 1997, pp. 1–2. This paper was subsequently revised and published as part of *Medical Records and Genetic Privacy, Health Data Security, Patient Privacy, and the Use of Archival Patient Materials in Research* (Washington, D.C.: American Medical Association, 1997).

23. AAMC, "Patient Privacy and the Use of Archival Patient Material," p. 2.

24. *Ibid.*, p. 4 (emphasis added).

25. See, for example, Dave Wendler and Ezekiel Emanuel, "The Debate on Stored Biological Samples: What Do Sources Think?" *Arch Intern Med* 162 (2002): 1457–62; and Robert M. Sade, "Research on Stored Biological Samples Is Still Research," *Arch Intern Med* 162 (2002): 1439–40.

26. Clayton et al., p. 1787.

27. CORN, pp. 7–8.

28. George Annas, Leonard Glantz, and Patricia Roche, "Drafting the Genetic Privacy Act: Science, Policy, and Practical Considerations," *J Law Med Ethics* 23 (1995): 361.

29. Neil A. Holtzman, "Panel Comment: The Attempt to Pass the Genetic Privacy Act in Maryland," *J Law Med Ethics* 23 (1995): 367–70; and Philip R. Reilly, "Panel Comment: The Impact of the Genetic Privacy Act on Medicine," *J Law Med Ethics* 23 (1995): 378–81.

30. Eliot Marshall, "Playing Chicken Over Gene Markers," *Science* 278 (1997): 2046–48.

31. Emma Daly, "Hoping DNA Will Discover Columbus, Post-Mortem," *New York Times*, May 23, 2002, p. A8.

32. Andrew Pollack, "Company Seeking Donors of DNA for a 'Gene Trust,'" *New York Times,* August 1, 2000, pp. A1, C10. The Web site quoted was last visited by one of the authors on June 28, 2002.

33. Eliot Marshall, "Company Plans to Bank Human DNA Profiles," *Science* 291 (2001): 575.

4

Molecular Genetics: Tissue Samples in the Laboratory

> DNA banking involves the storage (with individual identifiers) of transformed cell lines, extracted DNA, cryopreserved blood or other tissue, or biological samples preserved by some other method, so that at some future date the DNA can be studied for some purpose or purposes. Academic and commercial facilities that bank DNA generally do so for either or both of two purposes:... (*1*) research (gene mapping) purposes or (*2*) as a service to those who are at risk for a particular genetic disease and who thus may be interested in family-based linkage testing.
>
> Jean E. McEwen and Philip R. Reilly, 1995
> ELSI Research Program, NHGRI; and Interluekin Genetics, Inc.[1]

> The drug companies and biotech firms pursuing the [chip] technology are hoping that DNA chips will prove to be a primary research tool in a genetic-medicine revolution. They expect that understanding the genes active in disease will spawn a new generation of therapeutic drugs that treat underlying causes rather than symptoms.
>
> Robert F. Service, 1998, Journalist, *Science*[2]

Clinical laboratories and research laboratories have a long history of handling biological materials derived from patients or participants in research studies. Extensive quality control procedures established over many years of experience ensure that samples are logged in, analyzed, and tracked in a way that helps generate high quality information and also ensures, when samples remain identified or identifiable, that results are identified with the originating patient with close to 100% accuracy.

In the age of DNA analysis, samples can have a long life span within a laboratory that includes analysis not only for their originating purpose—the measurement of the hemoglobin level in a blood sample, the sugar level in a sample of cerebral spinal fluid, or the protein level in urine—but for additional scientific purposes as well. Subsequent research studies sometimes were not and could not have been anticipated when samples were originally collected. Thus one important reason for long-term storage of tissue samples in laboratories is to facilitate research for multiple scientific purposes, with some studies being done concurrently with several portions of stored samples and others taking place months or years later and requiring subsequent DNA extraction from pertinent stored samples.

In this chapter we present information regarding the scientific work done with stored tissues in genetics and other laboratories using molecular techniques. In short, we focus on the widespread scientific practices collectively known as DNA banking in the United States, "DNA sampling" in Canada, and "biobanking" in some European countries.

References to "DNA banking," "DNA sampling," and, occasionally, "DNA databanks" are often confusing. Sometimes such references are to blood or other tissues that are being stored for future laboratory use. Other references are to stored samples that have been "transformed" or "immortalized" through laboratory techniques so that they provide an unlimited source of identical DNA. Still others are to the data derived from DNA samples, with that data being stored electronically for the purposes of current research analysis, future research studies, or the provision of demographic information about the person(s) from whom the samples came.

As noted in Chapter 2, we use "DNA banking" as an inclusive term referring to two kinds of storage of DNA-related information for possible future use. Most frequently, we refer to the *stored biological material,* including (*a*) tissue samples that have been obtained from patients or research participants by means of blood draws or other sampling techniques and, in some laboratories, (*b*) one or more cell lines that have been made from the original tissue samples. Sometimes we also refer to the *genetic data* derived from tissue samples and/or cell lines, including stored DNA sequence data as well as other relevant information about individual patients or research participants (or criminals, in forensic contexts) stored in databases. Our emphasis here is on the practicalities of how various kinds of tissue samples can be obtained, processed, stored, and analyzed.

Biological Sampling Methods

As is commonly known, DNA is contained primarily within the nucleus of the cell. Fortunately for scientific investigators, DNA is a relatively stable molecule and is obtainable even from tissues that have not been prepared directly with DNA isolation in mind. Unfortunately, genetics investigators necessarily have concerns about the quality of the DNA material that can be obtained from improperly stored tissues. Thus the methods of processing and storing tissue samples are very important considerations when programs or strategies are devised to carry out prospective DNA analysis. These considerations are equally important but even more problematic when retrospective studies have to rely on samples that were obtained months, probably years, earlier without any thought that the samples might later be used for DNA analysis.

It is also important to indicate that in some cases other components within the cell can also provide information that is genetically relevant or relevant for both genetic and environmental causes of disease. Messenger RNA and its derivative, cDNA, can provide information about specific expressed genes that have been identified within a given cell. In some cases, this material will be the most sought-after component for a particular form of analysis. In addition, the downstream product of messenger RNA, namely the proteins derived from the information contained within the messenger RNA and its parent DNA, may also be the analyte of most interest to a specific investigator. Genetic information is sometimes best identified from the products of the genes—the proteins—rather than from genes themselves.

The techniques of analysis are also very important to issues related to the storage of DNA. In the early years of DNA analysis, the primary form by which analytic strategies took place made use of a technique known as Southern blotting, or Southern blot analysis.[3] In this procedure, a relatively large quantity of DNA (DNA fragments having at least 10,000 base pairs) had to be derived from millions of individual cells. Southern blots were the methods used to detect restriction fragment length polymorphisms (RFLPs), the first form of variant detectable at the DNA level. The identification of RFLPs led to many early genetics studies that provided chromosomal localizations for inherited diseases. They were also used for years as a diagnostic tool to make predictions about the likelihood of a genetic disease being passed from parent to child.

Although Southern blot analysis is still used in some settings, including both clinical diagnosis and forensic identification, it has been increasingly replaced in the last few years by (1) polymerase chain reaction analysis (PCR) and (2) direct DNA sequencing protocols. In some cases, direct DNA sequencing protocols may also rely on PCR analysis as an initial preparatory procedure, but there are also an increasing number of strategies available to carry out DNA sequencing that do not need to be connected directly to PCR.

Following its initial description in the mid-1980s, laboratory use of PCR revolutionized the way in which DNA can be analyzed.[4] The greatest strength of the PCR method lies in its ability to make use of very short lengths and very tiny amounts of DNA, so that even the amount of DNA found in a single cell can be practically analyzed using PCR. This method of analysis relies on the use of a recognized and identified DNA sequence and then the construction of a series of oligonucleotide primers that serve as reference points on either side of a DNA sequence of particular interest, usually a stretch of DNA having a mutation or base pair change in which the detection is targeted. These oligonucleotide primers, or DNA reference points, serve as one component of a reaction technique in which large quantities of DNA from the specific region of interest can be generated and then analyzed using a number of laboratory-based strategies, including gel electrophoresis and/or DNA sequencing. Gel electrophoresis allows DNA fragments to move through a gel-like material under the influence of an electric field, with larger, slower DNA molecules being separated from smaller ones. Because very short stretches of DNA can serve as an initial template or reference point for these reactions, the requirements for storage of the DNA samples are minimized.[5]

In addition, since very tiny amounts of DNA can be used in PCR analysis, the number of assays that can be carried out from a particular sample greatly increase and the methods by which samples can be stored are simplified. Although, typically, only a few individual sites along the genomic material of approximately three billion (3,000,000,000) nucleotides, or bases, can be analyzed in a specific PCR, analytic strategies now exist that conceivably can allow the DNA from even a single cell to be analyzed in hundreds, or even thousands of reactions by amplifying not just a few regions of interest, but the entire quantity of DNA isolated from that specific cell. In the future these technologies will have the ability to characterize enormous numbers of DNA variations so that very specific information about a particular individual will be developed, stored, and analyzed in laboratories.

Tissue Types

Viable Tissues. A variety of tissues are available for DNA banking purposes. The most complex tissues are living, or viable, tissues that exist in laboratories in two related but different forms. The first type of living tissue available for study are tissues such as skin cells (fibroblasts) that have been obtained directly from individual patients or research participants, processed and stored in the laboratory, and then grown in the laboratory in culture media. A parallel form of living tissue are cells obtained at the time of prenatal diagnosis, including amniocytes and chorionic villi cells, that may also grow for a limited time in the laboratory. These types of cells can be grown alive in lab dishes using culture media containing salts and growth factors similar to those in the human body. These cells can also be frozen, stored for an indefinite period of time (years or even decades), and then be thawed and grown again. While frozen, they are stored in ways that do not produce ice crystals, usually at $-135°C$ in liquid nitrogen.

The second type of living tissue available for study are cells that have been modified in some way to continue growing, either as part of an abnormal bodily process (e.g., cancer cells) or through modification that takes place in the laboratory. The modification of cells is typically accomplished by using one or more viruses to infect the cells and thereby to confer on the cells the ability to live almost indefinitely in laboratory conditions. The resulting products are "immortalized" or transformed cell lines. The most commonly used cell lines are lymphoblastoid cell lines, which are white blood cells taken from a blood sample, collected in a laboratory, and infected with the Epstein-Barr virus. The modified cell lines are then either maintained as indefinitely dividing cells in culture media, or (as with the fibroblasts described above) frozen for indefinite periods of time, subsequently thawed, and allowed to grow again.[6]

Living cells, such as these cell lines, provide scientific investigators opportunities for genetic analysis beyond that provided by the DNA contained within the cell lines. Thus, for example, transformed cell lines give genetic researchers opportunities to analyze expressed genes in the form of the messenger RNA, its derived complementary DNA (cDNA), or the proteins made from these messages. Current laboratory techniques can sometimes make more cost-efficient use of messenger RNA or protein than the DNA itself, although it is possible that in the future these current technologies will be supplanted by more powerful direct DNA sequence analysis.

Use of RNA from a tumor cell line, however, may provide more direct information about how that tumor might respond to certain therapies and thus be used in planning treatments. This use of RNA extracted from tumor cell lines is an increasingly common use for material obtained from individuals. In these cases, a genetic profile that is specific to the tumor rather than the individual patient may be derived. Such tumor-specific profiles are already being used to target changes in surgical, radiation, and chemotherapy approaches to treating cancer. Thus, although the biological material itself is derived from an individual, the genetic analysis takes place on the disturbed cells contained within a cancer of that individual, and the results are not specific to that person, but to a type of cancer.

Living cells can also provide an opportunity for testing the effectiveness of interventions on those cells. Such interventions may involve attempts to cure a genetic defect present in those cells. By treating the cells themselves with medications or with modified genes in a form of gene transfer, researchers may be able to evaluate the cell's response prior to testing that same medication or gene transfer protocol on the human being from which the cells themselves came. These kinds of interventions have the advantage of providing a test system without any direct risk to the affected individual.

As DNA is passed under stable conditions from one dividing cell to another, including cells that have been modified abnormally by tumors or intentionally through virus infections, the vast majority of the DNA remains a faithful copy of the DNA that was initially conferred on the fertilized embryo from which the cells began. In the case of some tumors, rearrangements do occur, but these changes are often at the chromosomal level, not at the level of most individual genes or DNA sequences. Nonetheless, there is always a risk that cells dividing in the laboratory may undergo some changes in their DNA. This possibility must be taken into account whenever any analysis has been carried out on cells that have been allowed to grow and divide many, many times under laboratory conditions.

Nonviable Tissues. Dead, or nonviable, cells that can be stored in a number of ways for long periods of time are a second type of tissue used for research purposes.

One way to store dead cells is to freeze them in a way that preserves the integrity of the DNA (usually to $-80°C$, with the cells having ice crystals). This method prevents the cells from growing and dividing in the laboratory, but still provides a stable source of DNA, RNA, and protein. Although the RNA and protein is limited to the amounts contained within the specimen obtained from an individual patient or research participant, it nonetheless provides some of the same opportunities for genetic analysis as outlined above. Since these cells are dead, however, they cannot be used for the same therapeutic testing protocols. Still, the cells contain DNA, RNA, and protein that apparently remain stable for many years when preserved in a frozen state. Indeed, samples of DNA have been analyzed from frozen human beings several thousand years old (e.g., see the Iceman case in Chapter 5). DNA samples have also been analyzed from frozen nonhuman creatures more than 10,000 years old.

In fact, however, freezing is not even essential for extracting usable DNA. Samples from humans or animals that have been buried, but remained unfrozen, have also provided a useful source for DNA analysis. This analysis has focused primarily on DNA contained within the mitochondria of each individual cell. Mitochondria are energy-producing structures within the cell that lie outside the nucleus and have a tiny portion of unique DNA material located within them. Mitrochondrial DNA is unusual in several ways, including the fact that it is passed directly from a mother to all of her children, but is not passed on by a father to any of his children. Moreover, the number of copies of DNA contained within each cell is often several thousand as compared with one copy of the nuclear DNA. Thus a higher proportion of mitrochondrial DNA samples can be analyzed. Moreover, research has shown that DNA variation within the mitochondria is often specific to the geographical origin of a particular individual, thereby enabling genetic analysis of the mitochondria to provide important information about the historical origins and evolution of a particular person.

Tissue samples that have been obtained in the course of a pathologic examination of tissues removed from a patient as part of an operative procedure, or obtained after the patient's death during an autopsy constitute another form of storage for dead cells that still provides opportunities to analyze DNA, and possibly RNA and protein. Tissues collected in either of these ways are typically analyzed microscopically by professionals in a pathology laboratory using a variety of chemical stains to provide information about the types of cells contained within the samples and the nature of any aberrant proteins that the individual cells might contain. These specimens may be stored as frozen samples or as thin sections cut and imbedded in paraffin so that they can be examined under a microscope. They can also be stored in solutions that preserve the structure of the organ or tissue, such as would be found in an organ or even a whole individual body stored in various types of embalming fluid. Pathology laboratories have a long history of obtaining and saving such specimens. Consequently, there is a rich resource of such pathologic specimens located in hospitals and laboratories around the world, as partially indicated by the estimated 160 million pathologic specimens in the United States (see Chapter 2). Most pathology departments store tissue samples indefinitely, with the oldest archived tissues often having been stored 20–100 years.[7]

When stored as specimens in pathology laboratories, tissue samples can undergo change. The structural nature of the cells and tissues may be preserved, but the components of those cells and tissues (the DNA, RNA, and protein) may be substantially altered. Nonetheless, it has already proven practical to obtain DNA samples with relative ease from these types of stored pathologic specimens, and, to a lesser extent, also to carry out studies of the RNA or protein contained within these samples. When the samples are obtained at autopsy, the individual from whom the sample is obtained may, of course, have been dead for many years before the sample is a candidate for use in a scientific study.

Still another example of storing dead cells is the widespread hospital practice of using neonatal blood spot cards in connection with legally mandated newborn screening programs. Blood samples are obtained by pricking infants' heels, placing the blood sample on a filter card, and then allowing the blood to be absorbed and dried. A portion of the sample obtained from each infant is removed by a small paper punch and typically analyzed for several disorders (e.g., congenital hypothyroidism, phenylketonuria, sickle cell anemia). In some countries and in some states in the United States, these neonatal blood spot cards are placed in long-term storage and have, in some cases, remained available for scientific investigators decades after the blood samples were originally obtained. Identifiers, including names and other demographic information, are retained in some countries and states so that a connection may still be made between an infant and a blood sample many years later. In countries having national health databases, scientific investigators and physicians are thereby enabled, when medically desirable, to recontact the originally identified individual through medical records tracking.

Long-term storage of neonatal blood spot cards has figured prominently in studies of birth defects over the past two decades, at least in part because such studies would be considerably more expensive if done with blood samples collected contemporaneously. In many cases, established birth defects registries already had information on some types of congenital anomalies and risk factors, and this information has subsequently been linked through identifiers to samples stored through newborn screening programs. These research findings have established clinically significant relationships between smoking and alcohol use during pregnancy and DNA variations and congenital structural anomalies in certain infants.

The ultimate source of dead tissues, of course, is found in graveyards and burial plots around the world. Although most individuals who are buried undergo some form of embalming procedure, the techniques used for embalming (e.g., formaldehyde, formalin) often allow the DNA contained within tissue samples to be retained in a form that still makes it amenable to genetic analysis, particularly using the

PCR method. Except for individuals whose bodies are lost through fires or explosions or whose bodies undergo a destructive procedure such as cremation, this fact means that DNA tied to a specific individual is available on all individuals for whom an identifiable burial plot still exists.[8]

Material from burial plots has already served as a resource for genetics studies. To cite several examples, genetics studies have been made of the remains of the Romanov family killed in the Russian Revolution in the early 1900s; of Jesse James, who died in the late 1800s; and of a number of less famous individuals to determine whether they might have been carriers for particular genetic conditions. Suggestions have frequently been made to disinter politically significant figures for a variety of reasons, including possible paternity (Thomas Jefferson), possible identification of individuals as carriers of specific genetic disorders (Abraham Lincoln and Marfan syndrome), disputed identity (the Columbus case in Chapter 3), and possible forensic purposes (an accused criminal in France claiming to be the offspring of Yves Montand). Although these buried tissues are not as easily available to genetics investigators as tissues frozen in cylinders of liquid nitrogen, specimens located in pathology laboratories, or dried blood samples on stored neonatal blood spot cards, they are nonetheless a rich potential source of banked DNA material.

All stored human tissue samples can be placed in one of these categories, as either viable or dead tissues, depending on how they are collected, processed, and stored in the laboratory. Thus, blood samples can be viable or nonviable, depending on whether they are fresh, transformed into cell lines, made into slides, frozen, dried out on neonatal blood spot cards, or removed from a cadaver.

Other "Types" of Tissues

In addition to these general categories for human tissues, there are other "types" of tissues that we need to mention briefly, either because (*1*) the tissue itself stands in some sort of special category compared with other human tissues, (2) the tissue is collected in an unusual way, or (*3*) the tissue is stored for an atypical purpose. The first category, human tissues that are special in some way, has at least three examples: blood, cord blood stem cells, and cryopreserved human embryos. The second category is best illustrated by tissues taken from the inside lining of persons' cheeks by means of a buccal swab. The third category is represented by DNA samples that are stored for nonbiomedical purposes, with the most common practices involving long-term storage of DNA samples taken from criminals for forensic purposes and from military personnel for unplanned, but possibly necessary military identification purposes.

Special Tissues. We turn first to human tissues that are special in some way, using blood as our first example. Why do we suggest that there is something special about the bodily fluid that flows through our veins and arteries, naturally drains from our bodies when skin is cut or pierced, is frequently removed from patients and research participants by means of a "common blood draw," and is regularly stored in thousands of laboratories around the world? We select human blood as an example of a special type of tissue (compared with other tissues) precisely because it seems to be ubiquitous, especially in biomedical settings. Multiple diagnostic tests use patients' blood, diverse therapeutic interventions use donors' blood (e.g., transfusions, surgery), and numerous ongoing research studies use blood obtained from research participants and, sometimes, patients.

Consider the following points. First, as mentioned above, a widespread practice in much of the world involves obtaining a small amount of blood after the birth of every newborn infant and testing that blood for a variety of disorders through biochemical and molecular genetics screening protocols. Early identification of the congenital defects currently screened for can result in an effective treatment preventing early death and mental retardation. These legally mandated blood samples are obtained from 99% of the newborn population in most developed countries, often without parental consent, and placed in long-term storage on the neonatal blood spot cards discussed earlier. These banked DNA samples provide a resource for genetic analysis both in cases where identifiers have been retained on the samples and where identifiers have been removed but the samples represent an important resource for population-based data on gene frequency distributions.

Another widespread practice of blood sampling occurs in the course of blood donations to blood banks and hospital clinics for other laboratory investigations of patients. In addition to being used for transfusion purposes, donated blood has been commonly examined for over 100 years as a source of disease. As indicated in Chapter 1, much of this research in the United States is done in the institutions that comprise the American Association of Blood Banks.[9] In many cases, these donated blood samples are destroyed following their use, but some research-related blood banks retain a portion of the initial sample for a variety of long-term research investigations. If the blood samples are stored in an identified or identifiable form, the samples also serve as a source of potential DNA that could be tied to specific individuals should clinical reasons for so doing surface at a future time.

A third practice of biomedical research with blood samples, post-diagnostic research, is somewhat similar, but harder to quantify. Every day many persons provide blood samples to physicians, hospitals, medical clinics, managed care organizations, and health insurance companies for numerous diagnostic purposes, but with no assurance that the blood samples will be destroyed after the diagnostic work has been done. When such samples are provided in clinical contexts, patients usually do not sign any consent document (unless surgery is planned), nor are they informed about the possibility that their blood may subsequently be retained for years in research labs as identified, linked, or anonymized samples for biomedical research having multiple scientific purposes. Given these circumstances, a "common blood draw" is certainly a common practice, but one that possibly also exposes patients to a variety of psychosocial risks in the era of genomic medicine.

By contrast to conventional blood samples, umbilical cord blood stem cell samples are special not because they are ubiquitous, very common, and easily collected. Rather, cord blood stem cell (or hematopoeitic stem cell) samples are special because, whether collected *in utero* or *ex utero* after delivery of the placenta, they provide the possibility of autologous blood transfusion in premature or ill neonates. Perhaps of greater medical interest, they can be transplanted into the bodies of patients with abnormal bone marrow stem cells or who have lost their bone marrow following chemotherapy or radiation treatments for cancer. Most significantly, cord blood transplants are less invasive, less risky, and less costly than more common transplant procedures that involve getting bone marrow or procuring stem cells from peripheral blood. As a consequence, cord blood has become a valued commodity for transplant and research purposes over the past 10 years, with numerous private and community cord blood banks being established, cord blood from thousands of infants being banked for private and community use, and several thousand cord blood transplants being done.[10]

Our third example of a special type of tissue is an obvious one: human embryos created *in vitro* with technological assistance are special because they possess the capacity, if implanted into women's bodies, of developing into persons. Even when stored for years in cylinders of liquid nitrogen, cryopreserved human embryos represent possibilities unprecedented 20 years ago: treating problems of infertility, providing couples with new reproductive possibilities, and creating novel means of family formation through embryo donation and/or gestational surrogacy.

Cryopreserved embryos also present both reformulated and new ethical problems: informed consent (for patients, donor couples, and recipient couples), confidentiality, the moral status of human embryos created and stored technologically, the fair distribution of donated embryos, and the planned destruction of "extra," unwanted embryos.[11] Of equal importance, these embryos present serious ethical and legal challenges regarding the types of biomedical research that can and should be permitted to be done with them. These challenges have been addressed by the American Society for Reproductive Medicine and other biomedical organizations, federal and state governments in the United States, and governments in Australia, England, and other developed countries.

Easily Collected Tissues. Still another type of tissue is special only because of the ease with which it can be collected. In contrast to the invasiveness, physical risk, and specialized training required to collect most tissue samples (e.g., drawing blood, cutting skin, removing organs), collecting DNA samples from tiny amounts of tissue inside the cheeks is easy. In fact, with the exceptions of getting hair bulbs or urine samples, no other method of DNA sampling is as easy. The collection method involves using a buccal swab, a small swab rolled against the inside of the cheek for a minute or less, and onto which enough cells are exfoliated to provide material for DNA analysis. This noninvasive, or minimally invasive, sampling method is usually acceptable even to people who are reluctant to have their blood drawn and can be used as an alternative (or supplement) to blood sampling for the purpose of laboratory analysis.

The technical advance provided by cheek swab assays is not so much in the quantities of DNA that can be obtained (relatively modest, similar to the amount of DNA obtained from a blood spot), but in the extreme ease of the procedure. These DNA samples can be obtained at home by untrained individuals, unlike blood sampling, which generally requires someone with training and experience. In addition, in many countries these materials can be treated as a different class of infection risk than tissue samples obtained through fresh blood sampling. This technology therefore provides the possibility of large numbers of individuals sampling themselves in their homes or at work without the need to have any direct contact with a health-care professional. Such sampling protocols, of course, also introduce an additional potential source of error into the sampling process, namely the risk that this unobserved sampling will sometimes result in tissue samples that have been mixed up, mislabeled, or exchanged with another sample.

Tissues Stored for Nonbiomedical Purposes. The final type of tissue samples to be mentioned is unusual—and presents unusual problems—because of the atypical purposes for which these DNA samples are collected, processed, stored, and analyzed. DNA samples gathered for forensic purposes (e.g., blood, semen, or saliva left at a crime scene) or military identification purposes (blood samples and cheek swab samples) are unusual because they are obtained and studied outside clinical or biomedical research settings.

In the forensic sciences, for instance, a variety of DNA samples are increasingly being used in legal proceedings both to prosecute suspected criminals and to exonerate previously convicted innocent persons. Backed by federal and state legislation, the FBI and state departments of forensic sciences are working to use the analytical methods of molecular genetics in the pursuit of justice. For example, the press recently reported that an individual under observation for a prior series of rapes was seen to spit on a sidewalk. The observing police officer used a small piece of absorbent material to collect the saliva, and the DNA contained within it on subsequent analysis provided a match with previously obtained forensic samples from rape victims, sufficient evidence for police to arrest the suspected criminal. In another case, police detectives were following a suspected killer who was observed spitting in a parking lot outside his workplace. They swabbed up the spittle, subsequent DNA tests showed that the spittle DNA matched the DNA from hair and blood collected at the victim's apartment, and the suspect now faces trial.[12]

Perhaps even more surprisingly, tiny amounts of tissue left behind in such day-to-day activities as drinking from a glass or opening a door can leave a sufficient residue of DNA and/or cellular material behind to enable forensics investigators to collect a sample, use molecular techniques to analyze it, and prove that it matches the DNA of the individual who inadvertently left that material behind. Although gathering tissue in this way is not yet widely practiced and is only one reason for establishing DNA banks, such examples illustrate the ease with which DNA samples can be deposited, collected, and subjected to genetic analysis.

These samples collected for forensic analysis have been studied extensively by a variety of criminal justice organizations. Enormous databanks of DNA variation associated with these samples are already in place and have been used to establish patterns of DNA variation that can be attached to individuals of specific geographic, ethnic, or racial origin. (We return to this topic in Chapter 10.) From such a sample, it is already possible to predict, with high accuracy, the ethnic or racial background of the sampled individual. This analytic capability presents the theoretical possibility that some day DNA analysis might be used to help produce a picture of what an individual is most likely to look like.

Sample Storage and Processing

Depending on the nature of the sample and the purposes for which it has been obtained, some additional processing of a sample may need to be carried out before the DNA contained within it is secure for long-term storage. For example, blood samples can be frozen immediately, typically at $-80°C$, and they will provide a stable source of DNA for years to come. Some laboratories, however, prefer to extract the DNA directly and to store it unmixed with the cellular material in a pure and isolated form.

An example of the sometimes unpredictable research benefits of DNA samples stored for long-term purposes is a set of blood samples collected in the 1930s in central Africa as part of an ongoing study of malaria and G6PD deficiency that subsequently proved to be very helpful in identifying the origins of a new medical condition. These blood samples were stored frozen, as serum samples only and not as cellular material, but the samples contained sufficient DNA within the serum itself (probably from ruptured cellular material) that they were used to identify and sequence the HIV virus approximately 50 years later.

Other sampling techniques provide opportunities for obtaining samples that can be stored for very long periods at room temperature without the need for any additional post-sampling processing. Some protocols involve collecting blood onto filter cards; others have samples applied to a filter card impregnated with material that both lyses the cells and binds the DNA. These technologies provide opportunities for very low-cost analysis, both in terms of reagents and the number of personnel needed to obtain large numbers of samples on a population basis. Since time and expense are important considerations in obtaining samples when there is no immediate anticipated use of them, the availability of low-cost, low-tech, and low-personnel technologies provides an incentive for scientists to collect larger numbers of samples if there is at least some contemplated utility in having the samples available later. Such practices have important implications for the number and types of samples that may be stored and collected in the future.

Types of Information

A blood sample obtained for laboratory analysis can have a wide variety of information obtained from it. Standard laboratory values, such as the hemoglobin level, the hematocrit, the white blood cell count, vitamin levels, and the measurement of electrolytes such as sodium and potassium can all be derived from a particular sample. Some of this information, such as blood type, has a long history of association with genetic inheritance. Other information, such as the hemoglobin level, would have, at best, only a very small correlation with any genetic factors. Proteins present in the blood sample, as well as RNA, can also be analyzed, and may in some cases give at least indirect indications of the genetic background of a particular person. For example, the identification of the hemoglobin-S protein in a blood sample would imply that the person who provided the sample has the DNA mutation responsible for the sickle cell form of hemoglobin.

Most importantly, a blood sample contains white blood cells in which DNA is located. This DNA can be extracted and subjected to the many different kinds of mutational analysis described earlier. At the present time, genetic information is mostly focused on mutations that may predispose an individual to have a certain genetic condition or be associated with disorders known to have a strong, or even weak, inherited component. Single gene disorders, such as cystic fibrosis, Huntington disease, Fragile X syndrome, and sickle cell anemia are examples of this kind of genetic information. Genes and mutations in those genes associated with predispositions to disorders that are at least partially genetic, such as Alzheimer disease, breast cancer, and colon cancer, can also be detected. In these cases, the genetic information can provide one component of a larger package of risk assessment for an individual's likelihood of developing that particular disorder at some particular time in his or her life.

DNA samples can also provide some information about normal variation. Yet at the present time, the DNA mutation contribution to an understanding of normal variation of things such as skin color, eye color, and normal behavioral traits is extremely limited. Only a few examples, such as mutations in genes in which red hair is likely to be an outcome, are currently realistic possibilities. In the future, it is likely that additional genes and their variations will be identified that are more strongly associated with more common variants. The impact of this information on how individuals think about themselves, given the importance of genetic self-knowledge, and how this information is used in a broader societal sense is an important topic that has previously been addressed elsewhere.[13] At this time, however, most of these traits appear to be very complex and require the interaction of many different genes. It is therefore not yet practical to develop physical profiles or models of individuals based on particular mutations, but that day will come.

Having said this, geneticists already know from the example of monozygotic, or identical, twins, that persons having identical genetic make-up grow up to have almost identical facial features and body habitus. Consequently, it is clear that every individual's DNA constitution is enormously predictive of that person's later face, body size, and body shape. While this genetic pre-program can certainly be disrupted by environmental events, such as exposures to infections and various kinds of trauma that can disrupt normal physical appearance, each of us has a physical appearance without such intervening events that is almost entirely genetically based. It is therefore possible and fair to predict a time when an individual's genetic profile could be used to draw an exact replica of his or her likely facial image and body size at various times of childhood and adulthood. This predictive information could have enormous familial and forensic implications.

In addition to normal trait variation that will be identifiable through DNA analysis, we are already in an age when disease-based genetic traits are identifiable. Geneticists use DNA sequence technology to test blood samples for common genetic disorders—sickle cell anemia, cystic fibrosis, and others—in many people each day, particularly through the carrier identification tests that are carried out in newborn screening programs on several million newborns each year in the United States alone. Although the primary goal of these tests is to identify affected individuals who will benefit from early medical intervention, most of the positive results from the tests of these autosomal recessive diseases identify a child who is a carrier, meaning that at least one of the child's parents is also a carrier. This carrier status has implications for other family members as well, since any individual who is a carrier must also have carrier parents—and, statistically, half of their siblings are carriers as well. Thus, a simple laboratory test done for newborn screening purposes can quickly have implications that extend throughout a family, for each of the extended family members could discover that his or her own risk for a particular disorder has now increased above that of the general population.

While carrier status for a recessive disease does not confer a risk for the individual, other DNA tests can confer such risks. Given current knowledge about the genetic factors in various cancers, geneticists recognize that genetically identifiable risks for breast or colon cancer can be dominantly inherited. These risks can be ascertained through laboratory testing of blood and other tissue samples—and place both the identified patient at risk as well as other family members who may have inherited the same genetic trait. Because these risks of a serious genetic condition can be perceived by different family members in different ways, these diagnostic tests done in the laboratory sometimes lead to controversies in families over whether individual family members should be tested for the condition, whether they should be informed of the test results, and whether they should share their test results with each other.

Anonymized Samples

A considerable amount of current genetics research is done with blood samples and other tissues that originate from identified individuals (e.g., voluntary participants in a research study, hospitalized patients, or persons in genetic counseling), but are anonymized in the laboratory. The anonymization of samples in laboratories can be done in several different ways, with quite different implications for the individuals from whom the samples originally came. In some cases, samples are *only partially anonymized* so that individual identifiers such as names or hospital numbers are removed from the samples, but a portion of the demographic information (e.g., the gender of an individual; the state, county, or city of origin; age; disease status) is retained. We generally refer to such samples in this book as being *linked* samples, in the sense that the demographic information can subsequently be used to link the samples with the individuals from whom the samples came. These samples are also called *coded* samples in practice or *identifiable* samples in some of the literature.

In other cases, even this demographic information is stripped, and blood samples are maintained in separate tubes and identified as having come from a specific individual, but *without any connecting or linking information*. In still other cases, samples are more completely anonymized by removing all available demographic data from them and then *pooling the samples* by mixing them into a common tube with other samples. Mixing such samples into a common tube still allows for the characterization of the presence of DNA variants or mutations in one or more samples within those tubes, but prevents the identification of any specific individual from which that sample might have come. In our view, both of these practices result in anonymized samples, in the sense that nobody inside or outside the laboratory can link a particular sample with the specific individual from whom it came, even if the geneticists or other biomedical investigators in a laboratory should come to have good clinical reasons for wanting to make such a connection with an individual.

The pooling of DNA samples has been used since the mid-1980s to measure gene frequencies in populations and, more recently, has been shown to be an effective way of studying the genetics of individual families. From a scientific perspective, the disadvantage of pooling samples is that the accuracy of measurement may be somewhat lower than it would be if each sample were analyzed by itself; the advantage of pooling samples is that a far larger number of samples can be analyzed in the same time and for the same price as a single sample. Since many studies involving hundreds or thousands of individuals can be extremely expensive, the financial advantage of the pooling procedure can be substantial. As genome technology becomes more accurate and the measurement accuracy of pooled samples improves, this research procedure may be used with increasing frequency. For example, an individual could contribute a tissue sample to a common DNA bank where the anonymity of the sample would be more assured and research would be done on all of the samples pooled together, with the degree of anonymity of any single DNA sample perhaps being proportional to the number of samples contained within the pool. Some geneticists can, in fact, envision a time in the future when a DNA sample from every person on the planet will be placed into a common, global DNA bank. Research studies would then be able to provide a true average view of the human genome.

Whether absolute anonymization of samples can be done is a matter for definition and discussion, if by "absolute" one means that the biological sources of such samples could *never* be identified no matter what was subsequently done with the samples. Surely an individual who provided a blood sample to an investigator or physician that subsequently has had all identifiers removed from it in the laboratory is not likely ever to be identified with that sample—unless a genetics investigator already has or subsequently acquires another blood sample from the same person and accidentally or intentionally produces a match. But since a sample from a particular individual might be reobtained in the future and matches made between that individual and a sample that was presumed to have been anonymized, it is always possible, though unlikely, in the absence of pooling, that such reidentification could be undertaken.

Short of such active reidentification, however, it is both possible and practical to be able to remove all known identifiers from a sample in a way that would make it extremely difficult to identify one particular individual out of more than a few tens or hundreds in a reliable way. Whether such anonymization practices in the laboratory remove all of the ethical problems involved in stored tissue research, as some persons think, is another question, one that we will address later. At the very least, laboratory practices of anonymizing tissue samples involve an important trade-off, producing virtually absolute protection of the identity of the person who provided a tissue sample at the cost, when all demographic data is removed, of never being able to track that person down in the event that clinical follow-up of that person might be beneficial.

New Technologies for DNA Testing

Two recent advances in DNA testing will provide improved opportunities in the future for cheaper and potentially quicker, more effective, genetic analysis of stored tissue samples. The first is the much-discussed DNA "chip," or DNA microarray, a diagnostic and analytical tool about the size of a computer chip.[14] DNA chip technology offers unprecedented possibilities for multiplex genetic testing, or testing a single tissue sample for multiple genetic mutations and genetic disorders at the same time.[15] The most common type of DNA chip contains on its surface a number of oligonucleotides, each of which has the potential for identifying an exact match from a sample of DNA amplified typically by the PCR reaction. The larger the number of such oligonucleotides present on the surface of a chip, the more DNA sequence that can be analyzed.

Improvements in chip technology now suggest that in the near future it is likely that many genes, including potentially hundreds of thousands of letters of DNA sequence, will be evaluated simultaneously on a single chip. At present, several biotechnology companies, including Affymetrix and Agilent Technologies, claim to have placed the entire human genome (with approximately 30,000 genes) on a single DNA chip.[16] This development means that multiplex genetic testing will become a practical option in the laboratory, raising the possibility that geneticists will be able to focus in some cases on a wide variety of batteries of genes associated with cancer or, more generally, a wide battery of genes associated with almost any disorder recognized to have a genetic predisposition.

Another possible use of chip technology will be genetic testing that involves RNA, not DNA. RNA, the expressed form of DNA that frequently differs from cell to cell, can also be assayed, and different expression profiles may have important implications for helping geneticists diagnose certain types of genetic diseases, such as particular tumor types, as well as implications regarding how particular genetic disorders might be treated. Chip technology has already been practically applied to the analysis of gene expression, and using diagnostic chips with RNA will be another important use of this technology in the future.

A second type of technology, mass spectroscopy, is competing with DNA chips to replace the more traditional and currently dominant "gel-based technologies" described earlier (Southern blot analysis, PCR, direct DNA sequencing, etc.). Mass spectroscopy makes use of the separation of charged molecules, based on both their electric charge and their mass or weight, for the purpose of identifying subtle differences in DNA sequence. This technology may allow much faster analysis of more samples than gel approaches.

It is not clear which of these new technologies will prove to be the most effective, either in terms of cost or reliability. Advances in gel technologies may still prove to be the best way to go, although DNA chips and mass spectroscopy may continue to receive considerable attention. While it cannot be predicted which technology will most likely be in widespread use five years from now, it is likely that new technologies will play an extremely important role in both bringing down the cost and improving the spectrum of screening for genetic mutations and the wide variety of genetic conditions that exists in the human population.

DNA Sequence Storage

Thus far, we have been discussing various aspects of the first kind of DNA banking mentioned earlier, namely the actual biological materials stored in the laboratory for long-term research use. The second kind of DNA banking is the storage of genetic data that has been derived from tissue samples and/or cell lines. This data includes DNA sequence information, which can be banked in two ways. First, an *individual DNA sequence variant,* such as a mutation that underlies cystic fibrosis, sickle cell anemia, or some other genetic disorder, may be identified in the course of a DNA analysis. This information can then be stored in a database to provide a record of which mutation was found. In this approach to banking DNA data, only one, or perhaps a very small number of base pair changes from a reference sequence would be identified for the individual whose DNA had been studied.

These DNA sequence variations often occur in single nucleotides and are referred to as SNPs, or single nucleotide polymorphisms, as mentioned in a case at the end of Chapter 3. Since polymorphisms represent common and normal variation, several large international projects are now underway to identify a comprehensive set of SNPs in humans. Their identification can provide powerful information that can distinguish one individual from another and also identify individuals at risk for particular genetic traits. Their use has been aggressively pursued in the area of pharmacogenetics.

In pharmacogenetics, pharmacologists, geneticists, and others know that variations in the genes involved in drug metabolism can confer widely differing metabolic profiles in particular individuals.[17] Thus, one person may respond very favorably to a certain chemotherapeutic agent, while another may suffer substantial side effects with limited therapeutic benefit. Well recognized for over 50 years, these kinds of variants can be easily tested for and are already playing an important role in targeting specific drug therapies and doses in the treatment setting. Their use has already improved cancer treatment by allowing some patients to minimize or avoid otherwise problematic side effects associated with some chemotherapeutic agents. In the future, increased knowledge about SNPs and other variations in genes will, we anticipate, evolve into a personalized medicine in which it will be the individual who is treated, not the disease. As one example, doses of medications will be modified to fit each patient's age, body weight, genetic profile, and predicted response to the medications. This new knowledge will afford substantial improvements in the efficacy of treatment options for patients, physicians, and pharmacists and further divide individuals into particular genetic groups.

A second approach to banking DNA data is increasingly being used to store more complex and comprehensive information in databases. Not limited to the storage of information about individual sequence variants, this methodology involves storing long stretches of DNA sequence information *from multiple research participants,* with that information consisting of hundreds to millions of base pairs of DNA. This approach, in fact, is being used in the sequencing of DNA information from the individuals whose DNA is being studied as part of the HGP. Although much of the DNA sequence comes from specific individuals whose anonymity is being protected, the amalgam of sequence being developed for the HGP also includes DNA obtained from dozens and, in fact, hundreds of individuals over the last two decades.[18]

DNA sequence is known to contain differences that occur approximately once out of every 1,000 base pairs. If sufficiently long stretches of sequences are available, this pattern of variation could be used to create a unique identifier for a particular individual. Although it is not yet technologically or financially practical to sequence many thousands of base pairs of sequence for a large number of individuals, the technological means of doing so is increasingly becoming available. As a result, it is likely that some day an individual's entire genome could be sequenced and stored in a databank.

This information is typically stored in databases in three different forms: (*1*) colored blobs of information on a computer screen, (*2*) electronic lines on the screen, and (*3*) extremely long lines of letters representing the ordering of the nucleotides, or bases (A, G, C, and T, for adenine, guanine, cytosine, and thymine) on the screen. Each of these forms of computer-generated information can, of course, also be printed in written form.

Most research genetics laboratories retain DNA sequence information for mutations that might predispose to genetic disorders in password-protected computer databases and also in closed, limited-access offices. When DNA sequence information is obtained to determine the normal sequence of a gene or genome, however, it is often placed into publicly accessible databases (e.g., GenBank) available to qualified scientists via the Internet. The identity of any individual from whom a sequence came is not, of course, placed in such databases, but the DNA sequences of numerous individuals are placed there. Although highly unlikely, it is therefore at least conceivable that subsequent identification of a specific DNA sequence with specific variations could be used to isolate a small number of individual DNA sequences in the database. It might even be plausible, for example, that one or more individuals whose DNA sequence resides in the database might be identified in the course of a forensic study making use of that database.

Many current genome projects daily identify sequences in their laboratories, with some labs generating hundreds of thousands of letters of DNA sequence per day. In the interest of scientific collaboration, cooperation, and advancement, these sequences are also often delivered to public databases on a daily basis. Thus enormous amounts of DNA sequence, each of which must have been derived from a single individual (even when that individual is now anonymous), are placed into databanks each day. There are, consequently, many billions of letters of DNA sequence derived from many thousands of specific human beings already stored in publicly accessible databases in many countries (e.g., Centre d'Etude du Polymorphisme Humaine, or CEPH, in France) and available to qualified investigators. This number will only increase in the future, thereby also raising the kinds of ethical and legal concerns we will address in subsequent chapters.

The Impact of Molecular Genetics on Scientific Research

Biomedical research has, without question, been transformed by molecular genetics. Consider two aspects of this transformation. First, the John Moore case, the NHANES III study, and the DeCODE database (see Chapter 1) illustrate that the work of geneticists and other investigators using molecular techniques has revo-lutionized many traditional research practices, as regularly indicated by the ways in which tissues from patients and research participants are now stored for long periods, analyzed, copied, transformed into cell lines, and then studied again for multiple scientific purposes. Second, molecular genetics has produced significant changes in traditional tissue-based research disciplines (e.g., pathology, anatomy) and elevated some fields (e.g., epidemiology, hematology/oncology, pharmacol-ogy, the forensic sciences) to a level of prominence they have not had in the past.

We turn briefly to each of these developments. To illustrate the multiple ways the era of molecular genetics has revolutionized many scientific practices, we consider NHANES III. Evaluation of blood samples obtained in projects such as the NHANES study are evolving from the tests that were carried out slightly more than a decade ago, with more changes to come in the near future. A large amount of DNA analysis is now available that was only beginning to be available in a practical way in 1990. This includes detection of specific mutations in a large number of disease-based genes, such as those that confer susceptibility to breast cancer, colon cancer, diabetes, and other conditions, and also for detection of mutations in individual genes that may, for example, confer susceptibility to drug metabolism differences. Genes such as those found in the P450 system have differential abilities to metabolize drugs or environmental toxins and can therefore affect an individual's susceptibility to drugs or chemicals.

A number of such genes are already identified and well characterized. It is now possible to carry out mutation searches on at least a handful of genes known to confer common susceptibilities to some cancers, as well as for some drug-metabolizing genes. Each of these individual assays is still quite expensive and might cost several hundred dollars when done commercially. Over the next five years, it is likely that this technology will improve. The completion of the HGP will, we hope, allow many genome scientists to focus on identifying a large number of additional genes that may play a role in human health. While not all such genes will be identified within a few years of the completion of the human DNA sequence, there will likely be rapid expansion of the number of genes that are suspected of playing a role. Though there is an increased cost associated with analysis of larger numbers of genes, the availability of new technologies (e.g., DNA chip analysis, mass spectroscopy) will likely lower the cost and also increase the number of such genes that can be analyzed from a relatively tiny sample.

In addition, scientists using molecular biology techniques in the early 1990s were just at the beginnings of the widespread use of the PCR assay. This technol-ogy continues to evolve and improve. Soon many genes will likely be able to be identified from even a tiny portion of a tissue sample obtained in a study such as NHANES.

As to changes produced in various scientific disciplines, two such fields—pathology and the forensic sciences—are examples of changes brought about by the scientific technologies now available in molecular genetics. Both fields are deeply involved in human tissue research; each has leaders with active roles in the debate about research with banked DNA. (Additional discussion of pathology specimens and the use of tissue samples in the forensic sciences occurs later in the book.)

That much of the work done by pathologists has been transformed by molecular genetics is most easily illustrated by the development of molecular pathology as a subspecialty within the discipline. The investigative methods of molecular biology and genetics means that long-archived samples in pathology laboratories can now, in some cases, provide two potential sources of information. First, these samples, often stored for decades, are reservoirs of DNA. Extracting DNA from such samples is not easy, but it is feasible and provides the possibility of gaining information about the genetic background of an individual long after that person died. Some particular pathologic samples, particularly those that might have been derived from tumors, may also contain information specific to the exact nature of the tumor type (e.g., colon cancer can be divided into many molecular subtypes). Such information may be extractable and have important consequences for the familial nature of some individual cancers.

Second, pathologic samples are also a potential reservoir for RNA. Although the extraction of RNA presents even greater challenges than extraction of DNA, it may also be feasible in some cases, depending on the storage methods used. RNA can give additional information as to how specific genes are expressed in a sample, again with emphasis on its utility in analyzing tumor samples.

Moreover, the nature of any pathologic sample has changed because the sample itself can now be subjected to more sophisticated interpretations than were possible in past decades. New information about how to view a histology slide, including new ways of interpreting the particular characteristics of the cells and tissues under the microscope, have undergone significant changes in recent years. The result is that pathologists, geneticists, and other biomedical scientists, using molecular techniques, are able to do research on archived samples that could hardly have been imagined when the samples were originally stored.

Tissue samples analyzed by professionals in the forensic sciences have also changed. Now, the traditional approaches used to try to establish the guilt or innocence of specific persons have been supplemented by the investigative methods of molecular genetics. The possibilities of such genetics analysis have had, and will continue to have, tremendous implications for police, judges, prosecuting and defense attorneys, forensic sciences experts in state and national governments, individuals arrested as suspects for an expanding list of crimes, individuals wrongly convicted and imprisoned for crimes they did not commit, and, indeed, for all citizens in developed countries worldwide.

The reason for these dramatic societal changes is fairly straightforward. Analysis of DNA for forensic purposes can result in two general outcomes. The most powerful outcome providing the most complete information is when a DNA sample isolated from an individual (e.g., a blood or semen sample) is shown not to be a genetic match for a DNA sample isolated from a specific crime scene. While in the long run, guilt or innocence of an individual depends on much more than genetic matching, it can nonetheless be true that if a sample found at a crime scene is that of the perpetrator and is clearly shown not to match that of the suspect (or defendant), this finding can be a strong indication of innocence. Several individuals, convicted of rape or murder and already serving prison terms, based on evidence outside of biological sample matches, have been exonerated when small quantities of biological material have been analyzed, showing no match between a crime scene sample and the convicted individual.[19]

The alternate strategy, proving that a sample does match an individual, is also powerful, but more problematic. Any such matching can only be based on the number of matches identified at the genetic level between a sample drawn from a specific individual and a sample obtained at the crime scene. Since any given individual may have several million different genetic variants and current technology is not even close to being able to analyze more than a few hundred at most, a complete genetic profile of an individual sample is not currently possible. Nonetheless, the assaying of even a dozen or so individual genetic variants can provide very strong evidence that a particular individual is likely to be matched with a particular sample (excluding the problem of monozygotic twins). All of these arguments are statistical, but powerful odds of a million to one, or even a billion to one, for matches between samples can easily be reported by geneticists.

But, if there are malicious or inadvertent sample mix-ups or contamination, sample matches may not represent reality. In fact, it is likely that malfeasance or incompetence rates may exceed, even in carefully regulated laboratories, the types of odds that can be generated from sample analyses themselves. In the end, avoiding such forensic problems requires careful law enforcement practices, combining good evidence-seeking and evidence-gathering protocols with the use of DNA information as a supplement to other information.

From the HGP to Genomic Medicine and Public Health

Much has been written about the HGP.[20] We will not provide a summary of this diverse literature. Rather, we celebrate the HGP's completion by (*1*) highlighting the unprecedented accomplishments of this international, large-scale biology project, (*2*) noting the achievements of affiliated genome projects with nonhuman organisms, (*3*) describing the HGP's recent expansion in several new directions, and (*4*) expressing our hope that many genome scientists worldwide will now redirect their research studies toward discovering, in ethically responsible ways, the genetic and environmental causes of human illness and abnormality so that the children and grandchildren of all the world's peoples will have better, healthier lives.

The HGP's major goal was to develop a complete scientific description of the human genome. This multidisciplinary project was designed to provide detailed information about the individual nature of all the nucleotides in human genetic material as a first step in a longer-term project to use that information to understand, prevent, and treat human inherited disorders. That first step has now been achieved, although not without considerable competition and controversy.

The success of the consortium comprising the HGP was due, in part, to the loosely coordinated work of scientists in a collection of organizations in many countries (e.g., the Human Genome Organization, or HUGO) who were willing to attend forums and develop mechanisms by which scientific information relating to the human genome should be obtained, stored, shared, and distributed. Also in part, the success—and increased speed—of the genome scientists working on the HGP was due to the competition provided by Craig Venter and other scientists at Celera Genomics.

The realization of one of the primary goals of the HGP—to identify a reference sequence for humans—was publicly announced as being virtually completed in June 2000. The results of the work accomplished by the publicly funded, international consortium of scientists were published in *Nature* in February 2001; the results by the competing, privately funded scientists at Celera Genomics in the United States were published in *Science* the following day.[21]

Two years later, in April 2003, the international consortium announced that it had largely finished its work, fittingly marking the 50th year anniversary of the description of the DNA double helix by James Watson and Francis Crick. The public consortium thus declared that the HGP—estimated in 1990 to be a 15-year project—had been completed two years ahead of schedule. The sequencing work by genome scientists in the United States accounted for roughly 53% of the three billion nucleotides in the composite human genome, and cost $2.7 billion.[22]

As of this writing, 99.9% of all DNA sequence in the human genome is completed, with a high level of quality. Only approximately 400 small gaps still remain to be filled for a totally complete sequence. The April 2003 report was a remarkable improvement on the publications two years earlier, both in terms of the additional sequence now stored in publicly available databases and the greatly improved annotation of that sequence that includes descriptions of genes, their structure, and their regulatory elements. The determination of the sequence at this level of completeness is a major milestone in human biology.[23]

In addition to scientific work on the human genome, the HGP has incorporated many other genome projects involving plants, animals, and microorganisms. The genomes of plants and animals of commercial interest, such as corn, rice, cow, and pig, have been studied as a way of better understanding the growth and development of these organisms, with the hope of improving their utility as food and clothing resources. The genomes of selected microorganisms have been studied so that scientists can better understand how various bacteria and viruses induce infectious diseases in humans. Several notable successes have already occurred in the sequencing of microorganisms, as illustrated by these microorganisms and the human disorders they cause: *H. influenza* (causes pneumonia and meningitis, DNA sequence completed in 1995); *H. pylori* (stomach ulcers, DNA sequenced in 1997); *M. tuberculosis* (tuberculosis, 1998); *N. meningitidis* (meningitis, 2000); *P. aeruginosa* (pneumonia, 2000); and *E. coli* (diarrhea and blood infection, 2001).[24]

Continuing projects are also intended to complete the sequencing of "model organisms" that have been studied for many years by scientists. Each organism provides some basic underlying biological principles that also serve as reference points for understanding human conditions. Moreover, studying model organisms has a number of advantages compared to studying humans: they usually reproduce substantially faster than do humans, they have considerably shorter life spans, and they can be manipulated in labs in ways that would be unethical with human research participants. Model organisms currently under study include yeast (with a genome size of 19.1 million nucleotides), the worm (97 million nucleotides), the fruit fly (180 million nucleotides), and the mouse (3 billion nucleotides, approximately the same as in the human genome).[25]

As indicated by these genomes, the HGP has expanded in several directions in recent years, with some of the additional scientific work focusing on other "omes." (In general, the suffix "ome" refers to global studies of a particular class of biological studies. Thus the "genome" refers to global studies of genes, the "proteome" to global studies of proteins, and the "glycome" to global studies of sugar modifications of proteins.) Recently, the proteome has received increased attention, given that proteins are the workhorses that carry out the structural and functional roles whose information is contained within genes. We anticipate that proteomic studies will contribute directly to new ways of preventing, diagnosing, and treating human diseases.[26]

Additional scientific work is being done in a number of other disciplines that are increasingly related to new discoveries coming from HGP-funded studies. Pharmacogenetics, for example, has been strengthened by work being done in pharmacogenomics and environmental toxicology, with all of these disciplines studying the interactions between genetics and the environment on human health and illness. The results are promising. Some of the work funded in the United States by the Environmental Genome Project, now in its sixth year, involves the complete resequencing of hundreds of genes in the human genome in an effort to find SNPs that have a role in environmentally related diseases in the U.S. population.[27] UK BioBank, the planned database in Britain, will include environmental data pertaining to the 500,000 participants in this national study.[28]

Finally, we hope that genome scientists who have contributed to the success of the HGP will not be satisfied with the completed sequence of the human genome. We encourage them to move beyond this first step to complete the related projects described above, namely, sequencing the genomes of relevant nonhuman organisms and improving the scientific understanding of the genetics/environment interactions on human health and disease.

We also hope that molecular geneticists and other genome scientists decide to apply their knowledge and skills to redirect the HGP so that it once again focuses on improving human health through personalized genomic medicine and public health genetics, rather than pursuing other scientific goals such as the sequencing of a virtually endless list of questionably relevant nonhuman organisms.[29] Moreover, we hope that they, joined by other investigators, change some traditional research practices so that the next period of human tissue research will be more collaborative in nature, whether the tissues being studied are obtained in developed countries or from indigenous people in remote parts of the world. We provide recommendations later in the book regarding several ways in which these changes can be made.

Scenario: Chapters in the Life of a Tissue Sample

The following account is one example drawn from many possible ways a tissue sample might be obtained during a normal clinic visit by a patient and then be utilized for multiple clinical and research purposes, with portions of the sample ending up in several DNA banks at the same institution.

An 82-year-old, female patient comes into a cancer center for ongoing treatment of her ovarian cancer. A blood sample is obtained to evaluate her white blood cell count in order to determine how she is responding to chemotherapy treatments. The oncologist, having previously obtained consent from the patient to carry out a genetic analysis on her blood sample, might, at the time of the blood draw, obtain an additional amount of blood on which a DNA analysis could be done. What happens to the blood after it leaves the woman's body will be indicated in this scenario as numbered chapters in the life of this particular blood sample.

The blood sample obtained during this clinic visit would later (*1*) be divided and examined in the pathology laboratory for the number of white cells it contains, and (*2*) the specific types of white blood cells would be studied to determine, for example, whether any leukemic cells are present. In some cases (*3*) additional microscope slides with the cells fixed on them might be stained with a variety of reagents to look for particular types of cancer cells important to treatment or prognosis. These slides themselves (*4*) might be stored in a hematology or pathology laboratory for many years, either for subsequent review for diagnostic purposes, teaching opportunities if the slides have particularly classic or interesting findings, retrospective research studies, quality-control reasons, or medico-legal reasons (e.g., an unlikely, but possible, legal case years later).

A portion of that same original blood sample (5) would also have been sent off to a genetics laboratory for DNA diagnostic studies. Such a sample itself might have been divided, but the portion sent to a research lab investigating new potential findings of DNA variants associated with cancer might have been anonymized and provided to the laboratory with only clinical or other rudimentary descriptors. An additional portion of the sample sent to the diagnostic laboratory (6) would be drawn off and stored as a reference for future studies, and (7) another portion would have the specifics of the DNA variants examined. The specifics of this DNA examination might include the setting up of not one but many different PCR reactions. These PCR reactions would themselves contain DNA from the affected individual and (8) might be stored in the laboratory in freezers or refrigerators for long-term comparative purposes.

Some additional portion of the sample (9) would undergo direct DNA sequence analysis. This DNA data analysis itself would be resident in the initial computer on which it was found, in hard copy forms that might be exchanged between patients and physicians to provide confirmation of a particular finding, and in information sent to other computer databases that might be collecting relevant information (e.g., on all ovarian tumors and their associated DNA variants) or to epidemiologists investigating such studies. In this way, different types of DNA databanks have been established from information contained in a computer or in hard copies that literally list A, G, C, and T letters in their order, and might be very specific to the particular woman under study if this portion of the blood sample is still linked to her (the same would be true for other patients with ovarian cancer who provided blood samples).

In addition, of course, numerous DNA banks would now exist at the institution, with portions of the original blood sample (10+) being stored on microscope slides and in freezers and refrigerators in several, potentially dozens, of different laboratories and/or investigators' offices. Thus, what might have seemed like a simple blood sampling procedure in a cancer clinic for a patient being evaluated for an ongoing chronic illness has provided samples that have been divided many times over again to provide resources for researchers and clinicians in a wide range of different sites in the institution. (The scenario could easily be extended to many other institutions, if one or more of the investigators used a portion of the blood sample to create a cell line and then shared the cell line with scientific collaborators in other parts of the world.)

Against this background, we next describe and assess the recommendations made by several multidisciplinary committees concerning some of the ethical and legal aspects of biomedical research with stored tissues. We begin Part II by examining some of the recommendations made about this issue outside the United States, then focus on developments in the United States by discussing the federal regulations for research, relevant legal cases and laws, and the NBAC report on this subject.

Cases and Vignettes

Scott Woodward, a microbiology professor at Brigham Young University, is directing the creation of one of the world's largest genetic and genealogical databases. To demonstrate that the world's peoples are "essentially one big family," the Woodward project begins with blood samples, four-generational genealogical charts, and informed consent from volunteers. Each blood sample and each chart is assigned a code number; all names are stripped from them to protect privacy. DNA is extracted from each blood sample in the lab, a tiny portion of DNA is separated for analysis, and the remaining DNA is frozen for future use. The DNA is analyzed by computer, which uses 250 genetic markers and produces a color graph of the results of the analysis. In a parallel step, information from each genealogical chart is entered into a database. In the final phase of the process, a supercomputer will combine the genetic and genealogical information to create a complex web of coded genes and geography. The project will cost tens of millions of dollars, include data from at least 100,000 volunteers worldwide, and be able to provide limited, coded genetic and geographical answers to persons in the future who are willing to provide a sample of blood, hair, or saliva for matching purposes.[30]

Scientific investigators in universities commonly share, on request, some of the tissues and cell lines in their labs with other investigators within their universities. They also share these tissue resources with collaborating investigators elsewhere, around the globe. The following quotes are two random e-mail requests received by a nonscientist faculty member at a research university: (1) "Does anyone have E9 cells (human immortalized embryonic cell line)? I need 1 ug total RNA to use as a control." (2) "We are looking for the human monocyte cell line U937. If anyone has it and can share it with us, please contact. . . ."[31]

The Cord Blood Registry, located in Arizona, is the largest private umbilical cord blood bank in the United States. The advertisements by the registry exhort expectant parents to pay to store a newborn's cord blood in case the child or a relative should ever develop cancer, certain genetic disorders, or other serious medical conditions that might be treated with stem cells derived from the cord blood. The registry indicates that cord blood is sometimes better than bone marrow in treating leukemia and some genetic conditions. The expense of storage: $1,200 for the collection and freezing of the cord blood, then $95 per year to keep it stored in liquid nitrogen at the University of Arizona's blood bank. Parental testimonials on the registry's Web site are enthusiastic: "This is the best life insurance our money could buy," and "We now have some peace of mind that if we have problems, we may have a solution." By contrast, critics raise questions about the value of storing a child's cord blood, the absence of meaningful informed consent, the types of research that might be done with the stored blood, and the cost involved.[32]

An author in the *New York Times Magazine* disclosed in 2001 that he had given a blood sample to Celera Genomics, possibly to be used by that company in their publication of the DNA sequence of the "basic" human genome. He wrote: "I can't be certain that I am one of the Celera Five, the group whose DNA makes up their genome sequence, but there's a good chance. Along with 20 other men and women from a variety of ethnic backgrounds, I gave [Craig] Venter my DNA last year to do whatever he wanted with it. . . . I'll probably never know whether I'm one of the Celera Five. Donors' DNA samples are identified with only a seven-digit code, and the key is locked away."[33]

When scientists at Celera Genomics announced in 2000 they had decoded the human genome, they said the genetic data came from anonymous donors; and they presented the map as a universal human map. More specifically, they indicated that the Celera map had been drawn from a pool of 20 donors from five ethnic groups, represented specifically by five individual donors whose DNA was marked by separate codes. Then, in 2002 Craig Venter disclosed that, actually, the human genome decoded was largely his own. While some DNA from each of the five individuals was included in the genome map, most of the map was based on Venter's DNA. This announcement was met with a wide range of responses, including surprise, disappointment, and criticism. The Celera Board of Advisors expressed regret that the process they had approved for choosing anonymous donors had been subverted by the scientist who directed the project.[34]

Notes

1. Jean E. McEwen and Philip R. Reilly, "A Survey of DNA Diagnostic Laboratories regarding DNA Banking," *Am J Hum Genet* 56 (1995): 1477.
2. Robert F. Service, "Microchip Arrays Put DNA on the Spot," *Science* 282 (1998): 396.
3. For more information about Southern blotting and other laboratory tools of molecular genetics, see Robert Nussbaum, Roderick McInnes, and Huntington Willard, *Thompson & Thompson Genetics in Medicine*, 6th ed. (Philadelphia: W.B. Saunders, 2001), pp. 33–50; and Thomas Gelehrter, Francis Collins, and David Ginsburg, *Principles of Medical Genetics*, 2nd ed. (Baltimore: Williams & Wilkins, 1998), pp. 61–89.
4. Kary B. Mullis, "The Unusual Origin of the Polymerase Chain Reaction," *Sci Am* (April 1990): 56.
5. See Carl Dieffenbach and Gabriela Dveksler, eds., *PCR Primer: A Laboratory Manual* (Cold Spring Harbor, N.Y.: Cold Spring Harbor Laboratory, 1995).
6. Nussbaum, McInnes, and Willard, pp. 135–36.
7. Elisa Eiseman and Susanne B. Haga, *Handbook of Human Tissue Sources* (Santa Monica, Calif., RAND, 1999), p. 105.
8. Susan C. Lawrence, "Beyond the Grave—The Use and Meaning of Human Body Parts: A Historical Introduction," in Robert F. Weir, ed., *Stored Tissue Samples,* pp. 111–42.
9. Eiseman and Haga, p. 128.
10. Dorothy E. Vawter, "An Ethical and Policy Framework for the Collection of Umbilical Cord Blood Stem Cells," in Weir, ed., *Stored Tissue Samples,* pp. 32–65.
11. Amy E.T. Sparks, "Human Embryo Cryopreservation: Benefits and Adverse Consequences," in Weir, ed., *Stored Tissue Samples,* pp. 66–81.
12. "Suspected Killer Spits, and DNA Brings Arrest," *New York Times,* March 24, 2001, p. A12.
13. See Robert F. Weir, Susan C. Lawrence, and Evan Fales, eds., *Genes and Human Self-Knowledge: Historical and Philosophical Reflections on Modern Genetics* (Iowa City: University of Iowa Press, 1994).
14. For basic information about DNA chips, see this Web site: http://www.science. education.nih.gov/newsnapshots/TOC_Chips/toc_chips.html. For information provided by Affymetrix, one of the leading producers of DNA chips, see http://www.affymetrix. com/index.affx. For information about the possible clinical applications of DNA chips as diagnostic tests, see http://www.physweekly.com/archive/97/11_17_97/twf.html.

15. Philip Reilly, "Panel Comment: The Impact of the Genetic Privacy Act on Medicine," *J Law Med Ethics* 23 (1995): 378–81.
16. Andrew Pollack, "Human Genome Placed on Chip; Biotech Rivals Put It Up for Sale," *New York Times,* October 2, 2003, pp. C1, C10.
17. See Consortium on Pharmacogenetics, *Pharmacogenetics: Ethical and Regulatory Issues in Research and Clinical Practice,* Spring 2002, np.
18. See Craig Venter et al., "The Sequence of the Human Genome," *Science* 291 (2000): 1304–51.
19. See, for example, Ross Milloy, "Some Prosecutors Willing to Review DNA Evidence," *New York Times,* October 19, 2000, p. A15; and Francis X. Clines, "Access by Inmates to Tests for DNA Gains Ground," *New York Times,* December 19, 2000, p. A18.
20. See, for example, James D. Watson, "The Human Genome Project: Past, Present, and Future," *Science* 248 (1990): 44; Daniel Kevles and Leroy Hood, eds., *The Code of Codes: Scientific and Social Issues in the Human Genome Project* (Cambridge, Mass.: Harvard University Press, 1991); Thomas Lee, *The Human Genome Project* (New York: Plenum, 1991); Robert Cook-Deegan, *The Gene Wars: Science, Politics, and the Human Genome* (New York: Norton, 1994), and Francis S. Collins and Victor A. McKusick, "Implications of the Human Genome Project for Medical Science," *JAMA* 285 (2001): 540–44.
21. The landmark publications are the issues of *Nature* 409 (February 15, 2001) and *Science* 291 (February 16, 2001).
22. Elizabeth Pennisi, "Reaching Their Goal Early, Sequencing Labs Celebrate," *Science* 300 (2003): 409.
23. For a more comprehensive assessment of this achievement, see Francis S. Collins, Michael Morgan, and Aristides Patrinos, "The Human Genome Project: Lessons from Large-Scale Biology," *Science* 300 (2003): 286–90.
24. This information comes from the Web site of TIGR: The Institute for Genomic Research. The Web site for this not-for-profit research institution is http://www.tigr.org.
25. This information, along with an enormous amount of additional information, can be found in the public consortium's database. See their Web site: http://www.nih.gov/science/models/.
26. Robert F. Service, "Recruiting Genes, Proteins For a Revolution in Diagnostics," *Science* 300 (2003): 236–37, 239.
27. Jocelyn Kaiser, "Tying Genetics to the Risk of Environmental Diseases," *Science* 300 (2003): 563.
28. Melissa Austin, Sarah Harding, and Courtney McElroy, "Genebanks: A Comparison of Eight Proposed International Genetic Databases," *Community Genetics* 6 (2002): 39–41.
29. Jeff Murray, "Reinventing the Genome Project," *Iowa City Press-Citizen,* April 27, 2003, p. 13A.
30. Hannah Wolfson, "Histories found via blood," *Des Moines Sunday Register,* March 4, 2001, p. 21.
31. These e-mails were received by one of the authors.
32. Rita Rubin, "Parents Banking on Umbilical Cord Blood," *Iowa City Press-Citizen,* December 10, 1998, p. 4C.
33. Thomas Hayden, "Quantifiably Normal," *New York Times Magazine,* March 4, 2001, p. 15.
34. Nicholas Wade, "Scientist Reveals Genome Secret: It's Him," *New York Times,* April 27, 2002, p. A1.

II

CURRENT LAWS, POLICIES, AND RECOMMENDATIONS

5

Recommendations and Policies
in Other Countries

> Broad social acceptance of the [research] use of human tissues
> requires in the first instance that the public be aware of its extent
> and importance. Our impression is that this is not yet sufficiently
> the case: in our view openness and information regarding
> the practice is the least that people are entitled to expect given
> current social attitudes. Such openness will increase people's
> acceptance and confidence.
>
> Health Council of the Netherlands, 1994[1]

> We need first to consider what makes a use of human tissue
> ethically acceptable. Some uses can, it seems, easily be judged
> unacceptable: cannibalism (except *in extremis*) or the production of
> human leather or soap (even in abnormal circumstances) are uses
> that can seemingly be judged unacceptable without detailed ethical
> argument. Other uses are more difficult to evaluate. Would it be
> proper to buy and sell human tissue? Do those from whom tissue
> has been removed have any rights or say relating to its further use?
>
> Nuffield Council on Bioethics, 1995[2]

The extraordinary successes of molecular biology and genetics in recent years have transformed the ways many of us think about ourselves, our families, and other persons and organizations that may have genetic information about us—or might have such profoundly personal information about us in the future. The laboratory practices that are common to the field of molecular genetics have, when coupled with the multiple concerns of many potential research participants, contributed to the ongoing controversy about human tissue research, whether that research is done in university research labs, government research labs, a variety of specialized tissue banks, commercial DNA banks, or biotechnology companies.

Chapters 1–3 described this controversy primarily as it unfolded in the United States during the 1990s and early 2000s. This chapter examines similar interests and concerns (e.g., the benefits of biomedical research, the value of privacy, the right of self-determination, the importance of avoiding harm) as they have surfaced in other countries. As shown by the examples of Iceland, Sweden,

Estonia, Denmark, and England in Chapter 1, this controversy is not limited to the United States. Rather, it has been played out in numerous committee reports, policy directives, and multidisciplinary conferences in different parts of the world. Here we sample some of these multiple policy documents regarding human tissue research to illustrate how this continuing controversy has been handled in other countries.

We have selected five examples of recommendations produced over a seven-year period (1994–2001): comprehensive reports and recommendations made by multi-disciplinary committees in three countries (the Netherlands, England, and Canada) plus shorter philosophical and political statements issued by HUGO and the Council of Europe. With the possible exception of the HUGO Ethics Committee, all of these committees could be said to reflect a European-North American perspective on human tissue research. Nevertheless, we believe that, collectively, these documents are representative of a global perspective that is multidisciplinary in nature, strongly supportive of biomedical research yet critical of some research practices, reasonably objective, and not easily dismissed as too liberal, too conservative, or too opinionated.[3]

The Health Council of the Netherlands (1994)

We begin our sampling with the Health Council of the Netherlands, the scientific advisory body of the government in the field of public health. In 1991 the State Secretary for Welfare, Health, and Cultural Affairs wrote to the Health Council requesting a report on the uses of human tissue in the Netherlands. The letter pointed out that once tissue samples are collected in diagnostic and therapeutic settings, "any surplus can then be used for a variety of other purposes such as research, teaching, treatment of other patients, quality assurance, and pharmaceutical and industrial processes (among them cosmetics manufacture)." Given these various uses of human tissues, a number of interests are at stake: "on the one hand society's interests in the availability of samples for science, teaching, and health care, and on the other the interests of the individuals who provide [the tissues], including the protection of their privacy." The state secretary added, "What I seek is information on the nature and extent of current and future practice in relation to the collection, storage, and use of human tissues for various purposes . . . including the ethical and legal aspects of this practice."[4]

In response to this request, the Health Council appointed a multidisciplinary "committee on human tissue for special purposes." The result of the committee's efforts was the comprehensive report *Proper Use of Human Tissue,* published in 1994. Unprecedented in scope, the Health Council report provided extensive information about the "special purposes" for which human tissue is used in the Netherlands. Some of the themes of the report are formulated as a series of six principles that should govern the acquisition, storage, and use of human tissue, especially when that use (or uses) of tissue samples is secondary to the purpose for which the tissue was originally collected. As stated in the executive summary, the principles are as follows:

- The intended use must be morally acceptable in so far as its purpose is to promote human health.
- Human tissue should always be used with the greatest of care.
- The relationship between patient and doctor must not be undermined by the use of bodily material. The patient must rest safe in the knowledge that his or her own needs will continue to come first. The doctor should exercise openness regarding the storage and use of human tissue and must duly inform the patient thereof.
- People cannot be forced to cooperate with the use of material obtained from them, even if it is in a good cause.
- The privacy of those whose material is put to further use must be respected and protected.
- The Committee endorses the principle of noncommercialism which applies to donation and extends this principle to the collection of human tissue in general. Such material should not be handed over or transferred to a third party by anyone whomsoever (whether patient, donor, doctor, or institution) with a view to making profit.[5]

The report's most notable feature is the information provided about current practices with human tissues used for post-diagnostic research and other secondary purposes, grouped together as "further purposes." In order to provide a comprehensive overview of current practices, the committee sent a questionnaire to individuals and institutions "whose work involves the use of human tissues." The 148 recipients of the questionnaire were told that their responses would be kept confidential, that the focus of the survey was "on the use of human tissue for purposes other than that for which it was originally collected," and that the committee hoped the information gathered would help them to provide "a realistic picture of what patients know about what happens to material they have surrendered."[6]

The questionnaire asked recipients to provide information about the origination or acquisition of each type of tissue sample. They were given four possible options: (1) "material originally taken for diagnostic purposes" (e.g., tissues to be sent to clinical chemistry labs, pathology labs, or genetics labs); (2) "material originally taken for research purposes" (e.g., blood, urine, or sperm from living donors; brain tissue from cadavers; tissues from tissue banks); (3) "material removed for transfusion or transplantation" (but proved unsuitable for that purpose); or (4) "residual material" (tissues not collected for a particular purpose, but remaining for discard after surgery, abortions, childbirth, in vitro fertilization, diagnostic work, or autopsy; this option also included cell lines).

Other parts of the questionnaire asked recipients about the destruction of tissue samples (For what reason is the material destroyed?); the storage of samples (For what purpose? How long? How much of the stored material identifies the person from whom it was taken, or could identify the person, or is anonymous? Are the donors/patients informed?); the use of samples (e.g., treatment of the patient, treatment of other patients, research, quality assurance, teaching, industrial production for health-care purposes, or industrial production for non-health-care purposes); and the supply of tissue samples to third parties (To what type of institution? How much of the material supplied identifies the person from whom it was taken, or could identify the person, or is anonymous?).

Three other features of this questionnaire are worth noting. First, the survey was written in an effort to reflect the process of tissue collection, storage, and use—a process that is described as starting when a patient, donor, or cadaver "surrenders material for a particular purpose." This process motif is repeated throughout the survey instrument by means of a recurring question, "What *then* happens to the material?" Second, the questionnaire repeatedly inquires about the openness of communications with patients and research volunteers about "further purposes" for their tissue samples by asking if patients, donors, or their legal agents were (*a*) "informed that the material is [to be] stored?," (*b*) "given the opportunity of objecting to its storage?," or (*c*) "asked for their consent?" Third, the questionnaire uses the theme of openness in communication with patients and research participants in another way by asking at one point, "What intended uses were known when the material was surrendered for its original purpose?"

The committee had reasonable confidence that the data gathered in the survey accurately portrayed national research practices with human tissues. They therefore drew several conclusions regarding secondary or "further" use of tissue samples in the Netherlands in 1992: (*1*) such samples, however originally acquired, "are more commonly stored than destroyed"; (*2*) tissue stored for research use is usually coded or nonidentifiable, in terms of the person from whom the tissue came; and (*3*) the "ultimate responsibility" for all types of stored tissue is usually vested in one individual, who is called the "tissue manager."

Two other conclusions from the survey data are especially important: (*4*) secondary or "further" research with tissue samples is so common and widespread as a practice that "*it can be called normal,* although use solely for the original purpose also occurs"; and (*5*) patients and donors are so rarely informed (much less given opportunities for informed consent) about plans for storage and possible "further use" of their tissue samples that the "*general rule that emerges* is that patients and donors are *not aware that material taken from them is stored*" and used for other purposes.[7] To cite one example, only 15% of patients gave consent for the storage of their tissues for post-diagnostic research purposes.[8] The committee concludes with these comments:

[M]any of the advances made in patient care could not have been achieved if human tissues were always destroyed once they had served the purpose for which they were obtained. Unless and until alternatives are available with the same or better properties, human tissues will have a vital role in the treatment of patients with a wide variety of conditions. The use of tissue samples . . . is not merely useful but *indispensable in modern medicine.*[9]

Nevertheless, the committee also emphasizes that "as an intrinsic 'part' of man, the body has a high moral value." That value, according to the committee, is of the highest sort in that the body's value "must not be violated" for any other purposes. Not having merely *instrumental* value, nor being usable as a "means" only to society's beneficial "end," the body has value in and of itself, a value that is *intrinsic* to its very existence. The best, and most appropriate way of acknowledging this value is to respect persons, who, after all, do not just "have" bodies, but "are" their bodies. Traditionally, Dutch law has translated this ethical principle of respect for persons into certain permissions and prohibitions that pertain to human bodies even in death. As examples, the committee points out that individuals, while alive, can grant permission for their bodies to be dissected after death, and other persons are prohibited from doing "disrespectful" things to the dead, such as necrophilia and other acts that involve the violation of corpses.

The challenge is in resolving the tension that exists between personal autonomy and beneficence to society or, as the report puts it, the tension between (*1*) the knowledge that "people are entitled to a say in what happens to their body" and (*2*) the knowledge that "the use of human tissues can bring great benefits" to society. Given that the scientific use of human tissues brings enormous benefits to society, the committee asks, "How far does autonomy stretch?" The legal answer is that autonomy stretches quite far. Here the committee's view uses an updated interpretation of property law to say that persons continue to exercise ownership of their bodies even when tissues have been removed from their bodies in a health care setting:

As medical advances have increased the usefulness and value of such material . . . a refinement has been introduced: the removal of material does not imply that the doctor or hospital becomes its owner. In this view the *patient is considered to retain ownership* of any material removed at surgery, with surrender by the patient being assumed only in the case of material which is destroyed or which is to be *used in some way known to the person from whom it was taken.*[10]

So, how can the important societal interests at stake be served without violating individual rights, including the rights of privacy, physical integrity, and self-determination? The answer is twofold: (*1*) a process of "openness and information" regarding scientific practices with stored tissue samples, combined with (*2*) an affirmation of the right of persons "to a say in what is done" with them. Therefore, they encourage physicians and investigators to provide information to citizens about post-diagnostic research and other "further" uses of stored tissues, thereby increasing "people's acceptance and confidence" in these practices. They explain:

Citizens should know what will happen to material taken from them under various circumstances. Institutions where tissue is collected have a job here: they must provide

general information on the fact that material may be stored and used for various purposes such as the treatment of other patients, research, quality assurance, teaching, and
production.[11]

From our vantage point several years later, the Health Council committee is to
be commended for their comprehensive report and generally sound recommendations.[12] They were trailblazers, trying to walk a still-difficult line between affirming the undeniable importance of biomedical research with human tissues and
making recommendations about how that research can be conducted with greater
respect for the values and concerns of the persons from whom the tissues come.

The Netherlands committee's report has a number of substantive strengths. First,
having developed a thoughtful, comprehensive questionnaire for scientific investigators, its authors were able to provide an unprecedented amount of information
(based on 1992 data) about the process of biomedical research with human tissue
samples. Second, they documented that the "further use" of human tissues for post-
diagnostic research, quality control, and medical education is a common, regular
practice in medical schools and teaching hospitals that is largely hidden from and
unknown by patients. A third strength of this report is the call for more openness and more information so that patients and other citizens will understand and
support research with stored tissues. Rather than being defensive about research
practices with stored tissues, committee members recommend (correctly, in our
view) that scientific investigators and their professional societies be more forthcoming with information about various steps in the multiple-step process of doing
scientific research with stored DNA samples. Fourth, they properly emphasize the
importance of individuals being able to "have a say in what happens" with tissues removed from their bodies for diagnostic, therapeutic, and research reasons.
Their position is strengthened by their willingness to interpret property law in the
Netherlands so that persons continue to control their tissues even when the tissues
have been removed from their bodies.

Nevertheless, the Health Council committee report also has some weaknesses.
First, the authors sometimes appear more interested in protecting professional turf
than in raising important questions about some of the ethical and legal implications of this scientific work. Second, they do not give sufficient attention to the
interpretation of the ethical principle of respect for persons. (The discussion they
do provide about respect for persons, however, is relatively novel in its application
of this principle to the debate about research with stored human tissues.) Third,
they do nothing with the concept of harm or even suggest that there may be risks of
harm (e.g., psychosocial risks in genetics research) in some kinds of research with
stored samples. Finally, the executive summary of the report is problematic. The
six principles laid out in the executive summary are not supported by the report
itself. They read like a late add-on to the finished report, perhaps providing a type
of window dressing for public relations reasons.

The Nuffield Council on Bioethics (1995)

In England, the task of writing a report on the ethical and legal aspects of stored tissue research was taken on by the Nuffield Council on Bioethics. The Nuffield Foundation, a private foundation that promotes science education, established the Council on Bioethics in 1991 because numerous bioethical issues were in need of analysis by a multidisciplinary panel of experts and the British government had not established any kind of national bioethics committee. The 15-member Nuffield Council on Bioethics soon became, by default, a bioethics committee with national standing, even though it was and is an independent body without any kind of governmental role.[13]

Analysis of the ethical and legal issues involved in stored tissue research was one of the first projects by the Nuffield Council, in part because some of its members had been troubled by the 1990 *Moore* decision in California. Although a state court decision in the United States, this case seemed to signal a new age in the regulation of human tissue research in technologically developed countries. The council therefore appointed a multidisciplinary Working Party on Human Tissue.

The working party's report, *Human Tissue: Ethical and Legal Issues,* was endorsed and published by the Nuffield Council. The report begins with a modest statement: "This report examines the ethical and legal questions raised by new and more traditional uses of human tissue and, where possible, suggests a way forward."[14] Its authors examine, adopt, and sometimes reject the views of various other parties in the new age of human tissue research. Accordingly, their subsequent recommendations reflect an eclectic assortment of perspectives:

1. The claims by biomedical investigators, physicians, biotechnology firms, and pharmaceutical companies about the almost endlessly beneficial uses of human tissue
2. British laws governing the use of human tissues (e.g., the Anatomy Act of 1832, the Human Tissue Act of 1961, the Human Organ Transplants Act of 1989)
3. The "exceptional and atypical" *Moore* case in the United States
4. Reports by the United States Office of Technology Assessment (1987), the Health Council in the Netherlands (1994), and the Council of Europe (1994 guidelines on human tissue banks)
5. Earlier British reports, such as the Polkinghorne Committee's report in 1989 on fetuses and fetal tissue
6. Public opinion, which is described as having a different attitude toward human tissue than toward other objects, displaying "a reluctance to talk in terms of ownership of the body or of its parts," and viewing "with distaste attempts to make money out of the transfer of 'rights' in the body or its parts"[15]

Human Tissue contains a variety of data regarding the collection and use of human tissue in England for therapeutic and research purposes. For example, the report has a table about the sources and uses of human tissue (e.g., patients, autopsy specimens, donors for research purposes, fetal tissue, body wastes, and "abandoned tissue"); information about the types of human tissue banks in the U.K. (e.g., five cornea banks, six heart valve banks, five bone banks); a discussion of the multiple uses of human tissues, including use in surgery and in products derived from human tissue; and a discussion about the importance of research with "left-over tissue." On the last point they simply accept a statement by the Royal College of Physicians: "[T]he use of anonymized left-over tissue for research is a traditional and ethically acceptable practice that does not need consent from patients or relatives, and need not be submitted to a research ethics committee."[16]

For one nonscientist on the committee, this compendium of information about clinical and research uses of human tissue was impressive. Onora O'Neill, a philosopher and administrator at Cambridge University, commented about the discrepancy between the voluminous information available about the multiple uses of human tissue and the paucity of legislation and regulation governing such uses. She later reflected:

Those of us on the working party who were neither doctors nor scientists were impressed by the complex practices of tissue [use in] day-to-day medical practice. Those of us who were not lawyers were startled to find how patchy the legal regulation of most use of human tissue is in the United Kingdom. . . . The task was to try to distinguish appropriate use from abuse and to formulate workable guidelines that could be incorporated into actual medical and scientific practice. . . .[17]

The committee agreed that traditional approaches in ethics, such as duty-based or rights-based deontological theories and utilitarian theories, were not very helpful. Likewise, they found appeals to "bodily autonomy," "bodily integrity," and "property rights" either "too fuzzy" or contrary to Britain's common law tradition. Such theories and claims were helpful in distinguishing cannibalism from blood transfusions, but what about the many other hard cases?

In an effort to develop "a more practical ethical stance," the committee sets forth two ethical principles, or "ethical tests" to distinguish appropriate use from abuse: legitimate uses of human tissue (*1*) do not inflict "gratuitous injury," and (*2*) do not override the consent of the persons whose tissues are used. In contrast to the Health Council committee in the Netherlands, however, the Nuffield committee does not think that consent is the primary concern, and they certainly do not agree with the Dutch view regarding the ownership of tissue.

Rather, the primary requirement for any type of ethically acceptable use of human tissue is the "avoidance and limitation of injury." More specifically, they use the ethical principle of nonmaleficence (without labeling it) to reject any use of human beings, or more narrowly their bodies and their tissues, in harmful ways that, on balance, "destroy, damage, or degrade." As examples of such *harmful uses,* they mention the uses of human tissues as food, as earrings and other entertainment, or as raw materials for products without therapeutic purpose (e.g., human leather). All of these uses "treat human beings or their bodies in ways that are destructive, damaging, or experienced as degrading, without any therapeutic intent which outweighs the destruction, damage, or degradation."[18] By contrast, they seem to find acceptable, on the basis of their first ethical test, almost any use of human tissue that is done in a "therapeutic context."

The second ethical test is *informed consent,* which the working party thinks is important but limited in actual practice. Informed consent is important because even if the removal of tissue from someone is a generally "acceptable type of action" in a health care setting, "the removal of tissue may be wrong if the person from whom tissue is removed does not consent, since its removal without consent in these conditions would constitute impermissible injury."[19] The working party points out, however, that "fully informed consent" is an "unattainable ideal," for at least three reasons: variable situations (e.g., patients, donors in research studies, relatives of a cadaver), the recognized fact that "consent will always be to action that is incompletely described," and the realization that "the ascription of consent is *defeasible*" (e.g., by coercion, deception, lack of disclosure of material facts, or manipulation).[20]

Given their emphasis on the avoidance of gratuitous harm and their more limited comments about the role of informed consent, what kinds of practical ethical guidelines does the working party put forth? Not many, at least for most adults in clinical and research settings. As long as the removal of tissue from patients is "integral to medical treatment," the act is "covered by a direct therapeutic intention." By contrast, in clinical cases in which the removal of tissue from a patient "is not integral to medical treatment" and research settings where tissue is removed from volunteers, the tissue needs to be "explicitly donated" by those persons with more specific consent. In these cases "the uses to which the tissue may be put are determined by the terms of the consent given by the donor." They summarize their general ethical guidelines with three questions:

[I]s the removal of tissue governed by intentions which respect human beings and their bodies, in that gratuitous injury is avoided?

[I]f the removal of tissue was in the course of medical treatment, was consent given by the patient?

[I]f the tissue [from a cadaver] was donated either by a [previously] healthy volunteer or post-mortem, was the appropriate consent procedure followed?[21]

The committee is, however, concerned about three kinds of situations: legal minors in research situations, removing tissue from adults who lack decision-making capacity (DMC), and the problems involved with commercialization. With legal minors, the committee backs away from a prohibition of tissue donation by children under the age of 18, but puts forth three ethical criteria for such situations: (*1*) the procedures "should be of negligible risk and minimal burden," (*2*) the consent "of the person with parental responsibility should be obtained," and (*3*) the "children themselves, where appropriate, should be consulted and their agreement obtained."[22] They propose that the same guidelines be used with adults lacking DMC, although they acknowledge that current U.K. law "may not entirely coincide with this view."

The committee's greatest concern involves the threat to the traditional uses of human tissue by the increased "commercialization of the human body." As a result, they marshal their strongest arguments against physicians, biomedical investigators, and institutions that might join biotechnology firms in a commercial "trade in tissue." They maintain that removing human tissue specifically for commercial gain is immoral, that human tissue should not be treated as a commodity, and that a market for procuring tissue would undermine altruistic desires to donate tissues and organs. They also argue that the *Moore* case has set an unfortunate and misleading precedent: most biomedical research with human tissues uses thousands of tissue samples, the importance of one tissue sample compared with others is usually a matter of chance, and no reward system should be established that would offer "large incentives for a few whose tissue happens to play a particularly central role in developing profitable therapeutic products."[23]

The working party's position on commercialization is based on two additional, strongly held views. First, patients have no right to any financial reward from biomedical research done with tissue samples because, even in the unlikely event they can demonstrate that patents and commercial products can be traced to research done with their tissue samples, it is no longer "their" tissue once it has been removed from their bodies. The committee asserts that "a person from whom tissue is removed has not the slightest interest in making any claim to it once it is removed," but even if there were such a patient (e.g., John Moore), the claim has no merit. Why? British law (*1*) does not recognize any right of property in a body and (*2*) says that consent to the removal of bodily tissue entails an intention to abandon the tissue. It is true that "an appendix or gallstone may be returned to a patient who may refer to it as *her* appendix or gallstone," but according to the law "by her consent to the operation she *abandons* any claim to the appendix . . . on removal the appendix acquires the status of a *res* (a thing) and comes into the possession of the hospital authority prior to disposal."[24]

The committee's second reason for taking a strong anticommercialization position is that commercialization in biomedical research is avoidable, at least with research using tissues obtained from patients. Specifically, they call on physicians, hospital- and university-sponsored researchers, hospitals, and tissue banks to take on a role that they describe as "medical intermediaries": an intermediate person or institution standing between patients (and research participants) and commercial biotechnology companies, which "connects the market and the non-market structures." Such medical intermediaries can procure, store, and allocate tissue samples, but should not enter into any commercial relations with patients or donors.[25]

"Suggesting a way forward," the Nuffield working party offers a number of conclusions and recommendations. In terms of *ethical guidelines,* they conclude that (*1*) the use of human tissue for medical treatment and research is ethically acceptable; (*2*) using human tissue in ways that "destroy, damage or degrade" are "unacceptable because such uses show lack of respect for human beings and their bodies"; (*3*) uses of human tissues in medical treatment and research are "only ethically acceptable when the tissue has been removed with the consent of those whose tissue is used" or "by procedures that give equivalent protection" (they provide no example of such procedures); and (*4*) "there are strong arguments against the commercial acquisition and supply of human tissue." As to desirable *legal standards,* they recommend that (*5*) tissues removed in the course of medical treatment "be regarded as having been abandoned by the person from whom it was removed"; (*6*) "medical intermediaries should supply users of human tissue on a non-profit making basis"; and (*7*) the Government should join with other member states in the European Patent Convention in adopting an "immorality exclusion to patents in the area of human and animal tissue."[26]

In our view, the report has numerous strengths and weaknesses. First, it is notable for several distinctive contributions to the ongoing, international debate about human tissue research: the legal theme of tissue abandonment in clinical and research settings, the strong emphasis placed on avoiding a "market in tissues," the concern displayed for children in clinical research situations, and the strong interest the council had in formulating guidelines that would be sufficiently practical that they might actually influence the practice of physicians and scientific investigators. Second, the report demonstrates the multiple benefits to society from biomedical research with stored tissues. Third, committee members candidly admit that traditional ethical theory is sometimes limited in its practical significance, especially with an issue as complex as human tissue research. Having made that admission, they proceed to develop two ethical principles—no gratuitous injury, do not override consent—that they consider "of practical use." Fourth, they display unusual interest in and concern about vulnerable patients who lack sufficient DMC to be able to make decisions about providing tissues from their bodies for diagnostic, therapeutic, and/or research purposes. Finally, for a group that, modestly, only wanted to "suggest a way forward," the Nuffield Council ends up making more than 20 recommendations. Although we do not always agree with the council, we believe that the debate over human tissue research has been helped by their thoughtful and practical contributions.

Our disagreements with the Nuffield Council report are multiple. Some pertain to substantive aspects of this complex issue that they simply never addressed: the distinctions among identified, coded, or anonymized stored samples; the differences between retrospective and prospective research with human tissues; the ethical complications caused by secondary research; and the concerns that the general public seems to have about genetics research, DNA databanks, and the threats they pose to the privacy of personal and familial genetic information.

The council also gave inadequate attention to several substantive points. For example, they place considerable weight on the notion of gratuitous injury, but never address the underlying concept of harm and how it can apply to individuals, families, and groups that may experience psychosocial harm from genetics research. They give some attention to the role of informed consent, but, because there can never (in their view) be completely informed consent or perfect informed consent, they accept a fairly weak notion of general consent rather than trying to show how a more substantially informed consent might be a practical possibility in the real world of stored tissue research. In addition, they focus on the general problem of commercialization with stored tissue research, but, curiously, fail to address the multiple ways (e.g., private tissue and databanks, scientific investigators with conflicts of interest, premature patent applications for DNA sequences) in which the possibility of huge monetary gain may improperly influence the work of some biomedical investigators and, perhaps, the relationships between those investigators and the participants they recruit for their research studies.

Some of the council's positions are simplistic, if not wrong. These include the acceptance of basically all current research practices with leftover tissue; the unquestioning acceptance of statements by medical authorities (e.g., the Royal College of Physicians) regarding the applicability of traditional human tissue research practices to the modern era; and the extent to which they build much of the report around the legal theory of abandonment. To sum up, we disagree with the equation that underlies much of their report (consent to treatment = intention to abandon tissue) because its legal basis (in the United States) is tenuous, it fails to take seriously the concerns and interests that some people have about research that might be done with their stored tissues, and it is based on assumptions about personal preferences unsupported by empirical data. Our views on the council's claim about abandonment are supported by the professional literature published in response to their report.[27]

The Human Genome Organization (1996, 1998)

HUGO was established in 1988 as an international organization of genome scientists. With funding from private foundations in the United States, Britain, France, and Japan, HUGO set up offices as an international coordinating body for genome research in Bethesda (HUGO Americas), London (HUGO Europe), and Osaka (HUGO Pacific).[28]

HUGO has a number of permanent committees, including a multidisciplinary Ethics Committee. With members from nine countries, the Ethics Committee has discussed many international concerns over the years: the fear that genome research might lead to discrimination and stigmatization of individuals and populations; the realization that persons in developing countries might continue to be used in insensitive, coercive ways by scientists from industrialized countries; and the concern that patenting and commercialization of scientific discoveries might result in the loss of access to important scientific work. Based on these discussions, the Ethics Committee has adopted four principles for any recommendations it makes:

1. Recognition that the human genome is part of the common heritage of humanity
2. Adherence to international norms of human rights
3. Respect for the values, traditions, culture and integrity of [research] participants
4. Acceptance and upholding of human dignity and freedom[29]

This set of principles is part of a preamble to the 1996 document entitled "Statement on the Principled Conduct of Genetic Research." Sometimes called the "HUGO 10 Commandments," the statement makes these points about international collaborative genetics research, including research done with DNA samples:

That scientific *competence* is an essential prerequisite for ethical research. . . .

That *communication* not only be scientifically accurate but understandable to the populations, families, and individuals concerned and sensitive to their social and cultural context. . . .

That *consultation* should precede recruitment of possible participants and continue throughout the research. . . .

That informed decisions to *consent* can be individual, familial, or at the level of communities and populations. . . .

That any *choices* made by participants with regard to storage or other uses of materials or information taken or derived from them be respected. . . .

That the recognition of privacy and protection against unauthorized access be ensured by the *confidentiality* of genetic information. . . .

That *collaboration* between individuals, populations and researchers . . . in the free flow, access and exchange of information is essential not only to scientific progress, but also for the present or future benefit of all participants. . . .

That any actual or potential *conflict of interest* be revealed at the time information is communicated and before agreement is reached. . . .

That undue inducement through *compensation* for individual participants, families and populations should be prohibited. . . . This prohibition, however, does not include . . . the possible use of a percentage of any royalties for humanitarian purposes. . . .

That *continual review,* oversight and monitoring are essential for the implementation of these recommendations. . . .[30]

This statement is an important step toward a greater international recognition of human rights, including the rights of participants in genetics studies. The

10 statements about principles, while somewhat vague, address many important points about genetics research, especially when that research is done by scientists from industrialized countries using tissue samples obtained from citizens in developing parts of the world. The HUGO committee properly emphasizes that in these diverse settings for genetics research, as in all settings for scientific research, it is important that scientists tailor the informed consent process to fit the needs, interests, cultural values, and traditions of the group being studied, including, perhaps, supplementing the consent of individuals with some kind of approval by the group.

Likewise, it is important that the choices made by participants regarding DNA banking be respected, that their banked tissues and any derivative genetic information about them be handled in ways that protect their confidentiality, and that procedures for future access to any banked samples or stored data be established in ways that protect the interests of research participants as well as the needs of scientists wanting access to the stored materials for research and, possibly, therapeutic purposes. In addition, it is important that the persons who provide the blood, buccal smears, urine, or other tissue samples for genetics research be appropriately compensated in some way, lest they feel both harmed and wronged by the scientists doing research with their tissues. The Ethics Committee's suggestion of a percentage of any royalties being used for humanitarian purposes is an important step in the right direction.

In 1998 the HUGO Ethics Committee produced a document specifically regarding genetics research with banked DNA samples. Entitled a "Statement on DNA Sampling: Control and Access," this second document continues the committee's emphasis on the international ethical and legal standards that are needed for human tissue research in the era of genomic medicine. They make several recommendations:

1. Policies and practices regarding genetics research with banked DNA samples should distinguish between tissue samples obtained during "routine medical care" and during "a specific research protocol."
2. Research with "*routine* samples" should be done *only* after individual patients have been given "general notification" of an institution's policies regarding future use of diagnostic samples, the patients have been given an opportunity to object (as part of the consent process) to the research option, and the samples have either been coded or anonymized.
3. The practice of secondary research (which they call "other research" in the future) with "*research* samples" should be done *only* after research participants have been given notification of this possibility, individual participants have not objected, and the samples have been coded or anonymized.
4. Policies regarding third-party access to stored DNA samples and the personal and familial genetic information contained in the samples should limit such access to "immediate relatives."

5. Individuals' requests for the destruction of their DNA samples in genetics labs should be carried out *only* if immediate relatives have no need for learning their own genetic status and if the samples have not already been entered into a research protocol or provided to other scientific investigators.
6. These ethical requirements regarding "the control and access of DNA samples and information" should be standardized worldwide.[31]

The recommendations made in these two HUGO documents are significant contributions to the expanding literature worldwide on the ethical and legal aspects of research practices with stored tissues. They are especially notable because they contain several themes not usually found in policy documents on this subject: an emphasis on the personal *and familial* information contained in DNA samples; a recommendation that hospitals and other research institutions disclose common research practices in advance to patients as part of the process of informed consent; an emphasis on the interests, needs, and rights of present *and future* family members genetically connected with the individual sources of DNA samples; and a recognition that recommendations about ethical and legal research practices with banked samples must transcend national boundaries, just as the research practices do themselves.

The Council of Europe (1997, 1999)

The Council of Europe (COE) was established by 10 western European countries in 1949 in the hopes of establishing, in Winston Churchill's words, "a kind of United States of Europe" that would strengthen democracy, human rights, and the rule of law throughout its member states. It now has 43 member states that accept the principles of democracy, human rights, and the rule of law.[32]

The COE works to achieve greater political unity by trying to reform and harmonize member states' practices and policies in diverse areas ranging from human rights to the media to sports to environmental issues. The clearest, most practical evidence of the COE's influence is the existence of over 160 European "conventions," or commonly accepted political statements, that COE leaders claim to be the equivalent of more than 10,000 bilateral treaties. Each of these conventions gains legal force in ratifying countries as soon as five member states officially express their legislative consent to be bound by the convention.

One of these conventions, the one most pertinent to human tissue research, is the Convention for the Protection of Human Rights and Dignity of the Human Being with Regard to the Application of Biology and Medicine that was officially accepted by the COE in 1997. The convention gained legal force in 1999 when a fifth member state ratified the document. As of this writing, the convention has been signed by 19 countries and ratified by 11 legislatures.[33]

More simply called the Convention on Human Rights and Biomedicine, this document has the potential of being the first legally binding international text designed to preserve human dignity, rights, and freedom against the misuse of advances in biology and medicine. The document has 38 Articles on a wide variety of subjects including equitable access to health care, privacy, informed consent, protection of persons participating in biomedical research, and prohibition of financial gain. Several of these Articles are especially relevant to research with stored tissues:

Article 2: *Primacy of the Human Being:* "The interests and welfare of the human being shall prevail over the sole interest of society or science."

Article 5: *Informed Consent:* "An intervention in the health field may only be carried out after the person concerned has given free and informed consent to it."

Article 10: *Private Life:* "Everyone has the right to respect for private life in relation to information about his or her health."

Article 11: *Nondiscrimination:* "Any form of discrimination against a person on grounds of his or her genetic heritage is prohibited."

Article 21: *Prohibition of Financial Gain:* "The human body and its parts shall not, as such, give rise to financial gain."

Article 22: *Disposal of a Removed Part of the Human Body:* "When in the course of an intervention any part of a human body is removed, it may be stored and used for a purpose other than that for which it was removed, only if this is done in conformity with appropriate information and consent procedures."[34]

This convention has the possibility of being an extremely important political and legal document. Somewhat like the two HUGO documents just discussed, the Convention on Human Rights and Biomedicine is an attempt to give greater international recognition to human rights, including the rights of persons who participate in biomedical research. Unlike the HUGO documents, this COE convention currently has the force of law in 11 European countries, and the number of legislatures voting to ratify the document continues to grow.

Of course, it remains to be seen whether and how the various articles of this convention are enforced in individual European countries. Some of the articles quoted above are so vaguely worded (perhaps intentionally so) that their practical meaning is unclear and open to differing interpretations. By contrast, the wording of the articles on informed consent (articles 5 and 22) and the article on discrimination may be sufficiently specific that they may be enforceable. If so, the convention may have two important impacts on human tissue research done in Europe: (*1*) it may diminish the concerns that some people have about the possibility of genetic discrimination following their participation in genetics studies, and (*2*) it may give legal "teeth" to the right of persons (in the words of the Netherlands document) "to a say in what is done" with their banked DNA samples, including what is done with their stored tissues or cell lines in secondary research studies.

The Canadian Tri-Council Policy Statement (1998, 2001)

In Canada, the Parliament has created and funded three research councils to promote and regulate all federally funded research done with human participants. Biomedical research, including research done with DNA samples, is funded and regulated by the Canadian Institutes of Health Research (formerly called the Medical Research Council). Other types of research done with human participants are funded and regulated by the Natural Sciences and Engineering Research Council and the Social Sciences and Humanities Research Council. Each of these councils published guidelines in the late 1970s for the ethical conduct of research involving humans.

A Tri-Council Working Group was mandated in 1994 to formulate a joint policy statement regarding human participants research. After several years of work and considerable criticism from various interest groups, this group published the *Tri-Council Policy Statement: Ethical Conduct for Research Involving Humans* in 1998, but described the document as a continually evolving policy statement that will need to be updated on a regular basis.[35] The rationale for the joint policy statement is threefold: it seeks (*1*) "to articulate ethical norms that transcend disciplinary boundaries," (*2*) "to harmonize the ethics review process," and (*3*) "to avoid imposing one disciplinary perspective on others" by requiring a "reasonable flexibility in the implementation of common principles." As to "contentious ethical issues," the anonymously written policy document states that it will outline applicable ethical principles and identify points of consensus, but not try to offer definitive answers.[36]

The *Tri-Council Policy Statement* differs from the other documents we have discussed in this chapter, both in authoritative status and in substance. Unlike the publications of the Health Council of the Netherlands, the Nuffield Council in England, and HUGO, this Canadian document has binding authority with federally funded researchers in Canada; if they do not abide by the policies set forth in this document, they will not be funded to do research. Unlike the COE convention, the Tri-Council policy statement has no legal authority in other countries, but it will certainly affect the lives of investigators, members of Research Ethics Boards (REBs), and research participants in Canada.

The Tri-Council policy statement also differs from the other documents in terms of its content. In contrast to the Dutch and British publications, this document is not limited to the subject of research with stored tissues, and in contrast to the HUGO statements and the COE convention, it is not limited to fairly general statements of principle that may be difficult to interpret and enforce. Rather, this policy statement sets forth an instructive ethics framework for research with humans, then provides numerous policy directives in a range of research areas that are expected to guide the decisions and conduct of researchers and REBs.

According to this document, the ethical principles and federal regulations that govern research with human participants in Canada are part of an ethics framework characterized by two important, sometimes conflicting values. On the one hand, there is the ongoing *need for research* driven by "a fundamental moral commitment to advancing human welfare, knowledge, and understanding." On the other hand, there is the moral imperative of *respecting human dignity* through (*1*) "the selection and achievement of morally acceptable ends" as well as (*2*) the selection of "morally acceptable means to those ends."[37]

In addition, the ethics framework for research—correctly understood—consists of a "subject-centered perspective" by researchers, institutions, and REBs that is guided by eight ethical principles expressing the "common standards, values, and aspirations of the research community." These principles, most of which are widely accepted in international research ethics, are as follows:

1. Respect for human dignity
2. Respect for free and informed consent
3. Respect for vulnerable persons
4. Respect for privacy and confidentiality
5. Respect for justice and inclusiveness
6. Minimizing harm
7. Maximizing benefit
8. Balancing harms and benefits[38]

Within this general ethics framework for research, the Tri-Council policy statement has separate sections with policies regarding the membership and procedures of REBs, conflicts of interest, informed consent, privacy and confidentiality, clinical trials, and research with aboriginal peoples. It also provides recommendations and policies regarding research with stored tissues, first in a section on human genetics research, then in a section on research at the beginning of human life (research on gametes, embryos, and fetuses), and finally in a concluding section on human tissue research.

In terms of genetics research, the policy statement emphasizes the applicability of three of the ethical principles: respect for "free and informed" consent, respect for privacy and confidentiality, and the avoidance or minimization of harm. In fact, consent and avoidance of harm are dual themes for this section of the document. Investigators and members of REBs are told that free and informed consent is a necessary feature of any type of genetics research, whether it involves family linkage studies, DNA banking, gene alteration studies, or genetics research that is secondary to the original purpose of a research study. Suggested methods of ensuring that research participants have given consent are twofold: (*1*) comprehensive consent documents that enable research participants to choose from a number of options (e.g., "use of the material only in the present study, use restricted to the condition, or other clearly specified use"), or (2) a more limited consent form that "specifies arrangements to maintain contact with the subject regarding future uses." Either method "must be clearly explained during the free and informed consent process."[39]

As to the minimization of harm in genetics research, the document points out that psychosocial harm can occur as a result of genetics studies in several ways: changes in self-identity and feelings of self-worth, tension within families, stigmatization of individuals and groups, and discrimination against individuals and groups. To minimize harm, the policy statement prohibits eugenic studies, germline therapy studies, and genetic testing of children who may have adult onset conditions lacking current treatment. Also to minimize harm, it encourages the use of anonymized samples, calls for the "actual destruction of genetic material or research data" if such a step is desired by a person withdrawing from a genetics study, and requires that investigators discuss the possible commercial use of genetic material or research data with their REB and with any persons who may participate in a study having commercial implications. Regarding the issue of ownership of stored tissues, the document states that, even though concepts of ownership of samples vary from culture to culture, "it is unethical for a researcher to claim ownership of genetic material by claiming that the concept of private ownership did not exist in the community involved."[40]

What about stored tissue research using reproductive cells or cryopreserved human embryos? In the section on research with human gametes, embryos, or fetuses, the Tri-Council policy statement is quite specific. Any research on human reproductive cells, whether obtained as a part of clinical care or in a research setting, requires the free and informed consent of the persons providing the sperm or ova and the disclosure of information by investigators regarding the purpose of the research (e.g., infertility, improved birth control). The same requirement of free and informed consent applies to secondary research, which in this context means research that is to be done on "gametes [that] were originally provided for a purpose other than research." As to research with cryopreserved human embryos, the document prohibits the creation of human embryos specifically for research purposes. But when human embryos are created for reproductive purposes and not used for that purpose, research on the stored, "extra" embryos is ethically acceptable under specified conditions.[41]

The concluding section on stored human tissue research is relatively short. The section begins with a description of cultural pluralism, then emphasizes the importance of applying the "subject-centered perspective" to research with stored samples with this statement: "It is a fundamental ethical principle that researchers, in the collection and use of human tissue, respect individual and community notions of human dignity and physical, spiritual, and cultural integrity."[42]

Regarding privacy and confidentiality, the document distinguishes among four categories of tissue, using a label for the first two categories that differ from the terminology we use: (1) *identifiable tissue* can be immediately linked to a specific individual (e.g., "by way of an identifying tag or patient number"); (2) *traceable tissue* is "potentially traceable to a specific donor provided there is access to further information such as a patient record or a database"; (3) *anonymous tissue* is anonymous due either to the absence of an identifying tag or the passage of time (e.g., "tissue recovered from archaeological sites"); and (4) *anonymized tissue* has been permanently stripped of identifiers. Yet, by means of a short case example, the document indicates that research with anonymized tissue is not exempt from ethical considerations. The example has a pathologist seeking REB approval for research with "non-traceable tissue left over" from earlier diagnostic work. The Tri-Council's advice is that the REB should approve the research (because it presents no problems pertaining to privacy and confidentiality), but should also consider discussing the benefits of doing research with identifiable or traceable specimens with the investigator because research with such samples (1) may permit the source of the sample to give free and informed consent concerning "the new research project" and (2) makes it possible, perhaps, later to offer some of the benefits of the research study to the individual and his or her family.[43]

The centrality of free and informed consent in stored tissue research is evident when the Tri-Council policy statement turns to the ethical aspects of *prospective* research. Simply put, the document states that "*all relevant information should be provided* to enable the potential subject to decide whether to give free and informed consent" to participate in a research project and, again, "potential subjects will *be empowered to decide*" whether they want to participate in a research study that will involve storage of their tissue samples.[44] The policy statement also recommends using advance directives for the purpose of making tissue donors' preferences known in advance to investigators, while pointing out that some Canadian provinces have laws requiring that the free and informed consent of a participant in research be based on an understanding of the "specific uses of tissue" in the research study.

Then, quite specifically, the document states that "research proposing the collection and use of human tissues requires ethics review by an REB." Researchers are required to demonstrate to the REB that a research study will be undertaken only with "the free and informed consent of competent donors," with the free and informed consent by an authorized third party if the research will be done with incompetent donors, or with the free and informed consent expressed in an advance directive or by authorized third party if the research will be done with cadaver tissue. The same requirement applies to investigators who plan to carry out a research study with tissue that was "acquired incidentally to therapeutic interventions." In all of these situations, researchers who "seek to collect human tissue for research shall, *as a minimum,* provide potential donors or authorized third parties" with the following information:

1. The purpose of the research
2. The type and amount of tissue to be taken

3. The manner in which tissue will be taken and preserved
4. The potential uses for the tissue (including commercial uses)
5. The safeguards to be used to protect a participant's privacy and confidentiality
6. The identifying information to be attached to specific tissue
7. The ways in which research with the tissue could cause harm[45]

In terms of *retrospective* research on previously collected tissues, the document makes two policy statements. First, when the samples are either "identifiable" or "traceable," researchers are expected to adhere to the same consent requirements as with prospective research studies: obtain free and informed consent from individuals (or their authorized representatives) by disclosing the informational items listed above, thereby empowering them to decide whether the tissue specimens can be used in the research study. Second, when the collected tissues are either anonymous or anonymized, and when "there are no potential harms" to anyone (i.e., the unknown persons from whom the tissue came and their unidentifiable families), the requirement to obtain free and informed consent does not apply.

Yet even here, in the context of the one permissible exception to the consent requirement in stored tissue research, investigators and members of REBs are reminded that "other ethical issues may warrant scrutiny." Specifically, they are reminded, again, that doing research with anonymized tissue samples can still involve ethical problems of two sorts: (*1*) some individuals do not want their tissue used "for any research purposes regardless of anonymity," and (*2*) "the interests of biological relatives or members of distinct cultural groups" may be harmed through research uses of their anonymous tissue.[46]

Compared with the other documents discussed in this chapter, the *Tri-Council Policy Statement* stands out as being quite different. Its authors, presumably representing several disciplines, took on a daunting task: to produce a set of ethical and legal guidelines for research in Canada that would be accepted by geneticists, anthropologists, nurses, oncologists, psychologists, and other professionals whose research involves working with other humans willing to take on some personal risk as participants in research studies. They succeeded in placing the policy statement in the context of international research ethics, emphasizing important ethical principles, and addressing areas of research that have particular relevance in Canada (e.g., research with aboriginal peoples). Yet the relative brevity of the policy statement means that important areas of research were left out or handled in an overly simplistic manner (e.g., research with adolescents, persons with HIV, prisoners, students, elderly persons), and specific policies were sometimes written at a problematic level of generality.

As to research with stored tissue samples, the Tri-Council policy statement is, at the very least, notable for the attention it gives to the ethical and legal issues involved in doing this kind of widespread, common research. By comparison, the 1993 federal research guidebook produced by the U.S. Office for Protection from

Research Risks (now the Office of Human Research Protections) covers a number of research areas left out of the Canadian document, but it does not provide any guidelines for stored tissue research.[47] In addition, the Tri-Council document is important because of the emphasis it places on informed consent, the rights of research participants, genetics research, research with cryopreserved embryos, the avoidance of psychosocial harm, and ethical concerns with research done with anonymized samples.

Nevertheless, its policies on human tissue research would be more acceptable if they had been made in a broader, more substantive context. That context would have provided investigators and REB members with a greater emphasis on the importance of biomedical research, information about competing ethical positions regarding human tissue research, and more guidance on how advance directives and consent documents can help patients and potential research participants be "empowered to decide" about taking part in research with banked samples.

This Canadian document is unusual because the three research councils announced upon its publication in 1998 that they were not producing a document intended to stand the test of time. Rather, they correctly recognized that some of the subject matter of research ethics has to be revised and updated as new, rapidly evolving, and unprecedented developments occur in the research sciences. Accordingly, the presidents of Canada's three federal funding agencies announced in 2001 that they were establishing a new governance structure for the *Tri-Council Policy Statement*. Named the Panel and Secretariat on Research Ethics, the new 11-member committee has a mandate to promote, interpret, update, and implement the federal policies for research involving humans in Canada.[48]

Summary

As should be clear by now, these committee reports and policy statements differ in a number of ways. First, they differ in authoritative status. The documents produced by the Health Council of the Netherlands, the Nuffield Council, and the HUGO Ethics Committee contain helpful summaries of common research practices and recommendations regarding future research practices with stored DNA samples. Yet as important as these documents are, they have neither the financial and legal weight of the current Tri-Council policies on research practices in Canada, nor the legal authority of the COE convention on human rights and biomedicine since its ratification by at least 11 European governments.

Second, the documents differ in terms of the composition of the committees that produced them. The Health Council committee was comprised primarily of Dutch physicians and scientists who seem to have had a considerable amount of knowledge about human tissue research, the benefits of that research, and the problems that some of their recommendations (e.g., regarding informed consent, ownership of samples) might cause for investigators. By contrast, the Nuffield Council consisted primarily of British nonscientists who seemed awed by the complexity of the subject before them, unduly influenced by the pronouncements of the Royal College of Physicians, and inclined to take positions that favored investigators, hospital organizations, and pharmaceutical companies. (We lack sufficient information about the composition of the HUGO, COE, and Canadian committees to make comparative comments about them.)

Third, the documents differ in terms of their intended audiences. The Dutch Health Council report was written as an advisory report for the state secretary who had requested it, with the committee also hoping to persuade investigators to make self-regulatory changes and the government to pass regulations that might ensure "good practice" in the widespread secondary research being done with banked tissues. The report by the Nuffield Council seems to have been intended to demonstrate three things to a U.K. audience: the complexity of current bioethical issues, the need for a multidisciplinary national bioethics committee, and the quality of work being funded by the Nuffield Foundation. By contrast, the intended audiences for the HUGO Ethics Committee documents, the COE convention on human rights and biomedicine, and the Tri-Council policy statement were, respectively, geneticists and other professionals in HUGO, governmental bodies and citizens within the countries comprising the COE, and researchers and REB members within Canada, and, ultimately for all three groups, all persons worldwide who have access to the Web.

More importantly, what about the content of these documents? Do they represent isolated, possibly esoteric points of view, or are there some shared concerns and common recommendations that transcend national boundaries and normal disciplinary differences? There clearly are several common themes. First, all of these documents emphasize that human beings, somehow, are not reducible to their "parts" and that blood, cheek cells, muscle tissue, and even urine retain some kind of "special" quality precisely because they are DNA samples from genetically unique (with the exception of monozygotic twins) human beings. Sometimes this point is made with unavoidably vague references to the "dignity" of human beings, or the centrality of "respecting human beings and their bodies," or the importance of having "respect for persons." Thus, the Dutch Health Council stresses that "as an intrinsic 'part' of man, the body has a high moral value"; the HUGO ethics committee calls for the "upholding of human dignity and freedom"; and the COE convention declares that the "primacy of the human being" means that the "interests and welfare of the human being shall prevail over the sole interest of society or science."

At other times the claims about the special-ness of individual humans takes a quite specific form: the claim that individual patients and research participants (in contrast, say, to nonhuman animals used in research) *retain ownership of their tissues* after the tissues have been removed from their bodies in health-care settings. The report of the Health Council of the Netherlands contains the most explicit statement of this position, and the Canadian Tri-Council policy statement expresses agreement with this view. In sharp contrast, the British Nuffield Council report claims that when hospital patients consent to treatment, they automatically abandon their tissues and any claim to ownership of the tissues or control over what is subsequently done with them.

Subsequently, however, this Nuffield Council position was rebutted in a 2001 report from the British Medical Research Council (MRC), thus bringing Britain into closer agreement with several other nations regarding the ownership of tissues. Pointing out that in Britain it is "not legally possible to own a human body," the MRC report observes that "the law is unclear as to whether ... one can legally 'own' samples of human biological materials or whether donors of biological material [in research settings] have any property rights over 'their' samples." The report interprets all research samples as donated "gifts with strings attached" and the university or hospital where research is conducted with these samples as having "*custodianship* of human material donated for research."[49]

The second common theme in these documents is the importance of informed consent in clinical and research settings. All of the documents agree, with varying degrees of emphasis, that research participants and patients have the right to know what research purposes will be carried out with their tissue samples, and to consent (or refuse to consent) to have their tissues used in the achievement of those research goals. The Canadian Tri-Council policy document, for example, encourages the development of research advance directives and improved consent documents that will enable persons to be "empowered to decide" about research that might be done with samples of their tissues.

The Netherlands report goes further by calling for a process of "openness and information" about scientific research with stored samples. One of the results of such openness will, we think, be greater societal acceptance of and confidence in the research that is being done with banked tissues. An example of how such openness can be practiced is provided by the 1998 HUGO document when it calls for institutional notification to patients and research participants regarding the possibility that research may be done with "routine samples" (diagnostic samples) and that secondary research with different research purposes may be done with "research samples."

Third, all of the documents, with the exception of the Health Council report, express concern over the psychosocial harm that may occur in some individuals' lives because of the research done with their stored tissues. For this reason, several of the documents emphasize the importance of maintaining the confidentiality and privacy of personal and familial information derived from research with DNA samples. Also for this reason, several of the documents point out that research done with anonymous or anonymized samples avoids the problems of breaches of confidentiality and privacy that sometimes occur when tissue samples are identified with the sample source or coded so that they can be linked with the source of the sample. Yet the 1998 HUGO document provides a cautionary note, pointing out that even the practice of anonymizing samples can, at least in a general sense, cause a measure of psychosocial harm to immediate relatives and future family members. For example, such relatives could come to have an interest in knowing the familial information contained in the now-unidentifiable, anonymized DNA samples of a dead relative who participated in a large research study years earlier, such as any of several epidemiologic or population-genetics studies with adult participants.

Connected to these concerns about harm, most of the documents make substantial use of the ethical principle of nonmaleficence in their recommendations. The Nuffield Council emphasizes this principle when they maintain that legitimate uses of human tissue do not inflict "gratuitous injury," and when they reject any use of human tissue samples that "destroys, damages, or degrades" the persons from whom the samples came. The Canadian Tri-Council policy statement lists kinds of psychosocial harm that can result from genetics research with DNA samples and makes a point unmatched by any of the other documents, namely that specific cultural groups can be stigmatized by research findings even when individual tissue samples from the groups have been anonymized.

Both of the HUGO documents and the COE convention focus on the problem of discrimination that can accompany or follow the use of tissue samples for research purposes. The 1996 HUGO document highlights the discrimination that can occur when scientific investigators take blood samples from persons in other countries without being sensitive to the social and cultural context of the people with whom they are working. The COE convention on human rights simply declares, "Any form of discrimination against a person on grounds of his or her genetic heritage is prohibited."

The concern about the problems connected with the commercialization of research is a fourth theme running throughout these documents. With the exception of the Tri-Council policy statement, which does not address the problem, all of the documents adopt some version of a noncommercialization position. The Nuffield Council, the only committee clearly influenced by the *Moore* decision, is the most explicit. For them, removing human tissue specifically for commercial profit "is immoral," the idea of sharing research profits with research participants risks turning human genetic material into a commodity, and any physicians or biomedical investigators who take part in either of these activities are engaged in an unjustifiable "trade in human tissue." In a similar fashion, the COE convention makes a blanket prohibition of financial gain through human tissue research: "The human body and its parts shall not, as such, give rise to financial gain." The 1996 HUGO document, by contrast, takes a more moderate position by prohibiting "undue inducement" for individuals or groups to participate in research studies, but permitting the sharing of research profits with research participants through the return of "*a percentage of any royalties* for humanitarian purposes."[50]

Finally, all of these documents address the widespread practice of secondary research, whether it takes the form of post-diagnostic research with tissues obtained in clinical settings or the underreported form of additional research studies done with DNA samples obtained in research settings. The Health Council report does the most with this theme because, after all, the purpose of this report was to provide information and guidance about the "further purposes" for which human tissue is being used in the Netherlands. Based on their survey results, they conclusively document that post-diagnostic and other secondary research with stored tissues is an indispensable part of modern medicine.

The COE convention, in particular, addresses the problematic nature of secondary research practices with banked samples. The authors of this legal document declare that such research practices are justifiable only when done in the context of informed consent by the person who provided the tissue: "When in the course of an intervention any part of a human body is removed, it may be stored and used for a purpose other than that for which it was removed, only if this is done in conformity with appropriate information and consent procedures."[51]

In the next two chapters, we provide a description and analysis of the multiple approaches that have been taken to regulate human tissue research in the United States, including federal regulations, court decisions, and state laws. Then in Chapter 7 we analyze the ethical and legal positions taken by NBAC members in their 1999 report on human tissue research.

Cases and Vignettes

A group of pathology professors and medical students in Britain decided to find out what patients think about the ownership and uses of "diseased parts of the body" (i.e., tissues) removed during surgery. Following the publication of the Nuffield Council's report in 1995, they surveyed 384 adult postoperative surgical inpatients to find out their views. Regarding the ownership of the postoperative tissue after their surgeries, 103 patients (27%) thought it belonged to the hospital, another 103 patients (27%) thought it belonged to nobody, 77 patients (20%) thought it belonged to the pathology laboratory, and 39 patients (10%) thought it still belonged to the patient.[52]

A person writing a letter to the *British Medical Journal* responded to an article indicating that many patients think that tissue removed during surgery either belongs to the hospital or is simply abandoned. The writer said, "I suspect that most patients [in considering litigation after surgery] would consider that they had an unfettered right to the return of the tissue removed from them—that is, that they would consider such property to be theirs if they suspected that it had been removed from them inappropriately and they wished to obtain a further histological opinion in contemplation of litigation."[53]

In September 2000, scientists thawed out the Iceman called "Utze," the 5,300 year-old mummy housed in a refrigerated museum display case in Bolzano, Italy. The Iceman, who once lived as a Bronze Age hunter, had been discovered a decade earlier by tourists hiking in the Alps. According to news reports, the temperature in the refrigerated case was gradually raised for 12 hours; then Utze's body was taken into a sterilized laboratory where scientists removed frozen blood, scraped off bone enamel from his teeth, chipped away bone fragments in his arms and legs, and snaked an endoscope into his intestines in order to harvest other tissue samples. These samples will be studied by forensic experts, geneticists, and other scientists at several European universities. After the Iceman was returned to his chilled case, the scientists said they expected DNA tests to reveal considerable information about Utze's life and death long ago.[54]

A neuropsychiatric geneticist at the Shanghai Research Centre of Life Sciences stated: "The populations of Finland and Iceland have become valuable resources for geneticists because of their relative isolation. In China, we have several Finlands and several Icelands." The geneticist's point is that although 93% of Chinese are from a single ethnic group, the Han, the country also has 55 minority groups. Many of them live in remote border regions, such as Kunming, the capital of Yunnan, a province close to the Himalayas. Kunming, with 25 ethnic groups, is a genetics gold mine. The director of a molecular genetics laboratory in Kunming has collected over 10,000 blood samples in the last two years, without bothering with a Western-style informed consent process. He is now considering bids from foreign biotechnology firms to use these samples in their efforts to find disease-causing genes and new pharmaceutical products.[55]

The Mannheim (Germany) Museum of Technology and Work has an exhibition called "Human Body World." Among the displays are the Runner, the Muscleman, and the Expanded Body: three donated human cadavers that have been preserved through a process called "plastination," transformed into "anatomical artwork," and placed in a running, a standing, and a sitting position. The three dramatic, thought-provoking figures have stirred up a debate in Germany over the boundaries of science, art, and morality. Many persons denounce the exhibit as a breach of human dignity. Many others praise the exhibit for giving them a new appreciation of the human body.[56]

Notes

1. Health Council of the Netherlands, Committee on Human Tissue for Special Purposes, *Proper Use of Human Tissue* (The Hague: Health Council of the Netherlands, 1994), p. 51.
2. Nuffield Council on Bioethics, *Human Tissue: Ethical and Legal Issues* (London: Nuffield Council on Bioethics, 1995), p. 39.
3. Readers who want additional information about the debate over research with stored tissues outside the United States are encouraged to read an excellent paper on the subject by Bartha Maria Knoppers, Marie Hirtle, Sebastien Lormeau, Claude M. Laberge, and Michelle Lablamme, "Control of DNA Samples and Information," *Genomics* 50 (1998): 385–401, and their NBAC version of the same paper.
4. Health Council of the Netherlands, Appendix A, p. 108.
5. *Ibid.*, p. 13.
6. Health Council, Appendix C, pp. 113, 115, emphasis added. The subsequent quotations without footnotes come directly from the report.
7. Health Council, pp. 63–64, emphasis added.
8. *Ibid.*, Appendix D, pp. 130, 135.

9. *Ibid.*, p. 29, emphasis added.
10. *Ibid.*, p. 35, emphasis added.
11. *Ibid.*, p. 87, emphasis added.
12. For a comparison, see U.S. Congress, Office of Technology Assessment, *New Developments in Biotechnology: Ownership of Human Tissues and Cells* (Washington, D.C.: USGPO, 1987).
13. Claire O'Brien, "U.K. Panel Weighs Tissue Ownership," *Science* 268 (1995): 492.
14. Nuffield Council on Bioethics, p. 1.
15. *Ibid.*, p. 7.
16. *Ibid.*, p. 23.
17. Onora O'Neill, "Medical and Scientific Uses of Human Tissue," *J Med Ethics* 22 (1996): 5–7.
18. Nuffield Council, p. 43.
19. *Ibid.*, p. 44.
20. *Ibid.*, p. 45.
21. *Ibid.*, p. 49.
22. *Ibid.*, p. 47.
23. *Ibid.*, p. 51.
24. *Ibid.*, p. 68.
25. *Ibid.*, p. 53.
26. *Ibid.*, pp. 124–36.
27. R. D. Start et al., "Ownership and Uses of Human Tissue: Does the Nuffield Bioethics Report Accord with Opinion of Surgical Inpatients?" *BMJ* 313 (1996): 1366–68.
28. Robert Cook-Deegan, *The Gene Wars* (New York: W.W. Norton and Company, 1994), pp. 208–09.
29. Human Genome Organization Ethics Committee, "HUGO Statement on the Principled Conduct of Genetic Research," *Genome Digest* 3 (1996): 2.
30. *Ibid.*, p. 3.
31. HUGO Ethics Committee, "Statement on DNA Sampling: Control and Access" is available from one of the regional HUGO offices and on the Web site: http://www.hugo-international.org/hugo/sampling.html.
32. Information about the Council of Europe is available on the Web site: http://www.coe.fr/eng/present/about.htm.
33. See http://conventions.coe.int.
34. For the text of this COE convention, see this Web site: http://conventions.coe.int/treaty/EN/cadreprincipal.htm. Similar themes appear in a report on the "Ethical Aspects of Human Tissue Banking" by the European Group on Ethics in Science and New Technologies; the draft opinion was given to the European Commission in Brussels in 1998. See this Web site: http://europa.eu.int/comm/european_group_ethics/docs/avis11_en.pdf.
35. Medical Research Council of Canada, Natural Sciences and Engineering Research Council of Canada, and Social Sciences and Humanities Research Council of Canada, *Tri-Council Policy Statement: Ethical Conduct for Research Involving Humans* (Ottawa: Public Works and Government Services, 1998). The document is also available on the Medical Research Council's Web site: http://www.mrc.gc.ca.
36. Tri-Council Policy Statement, pp. i.2–i.3. The subsequent quotations without footnotes come directly from this Canadian policy statement.
37. *Ibid.*, p. i.4.
38. *Ibid.*, pp. i.5–i.6.

39. *Ibid.*, p. 8.7.
40. *Ibid.*, p. 8.8.
41. *Ibid.*, pp. 9.2–9.3.
42. *Ibid.*, p. 10.1.
43. *Ibid.*, p. 10.2.
44. *Ibid.*, pp. 10.2–10.3, emphasis added.
45. *Ibid.*, p. 10.3, emphasis added.
46. *Ibid.*, p. 10.4.
47. Office for Protection from Research Risks, National Institutes of Health, *Protecting Human Research Subjects: Institutional Review Board Guidebook* (Washington, D.C.: USGPO, 1993).
48. A news release entitled "Federal Funding Agencies to Launch New Panel on Ethics in Research Involving Humans" was published on November 9, 2001. See it on the NSERC Web site: http://www.nserc.ca/programs/ethics/news.
49. Medical Research Council, *Human Tissue and Biological Samples for Use in Research* (London: Medical Research Council, 2001), p. 8, emphasis added.
50. HUGO Ethics Committee, "HUGO Statement," p. 3, emphasis added.
51. Article 22 of the COE "Convention for the Protection of Human Rights and Dignity of the Human Being with regard to the Application of Biology and Medicine," p. 7 of the Web version of this convention cited in note 46 above.
52. Start et al., pp. 1366–68.
53. A. R. W. Forrest, "Some Patients May Want to Retain Ownership of Tissue Removed from Them" [letter], *BMJ* 314 (1997): 1201.
54. Brenda Fowler, "For 5,300-Year-Old Iceman, Extra Autopsy Tells the Tale," *New York Times,* August 7, 2001, p. D2; and "Scientists Thaw Iceman, Begin Testing Samples," *Iowa City Press-Citizen,* September 26, 2000, p. 6.
55. David Dickson, "Back on Track: The Rebirth of Human Genetics in China," *Nature* 396 (1998): 303–06.
56. Edmund L. Andrews, "Anatomy on Display, and It's All Too Human," *New York Times,* January 7, 1998, pp. A1, A4.

6

The Federal Regulations for Human Tissue Research: Summary and Assessment

Efforts to determine how best to pursue genetic research depend in part on achieving an accurate understanding of the personal and social benefits and risks that may accompany genetic research and of the costs and benefits of seeking consent. Society at large must decide how it wishes to weigh the value of respecting persons with the desirability of obtaining socially useful knowledge in a timely manner and of individuals' participating in such research, particularly if the personal risks to them are small.
NIH/CDC Workshop Statement, 1995[1]

Ethical researchers must pursue their scientific aims without compromising the rights and welfare of human subjects. However, achieving such a balance is a particular challenge in rapidly advancing fields, such as human genetics, in which the tantalizing potential for major advances can make research activities seem especially important and compelling. At the same time, the novelty of many of these fields can mean that potential harms to individuals who are the subjects of such research are poorly understood and hence can be over- or underestimated.
National Bioethics Advisory Commission, 1999[2]

This chapter discusses the federal policy governing research with human participants, focusing on application of the federal regulations to research with stored tissue samples, and placing the research practices described previously in the regulatory framework in which they are commonly conducted. The animating objective of the federal policy is to ensure that critical societal interests in expanding scientific knowledge and biomedical progress are bounded by ethically sound policies and practices that minimize the risks of harm for participants and value respect for persons. To this end, there are two commitments at the core of the regulatory scheme: (*1*) respect for autonomy through an appropriate process of informed consent to participation in research; and (*2*) a process for review and approval of biomedical research designed to ensure adherence to informed consent requirements and to protect participants from harm in the conduct of research. Informed consent and IRB oversight are often called the "twin protections" of the federal policy.

With these themes in mind, this chapter also grounds in extant regulation the normative analysis in subsequent chapters of the significant ethical and policy questions at stake in the debate over human tissue research. We identify many of the areas where the existing regulatory scheme leaves important issues unsettled, and research participants, investigators, IRBs, and others at sea. In the main, states have relied on the federal policy, adding little to the regulatory scheme governing tissue-based genetics research. Research with human participants is also conducted within a larger legal framework, most notably state law governing informed consent and regarding ownership of and rights in human tissue and genetic information. For the most part, our discussion of the larger legal framework, including more detailed analysis of *Moore* and its implications, privacy and confidentiality of genetic information, and law relevant to ownership of the body and its parts, appears in the next chapter.

It bears emphasis that the core concern of this book is with paradigm instances of human tissue research, that is, research involving tissue samples obtained from autonomous adults in a clinical or research setting, supported with federal dollars, and conducted under the umbrella of the Federal Policy for the Protection of Human Subjects. The vast majority of this research is conducted with funding through the Department of Health and Human Services (HHS), often through the NIH. Some of the ethical and policy concerns raised by other settings, involving particular types of research or populations, are noted at various points in this book, but do not receive separate focal attention here.

A Summary of the Common Rule

The Federal Policy for the Protection of Human Subjects, known as the "Common Rule," because of its joint and widespread adoption within the federal government, has been the subject of an extensive literature.[3] Here we summarize the core features of the Common Rule relevant to stored tissue research, with special emphasis on informed consent requirements and the role of IRBs. Since its adoption there have been few judicial interpretations of the federal policy. Known cases have raised issues peripheral to the central themes of this book; for example, whether IRB proceedings are subject to discovery in a court of law,[4] and whether a participant's advance release of researchers from liability for injury is enforceable.[5] Two recent cases that have attracted some considerable attention involved whether the researcher–participant relationship is a physician–patient relationship that can give rise to traditional malpractice claims (the University of Wisconsin cystic fibrosis study)[6] and whether parents may consent to enroll their children in a non-therapeutic study that involves a risk of harm to the children (the Johns Hopkins University lead abatement study).[7] Here our description of the federal policy is based on a close reading of the rules and pertinent commentary. The discussion also outlines features of the regulations implementing the Health Insurance Portability and Accountability Act (HIPAA) pertinent to this type of research, and reviews state law governing human participants research.

Scope and Jurisdiction. For decades, research involving human participants conducted or regulated by an agency of the federal government, or supported in whole or in part with federal funding, has been governed by federal regulation. Precursors to emergence of the prevailing regulatory framework can be found in the commitments of the NIH and the Food and Drug Administration (FDA) to rules for human research in the 1950s and 1960s, but it was not until the 1970s that more widespread and uniform federal policy began to emerge.[8] Major revision of the federal policy was embraced in 1981, spearheaded by HHS (formerly the Department of Health Education and Welfare) and the FDA. This policy, codified at 45 C.F.R. Part 46, was reaffirmed without substantive change in 1991, with the endorsement of 17 federal departments and agencies.

The federal policy sets forth the most significant and comprehensive legal requirements for the conduct of research involving human participants today. At the same time, it establishes the minimum requirements for all research to which it applies, but does not preempt the field entirely, permitting states and localities to impose additional research requirements as long as they do not weaken the protections of the federal policy.[9]

Although agencies possess the authority to adopt additional rules, few have done so. Further regulatory requirements apply to particular types of research involving potentially vulnerable populations or raising special concerns—fetuses, pregnant women, in vitro fertilization, children, prisoners, and disabled persons.[10] International research conducted, supported, or otherwise subject to federal regulation is governed by the same requirements,[11] but agency and department heads are also granted some measure of discretion to "approve the substitution of foreign procedures" if they are "at least equivalent" to those provided by the federal policy.[12]

The oversight system created by the federal regulations applies to a great deal, but not all, of human participants research. Strictly speaking, the federal policy only applies when there is federal funding or other support for research; it does not govern privately or state-funded research. It is not uncommon for research under private or state auspices to follow these same or very similar rules, but there is no specific legal requirement that uniformly requires adherence to the federal rules.[13] For many years the reach of the federal policy has been extended to some non-federally funded research through Multiple Project Assurances, whereby institutions agree to be bound by the federal rules in oversight of research conducted by their employees and institutionally affiliated researchers, even if the source of funding is private and the research is conducted off site or for a private company.[14] This agreement with the federal government has long been a common practice among academic health centers. (A good deal of private corporate research involving drugs and medical devices is regulated by the FDA, at least when the research and resulting products are likely to affect interstate commerce, rather than be for use wholly within state borders.)

The MPA was recently replaced by the Federalwide Assurance (FWA). All institutions and entities subject to the federal policy must file a FWA. Once filed, the FWA can (and should) be used to bind "unaffiliated" investigators, such as private practice physicians not employed by the institution, to the Common Rule and oversight of the institution's IRB. The FWA should also be used to formally spell out the relationship between IRBs at two or more institutions engaged in joint or collaborative research. For example, institution A may file a FWA seeking approval to rely on the IRB of institution B, if certain requirements are met. However, the FWA institution must ensure, and retains ultimate responsibility for, appropriate protections for human research participants, including compliance with the requirements of the reviewing IRB.[15]

On the whole, however, this framework still leaves a substantial amount of research, in particular private corporate-sponsored research, exempt from the federal policy's umbrella. Citing lack of a comprehensive and effective oversight system, some have called for express legislative extension of the federal policy to all human research to close this "gap." The argument is forcefully stated by the NBAC, which recommends extension of a uniform system to the entire private sector, both domestic and international: "Participants should be protected from avoidable harm, whether the research is publicly or privately financed."[16] Lack of a comprehensive policy has further important implications with regard to morally controversial areas of scientific inquiry. For example, one of the core issues in recent debates over the permissibility of embryonic stem cell research and/or human cloning is whether legislation should be enacted to impose a truly national moratorium on such research, including the private biotechnology industry. As of this writing, however, the federal policy remains applicable only to federally conducted or federally supported research.

The Office for Human Research Protections. The government entity with oversight authority for implementation of the federal policy is the Office for Human Research Protections (OHRP), located in the Office of Public Health and Science, Office of the Secretary of HHS. The OHRP is directly under the authority of, and reports to, the Assistant Secretary for Health. OHRP succeeds the Office for Protection from Research Risks (OPRR), which had been under the umbrella of the NIH since its establishment in 1972. The OPRR played a prominent role in the interpretation, implementation, and enforcement of federal policy for three decades; its guidebook, issued in 1993, is still considered an authoritative source frequently relied on by IRBs.

For many, this restructuring of the federal oversight mechanism was a long time coming. The role and authority of the OPRR had been a topic of discussion for some time and had often included the widely supported proposal to make OPRR an independent agency not under the auspices of NIH—the agency that funds the vast majority of human participants research.[17] Prompted in part by these calls for change, NIH convened the Office for Protection from Research Risks Review Panel ("Review Panel") to examine two important questions: Whether the organizational placement of OPRR under the auspices of NIH remained appropriate to OPRR's mission and future directions for research and whether OPRR should have additional delegated authority to accomplish its mission. The Review Panel's June 1999 report to the NIH Director's Advisory Committee made a series of recommendations and concluded that OPRR should no longer be directly accountable to NIH; rather, it should be relocated in the Office of the Secretary of HHS and report directly either to the Surgeon General or the Assistant Secretary for Health. The Review Panel concluded that OPRR should be moved out of NIH and elevated to HHS-wide status. This move would strengthen its "stature and effectiveness," ability to fulfill its mission, and to interact with other federal departments and other agencies within HHS.[18]

OHRP's specific responsibilities include (1) developing, monitoring, and exercising compliance oversight concerning regulation of human participants research; (2) coordinating regulations and policies across federal agencies; (3) negotiating project assurances; (4) providing clarification, guidance, and educational programs and materials; (5) evaluating the federal policy's effectiveness; (6) serving as a liaison and resource for various governmental bodies concerned with ethical issues in medicine and research; and (7) promoting development of ways to avoid harm in the conduct of human participants research.[19] In several respects OHRP is given somewhat greater authority and responsibility for oversight and development of both policy and practice, compared to its predecessor.

OHRP (like OPRR) has the power to enforce federal regulations through such actions as audits of IRBs, requiring that noncomplying aspects of research be corrected, or suspension of an investigator's or institution's authority to conduct federally funded research. Between 2000 and 2002, OHRP conducted high-profile investigations and temporarily suspended research activities at several major academic research institutions, including Johns Hopkins and Duke.[20] These actions may suggest a commitment to a more aggressive oversight and enforcement posture that had begun to emerge under OPRR.[21]

This restructuring of the federal oversight mechanism (including appointment of a new director to head the newly-minted OHRP) is part of a broader effort to strengthen protections for human research participants. In May 2000, HHS announced a series of initiatives to guarantee effective oversight of human participant research, efforts that OHRP will play a pivotal role in shaping. Among the initiatives are efforts to fortify the informed consent process, for example, by requiring that records be audited for evidence of compliance with informed consent requirements; improve monitoring of research activities; identify, manage, and disclose potential conflicts of interest; and strengthen authority to pursue civil penalties for research violations. As of October 1, 2000, all investigators and "key personnel" submitting NIH grant applications are required to document completion of educational training on the protection of human research participants, and all IRB members and IRB staff must complete a training course accessible on the Web site maintained by the NIH Office of Human Subjects Research.[22] Still, it is important to note that these initiatives fall far short of NBAC's call for federal legislation to establish a unified, comprehensive federal policy regulating all research involving human participants, in both the public and private sectors, headed by a single, independent federal oversight office.[23]

The Institutional Review Board. Within research institutions across the country, responsibility for implementing and assuring compliance with the federal policy rests with local IRBs. Most often the local IRB bears frontline responsibility for reviewing and approving biomedical research, considering the merits of the proposed research, evaluating the process of consent, and assessing the potential risks, harms, and benefits for participants. The IRB's charge is to approve, disapprove, or require modifications to proposed research.[24] IRBs are also directed to undertake continuing review, "at least once a year."[25] It is estimated that there are 3,000 to 5,000 IRBs in operation across the country; most are associated with a hospital, university, or other research institution.[26] (For research conducted by one of the 17 agencies bound by the Common Rule, the oversight mechanism involves internal agency review.)[27]

Institutions receiving federal research grants must provide written assurances that they have in place an IRB whose composition and function conforms with the federal rules. Because those assurances obligate each institution to protect the welfare of research participants whether or not the specific research study is conducted or supported by a federal agency or department,[28] institutions typically indicate that IRBs have local jurisdiction over all human participants research. Sometimes designated the Research Committee or Research Board (in larger institutions with multiple committees, the IRBs may be referred to as Committee A, Committee B, and so forth), the IRB is the fulcrum of the federal policy.

By design, IRBs are multidisciplinary bodies with a mandated minimum membership of five persons, including at least one person whose primary interests are in a scientific area, one whose primary interests are nonscientific, and one who is neither affiliated with the institution nor immediate family of anyone at the institution. IRB composition should reflect appropriate race, gender, and cultural diversity, and the board cannot be comprised exclusively of men or of women. Additional relevant expertise is to be included when the research under review involves especially vulnerable populations (e.g., children, the disabled).[29] Many IRBs are much larger than this requisite membership, perhaps having as many as 20 or 30 members. The regulations specifically prohibit conflicts of interest for IRB members (e.g., no member should be involved in the research study under review).[30] At the same time, the federal policy clearly contemplates institutionally based or affiliated committees, concluding that institutional relationships do not in and of themselves raise conflict-of-interest concerns.

Increasingly, genetics research (like other types of biomedical research) is a collaborative activity across institutions, often involving the sharing of banked tissue samples by scientists in several research labs. In situations of multiinstitutional collaborative research, each location is responsible for compliance with the federal policy. Subject to the approval of the department or agency head, this process may be streamlined to avoid duplication of effort through agreement for joint review, reliance by one institution upon the review of another institution's IRB, or other suitable alternatives, pursuant to a FWA.[31]

IRBs evaluate research protocols based on a number of criteria that assess the risks and benefits of the proposed research, the nature of the informed consent process, and investigators' approach to ensuring privacy and confidentiality. Under the federal rules, specifically enumerated criteria for review include that: (1) risks to participants are minimized, in particular with a sound research design; (2) risks are "reasonable in relation to anticipated benefits, if any, and the importance of the knowledge that may reasonably be expected to result"; (3) selection of participants is equitable;[32] (4) informed consent is sought and documented; (5) adequate provision is made for monitoring the data collected to ensure safety of participants; (6) adequate protections for privacy and confidentiality are in place, where appropriate; and (7) additional protections are in place where there is risk of coercion or undue influence, such as with more vulnerable populations.[33] We examine some of these criteria at various points in this book.

One can hardly discuss IRBs without acknowledging that they have been the subject of considerable scrutiny and criticism from commentators and governmental study bodies alike. Many of the common concerns about the IRB system are summarized in a series of recent reports from the Office of Inspector General (OIG), HHS, which undertook a comprehensive examination of IRBs and their effectiveness. The OIG found that IRBs (1) "conduct minimal continuing review of approved research" and often limit this review to the paper record; (2) review too many protocols, sometimes devoting too little time to each, and with too little expertise appropriate to the protocol being reviewed; (3) pay scant attention to self-evaluation; (4) provide minimal education and training for investigators and board members; (5) increasingly face conflicts that threaten independence, such as commercial sponsorship of research; and (6) face major changes in the research environment, including cost pressures from managed care and capitated payment, the lure of private commercial funding, more frequent use of multicenter trials and interinstitutional arrangements, and the increased complexity of genetics and other biomedical research, compared to years ago. These changes exacerbate concerns about IRB workload, expertise, and effectiveness. The OIG concluded that instances of abuse are not common, that the IRB system "has provided important protections ... for many years," and should continue to play a central role in oversight of research, but that it is "time for reform."[34]

We share many of these concerns, and agree that the current state of the IRB system warrants reform. At various points in subsequent chapters we offer some suggestions tailored to human tissue research. Our focus, however, is on substantive matters of what IRBs should be doing and doing better (e.g., paying more attention to informed consent and privacy); we do not undertake any systematic examination of IRBs themselves.

Informed Consent: The Basic Framework

The law's approach to informed consent in research is predominantly concerned with two sorts of questions: What information must a physician-investigator disclose to a patient or research participant? And what standard of disclosure should be used to answer this query and to assess whether the physician-investigator has fulfilled the requisite duties of disclosure? The Common Rule sets forth specific categories of information that are to be provided as part of the informed consent process in the research context. These are styled the "basic elements" of informed consent, what we might call the *core disclosures for research*. The federal policy offers no answer to the second question, deferring instead to the law of the state in which the research is conducted.

Under the Common Rule, mandated disclosures include: (*1*) a statement that the study involves research; (*2*) explanation of the purposes, duration, and procedures of the study, and identification of any interventions that are experimental; (*3*) benefits to the participant or others; (*4*) reasonably foreseeable risks; (*5*) the rules and safeguards to be followed to protect confidentiality; (*6*) whether there will be compensation and/or treatment for injuries from participation in studies involving more than minimal risk; (*7*) a statement that participation is voluntary; and (*8*) notification of the right to withdraw at any time without penalty.[35] Additional categories of information should be included if appropriate to the research study. Potentially most pertinent to human tissue research is express provision for "a statement that significant new findings developed during the course of the research which may relate to the subject's willingness to continue participation will be provided," as well as information about the consequences of withdrawing from the study.[36] Informed consent is to be documented by a signed consent form approved by the IRB.[37] Typically, the form recites these basic elements, often employing, in part, standard form language used for a variety of research studies. In some circumstances a "short form" stating that the elements of informed consent have been presented may be used, together with an IRB-approved written summary.[38]

Informed consent procedures must also comport with other law, in particular state law, "which require[s] additional information to be disclosed in order for informed consent to be legally effective."[39] It is state law, most often case law, that provides a *standard* by which to determine the requisite nature and extent of disclosures, a yardstick for evaluating which benefits and which risks would be relevant to research participants and reasonable to disclose, and some indication of which risks, benefits, or other elements of the consent process may be waived or altered. State law of informed consent also provides a benchmark for assessing whether there are other types of information not listed in the regulations that ought to be presented, and whether research risks are minimal (or, would be perceived to be minimal to the average person), a key consideration in determining whether consent should be waived or truncated or research exempted from review altogether (see below).

Standards of Disclosure. In the main, the research setting has followed the law of informed consent and its standard of disclosure as it has evolved in the clinical setting. In the context of patient care, it is commonly recommended that physicians disclose to their patients relevant information concerning the patient's diagnosis; the nature and purpose of the proposed treatment and of reasonable alternatives; and the prognosis, including risks and benefits of the recommended procedure or treatment and reasonable alternatives, including the option of no treatment. For the most part, the legal doctrine of informed consent has emerged from disputes in which patients have alleged that a risk of a treatment or procedure of which they were not aware at the time of consent later materialized, causing physical, psychological, or emotional injury. In short, the claim is that "if I had known about the risk, I would have chosen differently—I would not have given my consent." The posture of the patient's claim has pressed the law to focus on physicians' obligations of disclosure, in particular disclosure of risk information.

Framed under the rubric of negligence, a critical inquiry is whether the physician acted reasonably under the circumstances, and by what standard of reasonableness is the physician's conduct (i.e., the disclosures that were made) to be measured. Approximately half the states now hold that the physician must disclose information that a reasonable person in the patient's circumstances would find relevant (material) to the decision to consent to or refuse the proposed medical intervention—*the reasonable patient-oriented standard*. About half of states still follow the older *professional standard* under which physicians are required to disclose whatever information a reasonable practitioner would under the circumstances.[40]

In our view, the reasonable patient (or reasonable person) standard is the appropriate legal standard that should, and typically does, govern IRB practice. IRBs often employ something like a reasonable patient test even in states with a professional standard of disclosure for clinical care. We use the reasonable patient (participant) standard at various points in our discussion of informed consent later on—with one important clarification: The consent process should be tailored to the particular informational needs of the study population. For example, individuals with a family history of Huntington disease or Tay-Sachs may find certain information concerning research on the genetic bases of these diseases material, and the consent process should respond appropriately. We understand this approach as emphasizing *what a reasonable person contemplating enrolling in this study (these circumstances) would find material,* not a subjective standard for disclosure that would require drafting consent documents to meet the informational needs of a particular individual, a test that has rarely been embraced in the law.[41]

Perhaps influenced by the law's emphasis on disclosure as defining the professional's obligations, the federal policy places strong (and in our view, undue) emphasis on the consent form, both as the vehicle for (documented) disclosure and as evidence of the requirement for "legally effective informed consent."[42] Although the rules provide that the consent process should allow "adequate opportunity to read"[43] the consent document and "sufficient opportunity to consider whether or not to participate" and "[should] minimize the possibility of coercion or undue influence,"[44] there is little regulatory attention paid to the nature and quality of the investigator-participant interaction, most importantly the centrality of participants' understanding of the decision to be made. Informed consent should emphasize the ethical norm of an interactive model of the physician–patient and investigator–participant relationship that facilitates understanding on the part of patients and research participants. Yet IRBs have come to be increasingly focused on the consent form and with formal legal compliance, less so on the underlying process and a more robust notion of autonomous, informed consent in response to relevant disclosures. This state of affairs may also be due in part to the constraints of being overworked and understaffed that many IRBs feel. Still, IRBs have broad discretion to modify the consent form and process—to tailor the process to each research study—and should strive to do so when appropriate.

Surrogate Consent. Typically it is the autonomous adult participant who consents to his or her own participation. The regulations also address situations in which surrogate consent from the person's "legally authorized representative" would be appropriate.[45] But neither the federal regulations nor other federal law specify who counts as a legally authorized representative, nor is there any federal rule regarding prioritization of authority, such as within families. Here, investigators and IRBs must look for guidance to state law. Rules for surrogate decision making as well as priority of surrogates can be found in state laws governing health care consent, advance directives,[46] and organ donation[47] or some combination of these areas in every state. Most states also provide legal guidance with respect to parents' authority to consent to treatment for minor children as well as the authority of mature and emancipated minors to make their own decisions.[48] Arguably, IRBs may look to this body of statutory and local case law both for specific guidance and as a general expression of the propriety of surrogate consent. Few states, however, expressly authorize surrogate consent for research. (See the discussion of state laws, below.) Surrogate consent to research may, therefore, find stronger legal backing when it arises in the clinical setting—and is thus closer to the surrogate's role as health-care decision maker—or when, in unusual cases, there is possible therapeutic benefit for the research participant.

Exemption, Waiver, and Expedited Review

Some research is *exempt* from the federal policy and may be conducted without IRB approval and oversight.[49] Technically, this is a matter of the jurisdictional reach of the regulations (that is, whether they apply at all), but it is common for investigators to seek exemption from the IRB (the board's concurrence) rather than quietly rely upon their own judgment, a practice and expectation shaped in part by the FWA. Of special importance to research with stored tissues is the exemption for (*1*) research involving "collection or study of existing data, documents, records, pathological specimens, or diagnostic specimens" obtained from publicly available sources; and for (*2*) anonymous research that does not use identifiers linking the information with the subject.[50] The principal rationale behind this exemption (like others for research in educational settings and involving educational tests) is that when the risk of harm to participants is minimal, IRB review is not necessary. We return to this important theme at various points.

IRBs may lessen some of the researcher's burdens by *waiving or altering* "some or all of the elements of informed consent," whether on expedited review or by a convened board. A key consideration here again is whether the research involves *no more than minimal risk*. To grant a waiver or alteration the IRB must also determine that truncated consent "will not adversely affect the rights and welfare of the subjects." In addition, investigators must show that it would be impracticable to carry out the research without waiver or alteration and make a commitment to provide participants with "additional pertinent information" after their participation has begun, "when appropriate."[51]

Another form of waiver within the IRB's purview involves documentation of informed consent. A signed consent form may not be needed when "the only record linking the subject and the research would be the consent document and the principal risk would be potential harm resulting from breach of confidentiality." In such cases participants must be offered a choice of whether there should be documentation linking them to the research.[52] Alternatively, if the research would involve no more than minimal risk for participants *and* "involves no procedures for which written consent is normally required outside the research context,"[53] waiver may be granted. A common example would be a return-by-mail survey in which the identity of respondents is anonymous.

Waiver of documented consent does not entail a waiver of consent altogether; rather, consent may be obtained orally. When documentation of informed consent is waived, IRBs still may require that participants be provided with a written statement regarding the research study, thereby fostering a degree of informed decision making in the absence of more formal and extensive documentation.[54]

Investigators may request *expedited review* for research involving "no more than minimal risk, and for minor changes in approved research." If the IRB chairperson agrees that expedited review is appropriate, the process is streamlined, with the chairperson, or an IRB designee, authorized to review, request modifications, and approve the research without full committee involvement. Disapproval is not permitted on an expedited basis; this can only be done after more thorough committee review.[55]

HHS publishes a list of categories of research for which expedited review is deemed appropriate. Recent amendments, the first since 1981, expand the list to include nine such categories. Likely most pertinent to stored tissue research are provisions allowing expedited review for (*1*) blood draws in small amounts, within not more than an eight-week period and not more than twice per week; and (*2*) prospective collection of biological specimens for research purposes by noninvasive means. However, the regulations leave unclear what counts as noninvasive means of collection (buccal swabs? urine samples?). Continuing review may be expedited in several situations, including "[w]here the remaining research activities are limited to data analysis," a provision of special importance to DNA database research. In response to reviewers' comments on these amendments, explanatory information stresses that expedited review is not synonymous with waiver; investigators and IRB members should understand that determination of appropriate informed consent requirements is an entirely separate matter and must be undertaken whether review is expedited or by a convened board.[56] Significantly, the amendments expressly state that expedited review is not appropriate where identification of the participants would "be damaging to subjects' financial standing, employability, insurability, reputation, or be stigmatizing," unless the research can be conducted "so that risks related to invasion of privacy and breach of confidentiality are no greater than minimal."[57] We address these potential risks in the next chapter.

Privacy and Confidentiality

Another piece of the general framework concerns the privacy of information, records, and data generated by investigators. The federal policy makes duties of confidentiality clear, but is largely deferential to state law and local practice regarding the rules and methods for meeting this obligation. IRBs have broad discretion to modify procedures for assuring confidentiality of research and often rely on organizational or institutional policies to ensure the confidentiality of personally identifiable information, particularly when data is collected in the clinical setting.[58] These policies are in turn shaped by relevant law governing confidentiality and privacy of health information, sometimes specifically genetic information.

As we will see below, recently enacted federal law strengthens privacy requirements for researchers and IRBs. The next chapter shows that existing law is, nonetheless, fragmented, leaving significant gaps in coverage for individual participants. Thus, on the one hand, IRBs and investigators need to fill this gap by crafting appropriate protections into the research design; on the other, in many cases they cannot represent to participants that the research study poses no risks that privacy will be compromised. Nor can it be routinely represented that participants are without risk of discrimination should personal, identifiable information get into the "wrong hands."

Finally, the rules also establish a process by which investigators can apply to OHRP for a Certificate of Confidentiality. However, the utility of the certificate is questionable. Its intended purpose is to shield research from discovery in a court of law, not to prevent employers, insurance companies, or others from obtaining information about who is enrolled in a study, or the research data, through other mechanisms. Though rarely tested, at least one court has upheld the validity of a certificate of confidentiality.[59]

Research with Stored Tissue Samples Under the Federal Policy

The meaning of the federal policy for research on stored tissue samples has only begun to engender serious discussion and has yet to be tested in a judicial proceeding. The most comprehensive, critical analyses to date are two publications discussed in other chapters: (*1*) the NIH/CDC Workshop Statement (discussed in Chapter 3), and (*2*) the NBAC report, *Research Involving Human Biological Materials* (the subject of Chapter 8). Both documents are likely to be influential in shaping future interpretations and policy directions.

Some of the key policy issues framing the current debate are (*1*) whether anonymous or anonymized research is/should be exempt from federal regulation and IRB oversight altogether; (*2*) whether anonymous or anonymized research is/should be subject to IRB review but exempt from informed consent requirements; (*3*) the nature and scope of the informed consent process, including when informed consent should be waived or altered for research using anonymous or anonymized samples or data; and (*4*) the property interests of participants, as well as the potential commercial interests of investigators and the biotechnology industry, in stored tissues and the information that tissue-based research may reveal.

Is Research with Anonymous or Anonymized Samples Exempt from Review? Investigators need to know, and IRBs are called upon to decide, whether research involving anonymous samples or data is exempt from the federal policy, or whether IRB review should waive or alter the consent process. These same questions must also be asked about anonymized research. To see how the exemption and waiver provisions might work in practice, it is helpful to consider two ways that research activities involving use of existing samples might be conducted from the standpoint of a pathology lab.

It is common practice for specimens to be retained following pathologic examination as part of a patient's clinical care. Pathologic specimens "on the shelf" in hospitals and laboratories around the world are a rich resource of raw materials—like the NHANES III blood samples, a veritable "treasure chest."[60] In our first scenario, suppose samples have already been stripped of identifiers, cannot be linked to the sample source by researcher, institution, or anyone else, and are available to a research team that does not include any of the pathologists who conducted prior diagnostic or therapeutic examinations (hence, secondary research use of anonymous samples). By contrast, consider a secondary team of researchers that plans to anonymize the samples, but this has not yet been done (scenario 2). Both practices are sometimes referred to as retrospective research because they involve samples previously collected for a different purpose—in our scenarios, a diagnostic or therapeutic purpose.[61] Both scenarios may be understood as a form of DNA banking.

Under the federal policy, anonymous research may be exempted from the Common Rule when it involves:

[t]he collection or study of existing data, documents, records, pathological specimens, or diagnostic specimens if these sources are *publicly available* or if the information is recorded by the investigator in such a manner that *subjects cannot be identified, directly or through identifiers linked to the subjects.*[62]

Also of relevance, the operative definition of "human subject" states that in order for information obtained in research to constitute human subject research, the information must be "individually identifiable."[63]

The prevailing interpretation is that for human tissue research to come under this exemption, two conditions must be met. First, the samples (or data sets) must exist prior to beginning the research (that is, the research must involve secondary use); second, the samples must be anonymous.[64] The principal rationale for exemption is that research with anonymous samples poses minimal (perhaps nonexistent) risks of harm for the participant because little, if any, possibly identifying information can be disclosed when research records and findings cannot be linked to the individual. Additional practical concerns arise with secondary uses of samples and data—namely, whether it is practicable for investigators to obtain consent from sample sources. This is obviously not possible with samples that have already been stripped of identifiers, but may be feasible when secondary researchers *plan* to anonymize the samples or data. Not to be overlooked, anonymous research provides no direct benefit to participants who by definition cannot be contacted with new findings that they might otherwise want to know.

Scenario 1 presents the strongest case for exemption. If samples (or data sets) used by other investigators who did not participate in their collection are truly anonymous, the risks for participants appear to be minimal. Many would say that here the balance tips heavily, indeed decisively, in favor of the pursuit of socially useful knowledge. Not only is consent not necessary when samples are obtained, consent ("re-consent") would be impossible. To hold this type of research to the scrutiny of IRB review or to requirements of informed consent would unduly compromise our collective interests in human biological research without offering any meaningful protection to participants already at only minimal risk.

There is room for disagreement, however, as to whether the risks to participants are so minimal that no IRB review is needed. Some doubt whether research is truly anonymous, especially in an increasingly electronic age of information storage, retrieval, and dissemination.[65] If there is a chance that information may come to the attention of others (a health insurance company?) without the individual's prior knowledge and permission, but with the possibility of linkage to that individual, then the risks of compromised privacy, and perhaps discrimination, are not readily characterized as minimal. Even assuming complete anonymity of individual participants, those recruited (invited) to give tissue samples for research may have important interests in how their participation affects the welfare of others, and may be quite concerned with how information obtained from their tissue sample will affect others in their family, ethnic, or racial group. For example, some may object to participating in research on a particular genetic disorder prevalent among persons of the same race or ethnicity, if new findings might contribute to stigma or discrimination for the group. The Common Rule here, as elsewhere, is narrowly focused on the risks of harms to individual research participants and does not address group harm. (In these circumstances it may be more accurate to construe the interests at stake in terms of wronging rather than harming—the language of the federal policy.)

For these reasons it is open to question whether even truly anonymous genetics research categorically entails sufficiently minimal risks to warrant proceeding without any IRB scrutiny. We agree with the majority of the NIH/CDC workshop participants, who concluded that the *exemption should be strictly construed,* stating "samples are anonymous if and only if it is impossible under any circumstances to identify the individual source."[66] But we also question whether even truly anonymous research poses, by definition, truly minimal risks to warrant forgoing IRB review.

A critical distinguishing feature of scenario 2 is that it may be possible to contact sample sources for their consent, depending on the circumstances (e.g., were samples collected last month or 10 years ago?). If this is deemed impracticable (one of the four criteria for waiver of consent), samples might be fully anonymized or partially anonymized. Partial anonymity occurs, for example, where clinical information (disease status) or demographic data (gender, state, county of residence, ethnic origin) is retained in a form that allows identification of groups (e.g., patients with colon cancer, residents of Johnson County, Iowa), but not individuals as members of the group. Archival research materials may also be partially anonymous in another way, such as when they are coded and not identified, but remain individually linkable with additional efforts (for example, a separate database under the control of other investigators that matches coded samples with their source). On a strict reading, *anything short of complete anonymity does not qualify for exemption,* but would be a candidate for waiver.

Beyond the question of whether seeking consent is feasible, waiver is warranted only if the research involves no more than minimal risk, and if truncated consent "will not adversely affect the rights and welfare of the subjects." Again the baseline inquiry concerns the risk that privacy and confidentiality will be compromised, opening the door to stigma or discrimination. The fourth criterion, that investigators provide participants with additional pertinent information post-participation, "when appropriate,"[67] introduces a further complication. To meet this commitment, anonymized samples must be linkable in some way. But if they are linkable, should consent be waived? Again, are the risks minimal and rights protected? Do the value of the research and the challenges of obtaining consent outweigh the value of consent and the risks to participants? How these and other questions are answered will depend, among other things, on the nature of the research, the method used to anonymize samples or data, the confidentiality protections in place, and the privacy and nondiscrimination protections in force.

Voices of the research community contend that the exemption from IRB review should be liberally construed. The College of American Pathologists (CAP) asserts that not just anonymous, but also anonymized, samples should be exempt from IRB review, "whether existing or collected concurrently."[68] NIH/CDC workshop participants concur that the regulations permit research with anonymized samples without consent, but find that the regulations support either exemption or IRB review with a waiver of consent requirements.

As should now be evident, the federal policy does not expressly answer the questions raised by our scenarios. Applicable provisions are framed in terms of guiding principles and criteria to be weighed and measured in particular cases. At bottom, whether particular protocols for anonymous or anonymized research should be exempted from review or conducted under the auspices of an IRB with truncated consent also depends on the value attached to informed consent and what is at stake for participants in the consent process. The Common Rule takes an unduly narrow approach to what is at stake for participants in human tissue research, largely ignoring psychosocial concerns and the various ways information obtained from the research may impact the interests of participants' families, ethnic, or racial groups to which participants' belong, or be put to other uses that may be of concern to sample sources.

Informed Consent: What Disclosures Are Required? Linkable or identifiable genetics research with stored tissues requires IRB review and, absent a waiver, participant consent. The federal policy's core disclosures identify information that ordinarily should be part of the informed consent process. However, the regulations fail to mention, much less emphasize, two factors that frequently distinguish genetics research from many other forms of research. First, in most cases of human tissue research, physical risks are often minimal (taking a blood sample or a buccal swab). These risks are commonly explained as part of the patient's consent to a surgical procedure. Yet the sorts of risk most pertinent to participants' willingness to enroll are predominantly psychosocial, such as their concerns about privacy and discrimination. Second, and related, these concerns are not limited to the individual. Rather, genetics has important implications for families. Disclosure of a parent's genetic predisposition to colon cancer could be linked to a child's risk or to that person's siblings.

We argue later that respect for autonomy requires making the risks of unauthorized disclosure and of genetic discrimination a more common part of the informed consent process—at least until the law provides stronger, more uniform protections—and that there is good reason to believe that the average reasonable research participant would find these risks *material* to his or her decision whether to provide a tissue sample or allow already existing samples or information to be used by an investigator. The HIPAA privacy rules, discussed below, are an important step toward making it incumbent upon IRBs and investigators to develop a basic familiarity with issues surrounding genetic privacy and discrimination, including applicable law, so that they can provide more accurate information about the risks. Nevertheless, given the ambiguity and uncertainty of extant law (discussed in the next chapter), crafting the wording of consent documents remains an important challenge. Is it sufficient to say, "There may be some risk that your insurer or employer will obtain information about you," or "We cannot anticipate how information gained through research will affect your insurability"?

Consent to Future Anonymous Research. When investigators collect tissue samples, they sometimes, but not always, seek advance consent to possible future anonymous research, perhaps saying that if samples or data are later shared with other researchers, all personal identifiers will be removed. A standard consent-to-operate document used at one of our institutions provides in the eighth enumerated paragraph: "I hereby authorize disposal of and/or release of any tissue removed to be used for scientific purposes after all necessary diagnostic tests have been completed. I understand that before any such specimens are made available, all identifying information will be removed."[69] Whether this sort of general consent is sufficient (and whether later investigators may retrospectively rely on it) is another area where the regulations and related law offer limited guidance.

Some (e.g., the CAP) believe that since the risks from anonymous or anonymized research are minimal, such generalized consent is sufficient.[70] Others observe that consent now for unspecified, possible research (perhaps years) later raises a broader set of questions about what sorts of anticipatory interests potential participants may have in what happens to their anonymized tissues, and information derived from those tissues, in the future. Among the possible future-oriented interests that may surface are concerns about the potential meaning of some types of genetic information for the community to which one belongs (e.g., studies of the genetics of Tay-Sachs disease among Ashkenazi Jews). The nature of some future research studies may also offend some persons, if they should find out about them, even if no individually identifiable information is revealed. Other persons may be troubled, as a matter of principle, by the prospect of substantial monetary gain in the future for investigators, pharmaceutical companies, or others in the biotechnology industry.

The Prospect of Commercial Gain. Rapid growth of the biotechnology industry and the legacy of the *Moore* case have thrust to the forefront debate over commercialization of stored tissue samples and their products—and the rights of sample sources. It is reasonable to infer that participants may want to know whether their samples or genetic information may bring investigators monetary gain, such as through future development of a biomedical product. But do investigators have an obligation to disclose these possibilities? Should they be engaged in financial negotiations with individuals, families, or groups over the terms of participation? The federal policy is largely silent on these matters and deferential to other, currently sparse, law.

To the extent the regulations offer guidance, there are two points of connection; both concern requirements about informed consent. First, investigators may be required to disclose possible commercial ventures when this is a part of the original purpose of the research. But this is a rare occurrence with genetics research. When such possibilities do emerge, it is typically years, even decades, later in the life of a tissue sample. Second, the Common Rule directs IRBs to assure that participation in research is voluntary, not coerced. This suggests that if research studies call for any compensation to participants beyond modest costs of participation (or for injury from participation, really a separate matter), the arrangement should be scrutinized to assure voluntary participation. Is an individual agreeing to participate in identifiable genetics research and assuming the risk of discrimination in exchange for future royalties in a pharmaceutical product?

Beyond these two points of connection, the federal policy fails to address the extent to which, if at all, IRBs should require disclosure of commercial possibilities or examine matters of financial inducement to participate. The Common Rule takes no position on the prior foundational question raised by *Moore:* Do research participants have property interests in tissues obtained from their bodies that ground rights-based claims of ownership and entitlement to monetary gain in exchange for consent to relinquish a part of one's body to the research enterprise? As we will see in the next chapter, extant law offers some guidance, but largely by analogy to other areas where the idea of property rights in the body and its parts has been addressed.

Is Human Tissue Research Human Subjects Research? Perhaps some types of human tissue research are not governed by the federal policy because they do not count as human subjects research. Sometimes the contention is that the operative definition of the term "human subject" requires that the participant be "a living individual" about whom the investigator obtains data either "through intervention or interaction" or that the data be "identifiable private information."[71] As noted earlier, in some cases parsing the definition bolsters the argument for exempting anonymous or anonymized research from IRB review.

This question about the general applicability of the federal regulations to human tissue research is most pertinent to research studies with tissues previously obtained for another purpose from individuals who are now deceased, and to post-mortem research. These matters have received scant attention, and the Common Rule offers little guidance. Yet it seems clear that investigators should honor the previously expressed wishes of sample sources, if these wishes are known. (Is there an advance research directive?) And in general, it would be not only inappropriate but even illegal to harvest tissue samples without consent from relatives.[72] In rare instances another surrogate, such as a health care proxy or estate executor, may have authority to give consent.

Thoughtful exploration of these matters must also take into account whether potential research participants have interests in what happens to their tissues and personal genetic information after death, not unlike our interests in how our bodies and tangible property are treated after death; whether posthumous harm to the interests of research participants and their families is possible; and whether interests that survive death should play a role in shaping permissible research and consent practices.[73] (We return to this inquiry in Chapter 10.)

The HIPAA Privacy Standards

As discussed further in Chapter 7, the federal HIPAA law brings new rules for the privacy and security of health information. In general, under HIPAA and its implementing regulations (known as the "Privacy Rule"), adopted by HHS in August 2002, individual consent for the use and disclosure of "personally identifiable health information" (PHI) is required, unless the use or disclosure is for purposes of treatment, payment, or health care operations. PHI is defined as "any information, electronic or otherwise, which identifies, or reasonably could be believed to identify, an individual, which in any way concerns that individual's health status, healthcare, or payments for his or her health care." PHI may relate to the individual's past, present, or future health or health care,[74] and includes genetic information, whether derived from genetic testing or family history, if it otherwise qualifies as personally identifiable.[75] Information is not identifiable if it does not identify the individual *and* "there is no reasonable basis to believe that the information can be used to identify an individual."[76]

Nonidentifiable (anonymous) research information is not subject to the Privacy Rule. Following a parallel path to the Common Rule, the Privacy Rule sets forth a process for the creation of "de-identified data sets," listing up to 18 types of identifying information that must be removed to qualify the data as "de-identified."[77] Following these steps and the process that is further detailed in the rules would give investigators a "safe harbor" of exemption from the Privacy Rule. Though HIPAA is thus more detailed than the Common Rule in its approach to defining nonidentifiable research, it does not completely map the Common Rule's definition of nonidentifiable (anonymous) research, conducted in "a manner [such] that subjects cannot be identified."[78] Significantly, the Privacy Rule permits deidentified data to be linked by codes.[79]

A new requirement under HIPAA calls for patients and potential research participants to receive a "Notice of Privacy Practices" developed by the institution.[80] The Privacy Rule also sets forth the core contents of a mandated written "authorization" for disclosures of PHI.[81] An authorization can be combined with a consent under the Common Rule; HIPAA does not require double documentation.[82] And the Privacy Rule establishes an individual's right to receive an accounting of disclosures of PHI, including a statement of the purpose of each disclosure.[83] Collectively, these provisions should encourage more careful attention to both privacy and record-keeping.

HIPAA calls for oversight to be provided either by an IRB or by a "privacy board" established in accordance with the criteria set forth in the Privacy Rule, many of which parallel existing requirements for constituting IRBs.[84] Several provisions direct investigators and IRBs to attend to privacy matters. Investigators planning to use PHI must seek waiver or alteration of consent, and the review and approval process must take into account the privacy interests of participants, together with other factors such as whether use or disclosure of PHI "involves no more than minimal risk."[85] IRBs must consider whether "[t]he privacy risks to individuals whose protected health information is to be used or disclosed are reasonable in relation to the anticipated benefits if any to the individuals, and the importance of the knowledge that may reasonably be expected to result from the research."[86] Separate provisions call for limiting disclosure of PHI to that which is "minimally necessary" to the intended purpose of the disclosure.[87]

The Privacy Rule took effect April 14, 2003. It likely will bring more changes to some research practices than others. As just noted, HIPAA does not apply to anonymous research; thus, it may have limited meaning for a great deal of human tissue research and research with anonymous DNA databases. Its most significant impact on the conduct of research may lie less in the rules themselves than in the likelihood that HIPAA will press IRBs, and the research enterprise generally, to more carefully scrutinize access to personally identifiable information about research participants, filling some of the gap in the Common Rule. We discuss the HIPAA privacy rules in more detail in the next chapter.

State Regulation of Research

A significant number of state laws specifically address some aspects of biomedical research with human participants. A number have adopted rules that largely mirror the federal policy and impose few, if any, additional requirements. Many reinforce the twin protections of informed consent and IRB review.[88] Most states also narrowly regulate particular types of research, such as cancer registries.

One of the salutary features of state laws is that they typically govern the private as well as the public sector. But there are also exceptions. While some states place restrictions on researcher access to patient data or on redisclosure of patient information, many carve out exceptions that allow research with patient records maintained by private entities without patient consent.[89] This body of law is notably silent with respect to matters typically governed by the states, such as surrogate consent, the role of advance directives, or related matters, for example, whether the family's time-honored quasi-property rights in the body of the deceased includes the right to consent to retrieval of tissue samples for research.

Among the more extensive statutes, New York's regulates research not covered by the federal rules, including a requirement that research with human participants is authorized only with the individual's written informed consent. But the law likely has little relevance to human tissue research, for it expressly excludes from its reach research with body tissues and fluids removed "in the course of standard medical practice" and defines a "human subject" as an individual who may be exposed to injury as a result of participation, a provision that "arguably permits" research with anonymous and anonymized samples without consent.[90]

Other states, such as Virginia,[91] have also put in place protections for human research not regulated by the federal policy. A close look at these laws suggests that, like New York, they typically have little or no relevance to human tissue research and add little to the Common Rule in this area. Only a handful of states have enacted legislation specifically directed to genetics and tissue-based research, sometimes with rules that would apply both to research governed by the federal policy and to research done outside of its parameters. The most important, and controversial, feature of these laws is the effort to strengthen consent requirements by characterizing human tissue as the *property* of the individual. Chapter 7 discusses this issue and the larger matter of ownership of human tissues. State genetic privacy laws, also discussed in the next chapter, play an additional role in structuring the research environment.

To sum up, this chapter has described the basic framework of the federal policy for human participants research and has identified the important issues raised by application of this policy to genetics research with stored tissues. We have also identified areas of debate where the Common Rule leaves key questions unanswered. The latter part of the chapter has shown that while the federal HIPAA rules and state law fill in some gaps, many significant and unanswered questions remain ripe for policy reform.

We have not (and will not) proposed specific language changes to amend the federal rules, though we have indicated some of the ways that federal policy, if not the rules themselves, should be improved. We join with other voices in the debate who have concluded that IRBs have a useful role to play in providing *some level of review for research with both anonymous and anonymized* stored tissues. To make this a reality, federal policy should be modified or interpreted to require that rules for exemption for anonymous research be strictly construed. Some level of IRB review also should be mandated for research with partially anonymized tissues that are linkable to the sample source. Clearly, there are some circumstances in which consent should be waived or modified, but it should not be presumed that because research records and findings cannot be linked to sample sources, the risks are therefore minimal.

We also believe that research policy should straightforwardly establish *some rules for resolving the property issue,* focusing both on the rights of participants in their tissues and on the informed consent process. As we will see in greater depth in the chapters ahead, there is much disagreement about these points. Our policy positions and recommendations, and the basis for them, are spelled out in subsequent chapters. The next chapter takes a closer look at the *Moore* case, and turns to the current state of affairs regarding matters of genetic privacy, genetic discrimination, and the ownership of tissues.

Cases and Vignettes

The IRB coordinator for a state Department of Health Services sent out an e-mail request to a national list of bioethicists for feedback regarding a research proposal under review. The scenario was described as follows: An investigator wants to use identified specimens in a research study. The specimens have been collected over several years without patient knowledge or consent for storage and research use. Many of the specimens have been collected at the investigator's home institution, but other specimens were collected all over the state. The investigator wants to link identifiers from the specimens to two other DHS databases and include lab analyses of all collected specimens from patients with the health condition being studied and a sampling of specimens from other patients as controls. The protocol has been approved by the IRB at his institution. If his protocol is now approved by the DHS, he will end up with a research database connected to 50,000 banked specimens, all of them identifiable and originally collected for clinical purposes. But the state IRB has serious questions about the proposed study. Is a waiver of consent appropriate for prospective collection of identified specimens? If getting consent is impracticable, is it sufficient to notify patients at the time of specimen collection that identified leftover specimens may be used for research? If the state IRB approves even a limited linkage study, does this sanction a prospective repository of identified specimens without patient knowledge or consent?[92]

The National Birth Defects Prevention Study is a multistate, case-control study of major birth defects. Over 6,000 cases and more than 2,500 controls have been collected in eight states: Arkansas, California, Georgia, Iowa, Massachusetts, New Jersey, New York, and Texas. The CDC's Birth Defects and Pediatric Genetics Branch coordinates the NBDPS and maintains copies of the data collected in each state. One of the strengths of this large, complex study is the heterogeneity of the study populations in the various states, as well as the combined expertise of the multiple investigators. One of the difficulties of the study is the heterogeneity of the 12 IRBs that approved the protocol (some states had more than one IRB review, and the CDC's IRB also approved the study). Although the various IRBs technically follow the same federal regulations for research with human participants, the expectations and requirements of the IRBs vary because of differing committee memberships, institutional requirements, and state laws regarding genetic testing, informed consent, and the research use of identifiable data.[93]

Renata Pasqualine and Wadih Arap, biologists at M. D. Anderson Cancer Center in Houston, were convinced that if they could track which peptides—short strings of amino acids—are drawn to blood vessels in specific tissues, they would pave the way toward the development of targeted cancer drugs that would reach the blood vessels feeding particular tumors. They had done lab work with mice, but needed to take their research to the next level—human research participants. Yet they faced two problems: (*1*) the multiple biopsies needed to get human tissues—skin, muscle, bone marrow, prostate, fat, and liver—would be too invasive to do with conscious patients; and (*2*) their IRB had never approved a research proposal that targeted near-death patients or brain-dead bodies still on life supports. With the help of two clinical ethicists, they formulated a protocol to present to the IRB. The result: the IRB, with some reluctance, approved the controversial proposal (to infuse approximately 200 million different peptides into selected near-death patients and brain-dead bodies still on life supports) and its ethical requirements that prior family inquiries about organ donation or research are required, families must complete an extensive consent document for the research study, and families are warned that death could occur with a patient near death. The report about their first experiment with a brain-dead body was published in 2002.[94]

Notes

1. Ellen Wright Clayton et al., "Informed Consent for Genetic Research on Stored Tissue Samples," *JAMA* 274 (1995): 1786–92 (hereafter, NIH/CDC Workshop Statement).
2. National Bioethics Advisory Commission, *Research Involving Human Biological Materials: Ethical Issues and Policy Guidance* (Rockville, Md.: NBAC, 1999), p. i. (hereafter, NBAC report).
3. Among the many resources on the topic are the Advisory Committee on Human Radiation Experiments, *The Human Radiation Experiments* (New York: Oxford University Press, 1996); Robert J. Levine, *Ethics and Regulation of Clinical Research,* 2nd ed. (New Haven: Yale University Press, 1988); President's Commission for the Study of Ethical Problems in Medicine and Biomedical and Behavioral Research, *Implementing Human Research Regulations* (Washington, D.C.: USGPO, (1983); and National Commission for the Protection of Human Subjects of Biomedical and Behavioral Research, *The Belmont Report* (Washington, D.C.: USGPO, 1979). Also see Jeremy Sugarman, Anna Mastroianni, and Jeffrey Kahn, *Ethics of Research with Human*

Subjects: Selected Policies and Resources (Frederick, Md.: University Publishing Group, 1998) for related documents and resources.

4. *Esdale v. American Community Mutual Ins. Co.,* 1995 WL 263479 (N. D. Ill., May 3, 1995).
5. *Vodopest v. MacGregor,* 128 Wash. 2d 840, 913 P.2d 779 (1996).
6. *Ande v. Rock,* 2002 WL 992751 (Wis. App., May 16, 2002).
7. *Grimes v. Kennedy Krieger Institute, Inc.,* 366 Md. 29, 782 A.2d 807 (Md. 2001).
8. Ruth Faden and Tom Beauchamp, *A History and Theory of Informed Consent* (New York: Oxford University Press, 1986), ch. 6.
9. 45 C.F.R. § 46.101(f) (2002).
10. *Ibid.,* subparts B–D.
11. *Ibid.,* § 46.101(a).
12. *Ibid.,* § 46.101(h).
13. Jonathan Moreno et al., "Updating Protections for Human Subjects Involved in Research," *JAMA* 280 (1998): 1951–58.
14. 45 C.F.R. § 46.103.
15. See the OHRP Web site: http://ohrp.osophs.dhhs.gov/humansubjects/finreltn/faq.htm#TOP.
16. National Bioethics Advisory Commission, *Ethical and Policy Issues in Research Involving Human Participants,* Vol. I (Bethesda, Md.: NBAC, 2001), p. v. (hereafter, NBAC Report, *Research Involving Human Participants*).
17. *Ibid.*
18. Health and Human Services Fact Sheet, "Protecting Human Subjects" (June 6, 2000), available online at http://www.hhs.gov/news/press/20000606a.html; see also Carol Mason Spicer, "Federal Oversight and Regulation of Human Subjects Research—An Update," *Kennedy Inst Ethics J* 10 (2000): 261–264 (summarizing these initiatives).
19. *65 Fed. Reg.,* 37136–37 (2000).
20. Stacey Shultz, "Trials and Errors: A hospital takes a hit," *US News & World Report,* July 30, 2001, p. 19. For a longer account of the events at Johns Hopkins, see Dale Keiger and Sue De Pasquale, "Trials & Tribulations," *Johns Hopkins Magazine* (2002), available at http://www.jhu.edu/~jhmag/0202web/trials.html.
21. Office of Inspector General, Department of Health and Human Services, report, OEI-01-97-00197, "Protecting Human Research Subjects: Status of Recommendations" (April 2000), p. 2 (hereafter, OIG report).
22. The online tutorial can be found at http://ohsr.od.nih.gov/.
23. NBAC Report, *Research Involving Human Participants,* p. xii.
24. 45 C.F.R. § 46.109(a).
25. *Ibid.,* § 46.109(e).
26. U.S. General Accounting Office, *Medical Records Privacy: Access Needed for Health Research, but Oversight of Privacy Protections is Limited,* GAO/HEHS-99-55 (Washington, D.C.: USGPO, 1999), p. 5.
27. 45 C.F.R. §§ 46.101, 46.120.
28. *Ibid.,* § 46.103.
29. *Ibid.,* § 46.107(a).
30. *Ibid.,* § 46.107(e).
31. *Ibid.,* § 46.114.
32. This criterion has been especially important when there is a direct benefit to patients from participation (e.g., in AIDS clinical trials), but may be less important with many types of genetics research that contemplate no direct benefit to patients or participants.

33. 45 C.F.R. § 46.111.
34. Testimony of George Grob, Deputy Inspector General for Evaluation and Inspections, Before the Committee on Government Reform and Oversight, Subcommittee on Human Resources, U.S. House of Representatives, "Institutional Review Boards: A Time for Reform" (June 11, 1998), pp. 4–11; see the OIG report. See also Jonathan D. Moreno, "IRBs Under the Microscope," *Kennedy Inst Ethics J* 8 (1998): 329–37.
35. 45 C.F.R. § 46.116(a).
36. *Ibid.*
37. *Ibid.*, §§ 46.116(b)(4) and (5).
38. *Ibid.*, § 46.117(a)(2).
39. *Ibid.*, § 46.116(e).
40. See generally Jessica Berg, Paul Appelbaum, Charles Lidz, and Lisa Parker, *Informed Consent: Legal Theory and Clinical Practice,* 2nd ed. (New York: Oxford University Press, 2001), especially ch. 3.
41. See, for example, *Hartman v. D'Ambrosia,* 665 So.2d 1206 (La. App. 1995). Some courts have used different language to describe the standard for disclosure in human experimentation. Some early cases (preadoption of the federal policy) involved clinical procedures that were considered innovative or experimental at the time. For discussion of this body of law and an argument that research should not follow the standard established in the clinical context, see Karine Morin, "The Standard of Disclosure in Human Subject Experimentation," *J Leg Med* 19 (1998): 157–221.
42. 45 C.F.R. § 46.116.
43. *Ibid.*, § 46.117(b)(1).
44. *Ibid.*, § 46.116.
45. *Ibid.*, § 46.117(a).
46. See generally, Alan Meisel, *The Right to Die,* 2nd ed. (New York: John Wiley & Sons, 1995).
47. See Alexander M. Capron, "Reexamining Organ Transplantation," *JAMA* 285 (2001): 334–36.
48. See Robert F. Weir and Charles Peters, "Affirming the Decisions Adolescents Make about Life and Death," *Hastings Cent Rep* 27 (1997): 29–40.
49. 45 C.F.R. § 46.101(b).
50. *Ibid.*, § 46.101(b)(4).
51. *Ibid.*, § 46.116(d)(1–4).
52. *Ibid.*, § 46.117(c)(1).
53. *Ibid.*, § 46.117(c)(2).
54. *Ibid.*, § 46.117(c).
55. *Ibid.*, § 46.110.
56. *63 Fed. Reg.,* 60364-02 (1998).
57. *Ibid.*
58. GAO report, pp. 12–13.
59. *People v. Newman,* 32 N.Y. 2d 379, 298 N.E. 2d 651 (1973), *cert. denied,* 414 U.S. 1163 (1973).
60. Several CDC scientists referred to the NHANES III blood samples as a national "treasure chest" during the NIH/CDC workshop in Bethesda, Maryland, in July 1994.
61. American Society of Human Genetics, "Statement on Informed Consent for Genetic Research," *Am J Hum Genet* 59 (1996): 471–74.
62. 45 C.F.R. § 46.101(b)(4), emphasis added.

63. *Ibid.*, § 46.102(f)(2).
64. NIH/CDC Workshop Statement, p. 1787.
65. Latanya Sweeney, "Weaving Technology and Policy Together to Maintain Confidentiality," *J Law Med Ethics* 25 (Summer & Fall 1997): 98–112; and Renee M. Landers, Nancy Rice, and Beth Rubin, "'Research' in the Information Age," monograph (Washington, D.C.: American Health Lawyers Association, 2002).
66. NIH/CDC Workshop Statement, p. 1787.
67. 45 C.F.R. § 46.116(d)(1–4).
68. College of American Pathologists, "Uses of Human Tissue," unpublished manuscript (August 28, 1996), on file with authors (hereafter, CAP statement); see Chapter 3 for our earlier discussion of this document.
69. This form has been used at SUNY Upstate University Hospital.
70. CAP Statement, pp. 6–7.
71. 45 C.F.R. § 46.102(f).
72. See NIH/CDC Workshop Statement, p. 1790.
73. See Council of Regional Networks for Genetic Services, "Issues in the Use of Archived Specimens for Genetics Research: 'Points to Consider,'" unpublished manuscript (December 8, 1996), statement on file with authors (the statement notes that in some circumstances, research with tissues from deceased patients should either be rendered anonymous or consent from identifiable survivors should be sought); we discussed this document in Chapter 3.
74. 45 C.F.R. §§ 164.501, 164.502 (2002).
75. Joanne Hustead and Janlori Goldman, "Genetics and Privacy," *Am J Law Med* 28 (2002): 289 (quoting the December 28, 2000, final rules).
76. 45 C.F.R. § 164.514.
77. *Ibid.*
78. *Ibid.*, § 46.101(b)(4).
79. Thanks to Marti Benedict, IRB Administrator and Chief Compliance Officer for Research, SUNY Upstate Medical University, for her help with several of these points. Another basis for exclusion from HIPAA compliance for some genetics research is that the Privacy Rule only applies when the research has or may have some therapeutic benefit for participants. Some institutions, however, have chosen not to rely on the therapeutic benefit exception.
80. 45 C.F.R. § 164.520.
81. *Ibid.*, § 164.508.
82. See Mark Barnes and Sara Krauss, "The Effect of HIPAA on Human Subjects Research," *BNA Health Law Reporter* 10(26) (2001): 1030.
83. 45 C.F.R. § 164.528.
84. *Ibid.*, § 164.512(i).
85. *Ibid.*, § 164.502(b).
86. *Ibid.*, § 164.512(i).
87. *Ibid.*, § 164.514. For further legal analysis of HIPAA's application to research, see Landers, Rice, and Rubin (note that this monograph was published prior to adoption of the final Privacy Rule).
88. Jack Schwartz, "Oversight of Human Subject Research: The Role of the States," in National Bioethics Advisory Commission, *Ethical and Policy Issues in Research Involving Human Participants,* Vol. II (Bethesda, Md.: NBAC, 2001), commissioned paper, pp. M-1–M-20.

89. Joy Pritts, Janlori Goldman, Zoe Hudson et al., "The State of Health Privacy: An Uneven Terrain (A Comprehensive Survey of State Health Privacy Statutes)," *Practicing Law Institute, Patents, Copyrights, Trademarks, and Literary Property Course Handbook Series* 607 (June 2000), p. 650.
90. N.Y. Public Health Law, Art. 24-A (McKinney 2001). This interpretation can be found in The New York State Task Force on Life and the Law, *Genetic Testing and Screening in the Age of Genomic Medicine* (New York: NY Task Force, 2000), p. 199.
91. *Va. Code Ann.* §§ 32.1–162 et seq. (West 2001).
92. This e-mail request was sent to the Medical College of Wisconsin IRB mail list in 1999. It was forwarded to one of us by a member of the mail list.
93. Paul Yoon et al., "The National Birth Defects Prevention Study," *Public Health Rep* 116(Supplement) (2001): 32–40.
94. Jennifer Couzin, "Study of Brain Dead Sparks Debate," *Science* 295 (2002): 1210–11.

7

The Larger Legal Framework for Human Tissue Research: *Moore* and Beyond

> [T]he pertinent inquiry is not whether a patient generally retains an ownership interest in a body part after its removal from his body, but rather whether a patient has a right to determine, before a body part is removed, the use to which the part will be put after removal.
> Justice Broussard, concurring and dissenting in the California Supreme Court's decision in *Moore,* 1990[1]

> [A]s knowledge grows about the genetic basis of disease, so too does the potential for discrimination and stigmatization based on genetic information. Too many Americans fear that their genetic information will be used to discriminate against them and too often they are right.
> U.S. Department of Health and Human Services, 1997[2]

Federal policy for research with human participants establishes the core legal parameters for investigators and institutions, but it does not constitute the sum total of pertinent law. As we have seen, various provisions of the Common Rule defer to other law regarding such matters as informed consent and privacy. Moreover, the regulations do not offer answers to important related questions about the risks of genetic discrimination or ownership of removed tissues. This chapter places genetics research with stored tissue samples in its larger legal and, to an extent, social context. Our account of the existing legal landscape is descriptive, though various points of interpretation may have normative features. While legal remedies for violations of a sample source's rights are discussed at various points, this is not a central focus, and we refrain from theorizing about possible legal claims for alleged violations of participants' rights and interests.

The discussion is organized around four broad questions that loom large for research participants, investigators, IRBs and policymakers: (*1*) What does the law instruct regarding ownership of the body and biological materials? (*2*) What general rules govern patenting of human biological materials, and how does patent law view the relative contributions of sample sources and biomedical scientists? (*3*) To what extent does the law safeguard the privacy of genetic information, including the personal and familial information in DNA samples and accessible research databases? (*4*) Are patients/participants protected against the risks of

155

genetic discrimination? Along the way, we confront a number of subsidiary issues. We do not pretend to offer a comprehensive treatment of the diverse and dynamic bodies of law potentially relevant to genetics research, a task beyond the scope of this book. We do, however, hope to place important and controversial issues in the stored tissue debate in an informative legal context, one that also serves to set the stage for the analyses and recommendations in later chapters.[3] We begin with an expanded version of John Moore's story.

John Moore's Spleen

The tale of John Moore's spleen has generated substantial commentary and debate.[4] The 1990 decision of the California Supreme Court in *Moore v. Regents of California*[5] is widely viewed as a polestar for analysis of many of the legal, ethical, and policy issues fundamentally at stake in the patient/participant–physician/ investigator relationship.

The story began rather unremarkably. While employed on the Trans-Alaska pipeline, John Moore became ill and consulted a physician. Diagnosed with hairy cell leukemia, a rare and potentially fatal form of cancer, he consulted his father, a California physician, who in turn identified two specialists. Moore then contacted Dr. David Golde at the UCLA Medical Center.[6] At Moore's first visit on October 5, 1976, Golde confirmed the diagnosis, after "withdrawing extensive amounts of blood, bone marrow aspirate, and other bodily substances."[7] Several days later, Golde informed his patient that "he had reason to fear for his life" and recommended surgery to remove the 22-pound spleen (a normal spleen weighs about 7 ounces) as "necessary to slow down the progress of his disease."[8] Moore signed the requisite surgical consent form, and the splenectomy was successfully performed. As far as we are aware, Moore was generally pleased with the quality of clinical care he received at UCLA.[9]

Golde and his research colleague, Shirley Quan, had an additional agenda. Upon their first encounter with the patient, they quickly became aware of the potential commercial value of some of the unusual properties of Moore's cells. Approximately 10 days after the surgery, Golde directed that a portion of the spleen be taken to his research lab. The results confirmed the researchers' prior beliefs, and they set in place a research agenda, featuring Moore as the unknowing research participant. Moore traveled from his home in Seattle to the UCLA Medical Center many times between 1976 and 1983. Each time he was told that testing of additional samples of "blood, blood serum, skin, bone marrow aspirate, and sperm" was necessary to ensure his health, and he gave consent to withdrawal of these tissues from his body.[10]

Golde's instincts were sound, at least from the standpoint of science. As recounted by the court, due to the presence of a virus in his cells, Moore's T-lymphocytes (a type of white blood cell) overproduced certain T-lymphokines, which possessed potentially therapeutic properties. Excessive production allowed the research team to identify the genetic material that, in turn, paved the way to development of an immortal cell line. Because all human beings ordinarily produce the same lymphokines, identification of the genetic material is akin to a search for the proverbial needle in a haystack. But in this case, the nature of the removed cells simplified the researchers' task dramatically.[11] Development of the "Mo" cell line in the late 1970s led to a patent application process beginning in 1981, with a formal filing in 1983 for a "unique T-lymphocyte line and products derived therefrom." On March 20, 1984, patent # 4,438,032 was issued, naming Drs. Golde and Quan as inventors and the California State Regents as the assignee of the patent.[12]

The potential commercial value of the patent, which covered "various methods for using the cell line to produce lymphokines," was estimated at approximately $3.01 billion by the year 1990. With the help of the Regents, Golde negotiated lucrative agreements with two private companies (Genetics Institute and Sandoz) for commercial development of the cell line, including the rights to 75,000 shares of common stock in Genetics Institute and payments to Golde and the Regents of at least $440,000 over three years (some of which went toward a pro-rata share of Golde's salary and benefits).[13]

Throughout this seven-year period, according to Moore, he had no idea what was happening to his blood and other tissues following their removal and examination. Suddenly, on his last visit to UCLA in September 1983, he was "presented with a consent form that was different from most of the papers [he] had signed in the past." He was now, for the first time, asked to "voluntarily grant to the University of California any and all rights [he or his heirs] may have in any cell line or any other potential product which might be developed from the blood and/or bone marrow obtained from [him]."[14] He circled "I do not," and returned the form with his signature.[15] At his parents' house later that day, he received a telephone call from Golde saying that he had "missigned" the form. Several days later, after returning to Seattle, he received a package with a new consent form and a large sticker and an arrow saying "Please circle 'I do.' "[16]

Unwilling to comply and "bothered by the persistence of his doctor," he consulted a law firm. His lawyers discovered articles written by Golde about his work and his efforts to obtain a patent for the "Mo" cell line from a patient in Seattle.[17] Moore's landmark lawsuit was instituted on September 11, 1984, against Golde and Quan, the Regents, and the two pharmaceutical companies that had contracted for development of the cell line.

By the time the case reached the California Supreme Court, most of Moore's claims had been either dismissed or consolidated. Ultimately, the court ruled on two issues central to the physician/investigator–patient/participant relationship. The first was whether Golde's failure to disclose his research and commercial interests violated Moore's personal right to make an informed decision about permitting his tissues to be used for this purpose (and the related allegation that nondisclosure was a breach of the physician's fiduciary duty). The second was whether use of Moore's cells for research and commercial ends violated his property rights in the removed bodily tissues. Moore sought compensatory damages in the form of a share of the market value (the profits) from the "Mo" cell line.[18]

Informed Consent. As noted in the previous chapter, the legal doctrine of informed consent holds (in about half the states) that physicians are obligated to disclose information that a reasonable patient would find relevant to making an informed decision. California first embraced the "reasonable patient" standard in 1972 (among the first states to do so) in a case involving a series of internal injuries caused (at least in part) by premature absorption of a suture, the risks of which were allegedly never disclosed to the patient.[19] Thus, this was the prevailing standard of disclosure when Moore and Golde first met.

In his complaint Moore claimed that the physician "failed to disclose the extent of his research and economic interests in [his] cells,"[20] and that without this information, he was denied his right to make informed decisions in the course of his relationship with Golde. (He did not allege actual physical injury or harm.) Thus, the question to be decided was whether a reasonable patient in Moore's situation would find Golde's research and economic interests relevant to the consent process. Affirming the patient's fundamental right and interest in controlling decisions about his own body and the essential place of informed consent in securing this right, the court agreed that a reasonable patient would consider knowledge of a physician's personal research and commercial interests material to his or her decision. The court ruled that "a physician must disclose personal interests unrelated to the patient's health, whether research or economic, that may affect the physician's professional judgment...."[21]

The court's reasoning closely links informed consent with breach of fiduciary duty. With respect to research itself, one who acts as both treating physician and researcher "has potentially conflicting loyalties" and may, for example, "be tempted to order a scientifically useful procedure or test that offers marginal, or no, benefits to the patient."[22] (This was Moore's allegation about the postoperative removal of cells from his body.) With respect to the physician's economic interests, *Moore* relies upon two analogous precedents. The first, a California Court of Appeal decision upholding the constitutionality of a state law banning physicians from holding proprietary interests and co-ownerships in pharmacies, where the court stated (*in dictum*): " 'Certainly a sick patient deserves to be free of any reasonable suspicion that his doctor's judgment is influenced by a profit motive.' "[23] The second was California's law against physician self-referral without prior disclosure and written consent—further evidence of the importance of avoiding, or at least disclosing, potential financial conflicts of interest. Acknowledging that informed consent cases usually involve alleged failure to disclose medical risks, not the physician's personal interests, *Moore* held that "[t]he concept of informed consent . . . is broad enough to encompass the latter."[24] Thus, a physician's failure to disclose such interests exposes the physician to potential liability.[25]

Property and Ownership. Moore was less successful in his quest to recover a share of the profits from the "Mo" cell line. Though novel, the claim was straightforward in its logic. According to Moore, the cells removed from his body were his personal property. Since his informed consent had never been properly obtained, use of his cells in research constituted interference with his ownership interests. And since they had never been relinquished or transferred, his property rights, in effect, accompanied his cells throughout their travels. In legal parlance, Moore alleged the tort of conversion of personal property and asserted "a proprietary interest in each of the products that any of the defendants might ever create from his cells or the patented cell line."[26] From the court's standpoint, the issue was not only one of first impression, but was far more complex. In contrast to their view of informed consent, the justices were deeply divided over the conversion issue, with three of the seven justices writing separate opinions.

The Opinion of the Court. Justice Panelli, writing for the court, found that Moore's claim failed under established principles of conversion law. To maintain an action for conversion the plaintiff must show "actual interference with his ownership or right of possession." Since Moore had no expectation of retaining possession of the removed tissues (his expectation was that they would be discarded), his claim must rest on having an ongoing ownership interest in his removed cells.[27]

For the majority there were three "reasons to doubt" that Moore retained any such ownership interests. First, there was no precedent supporting Moore's contention, either directly or indirectly; this was a novel claim.

Second, California statutes drastically limit patients' continuing property-based interests in removed cells. For example, the medical waste law directing disposal of human tissues, remains, and waste "following conclusion of scientific use" in effect cuts off a host of property rights by restricting use of excised tissues and cells and directing their subsequent destruction. Analogous laws deem the procurement, processing, and distribution of blood to be provision of a service, not a sale of goods; provide for the disposition of the body and its parts following autopsy; and recognize rights of donation for purposes of transplantation, research, or education. All, in the court's view, embody the understanding that removed human biological materials are unique: "objects *sui generis.*" Each of these laws expresses policy judgments limiting individual property rights (e.g., sale of solid organs is prohibited; families have "quasi-property" rights in the body of the deceased for burial). Moreover, these laws collectively express the judgment that ownership of biological materials should not be governed by the general law of personal property.[28]

Third, the court found that the subject matter of the patent—the cell line and its products—was distinct, both factually and legally, from Moore's cells and therefore could not be considered Moore's property. Here, it was noted that the patented cell line has properties different from those taken from Moore's body, including an enhanced growth potential. The court's conclusion, however, rested not on scientific distinctions—but *on the bare fact that a patent for the cell line was granted.* The cell line is, the court held, factually distinct because, as recognized by the patent award, it "represents the product of 'human ingenuity' [and] 'inventive effort.'" It is legally distinct because the assertion of continuing ownership is "inconsistent with the patent, which constitutes an authoritative determination that the cell line is the product of invention."[29] Moore's contribution as the "supplier of raw materials" may have been unique in some sense, but it did not warrant ascription of property rights.

Taking these positions together, the court seemed implicitly to conclude that the general principle of statutes governing disposal of removed biological materials applies equally to Moore's situation, namely, that any ownership interest in his cells was abandoned when his tissues were removed with his consent. That the consent was not informed does not vitiate this conclusion.

Beyond this analysis, the most significant question troubling the court concerned public policy, as revealed in its discussion of whether conversion liability should be extended to offer a remedy in a case of this sort. Keenly aware that the issues before it were of first impression, the opinion embarked upon an extended discussion of the underlying policies and interests at stake should a cause of action for conversion be recognized.

The two most significant interests to be balanced, in the court's view, are the individual's right of autonomous choice and society's interests in medical and scientific progress through biomedical research. The language of the majority sharpens the issue: "The second important policy consideration is that we not threaten with disabling civil liability innocent third parties who are engaged in socially useful activities, such as researchers who have no reason to believe that their use of a particular cell sample is, or may be, against the donor's wishes."[30] For the majority, the scales seemed to tip easily in favor of protecting the research community. To extend the conversion theory would "utterly sacrifice" biomedical research; research with cell samples would be like purchasing "a ticket in a litigation lottery."[31] Justice Panelli reached a related and controversial conclusion: The legal requirement that research and economic interests be disclosed in the informed consent process provides sufficient protection for future patients. The court need not, and should not, go further.[32] Justice Arabian echoed these same themes in a separate concurrence, adding that as a matter of morality, to embrace Moore's position would be "to regard the human vessel—the single most venerated and protected subject in any civilized society—as equal with the basest commercial commodity.... [It would] commingle the sacred with the profane."[33]

Significantly, though it clearly came down on one side of the policy debate, the majority simultaneously suggested that extension of conversion law to biomedical research is a policy matter better left to the legislature: "If the scientific users of human cells are to be held liable for failing to investigate the consensual pedigree of their raw materials, we believe the Legislature should make that decision."[34]

The Dissents. The dissenters differed on several points, including the proper role of the judiciary in charting a course to guide future research with human biological materials. Justice Broussard, concurring and dissenting, contended that interference with Moore's rights to control disposition of his bodily tissue occurred before their removal, hence at a time when they were unquestionably his property. The wrong was done when information material to Moore's right of control was withheld, and damages for conversion should be the remedy. Taking issue with the majority's claim that recognition of such a remedy would be unfair to innocent researchers who only later became aware of the potential scientific or commercial value of the patient's cells, Justice Broussard would find conversion liability only in cases (like this one) where the researcher deliberately withheld relevant information. In effect, he would allow a claim for conversion and monetary damages in cases of fraud.[35] For Justice Mosk, also dissenting, to whom the principle that "every individual has a legally protectable property interest in his own body and its products" is profound and fundamental, it seemed unnecessary to determine when the conversion occurred. Dr. Golde's actions constituted a continuing misappropriation and conversion.[36]

The dissents offer alternative views of Moore's "unique" contributions. For Justice Broussard, since the conversion occurred at the time of removal, not with subsequent use, the question of uniqueness, central to the weight given the patent by the majority, was irrelevant. It matters not whether the patient's claim involves ordinary property or unique property. The "uniqueness" of Moore's contributions are relevant, if at all, only on the question of how much he is entitled to recover as damages (that is, relative to his contributions).[37] Justice Mosk insisted that Moore's crucial contribution of the raw materials requisite to invention ("an invention named, ironically, after him") could not be denied. To hold, as the majority did, that the judgment of the patent office cut off the individual's interests was unfair and made a patent "a license to defraud."[38]

The dissenters also offered different interpretations of at least two statutes to which the majority looked by analogy for guidance. Both found that the donative intent embodied in California's adoption of the Uniform Anatomical Gift Act (UAGA) affirms, rather than limits, the individual's right of control over his own body. Moreover, the UAGA does not preclude sale of body parts for research purposes. As stated by Justice Broussard, "[t]here is no basis to conclude that there is a general public policy in this state prohibiting hospitals or medical centers from giving, or prohibiting patients from receiving, valuable consideration for body parts which are to be used for medical research or the advancement of medical science."[39] Neither of the dissenting justices would sanction a legal presumption that the patient abandons surgically removed tissue and any rights to control its use, thereby giving researchers freedom to claim it for their own purposes. Legally authorized "scientific use" of excised tissue includes diagnostic and prognostic examination, but in the words of Justice Mosk, "[I]t would stretch the English language beyond recognition . . . to say that commercial exploitation of the kind and degree alleged here is also a usual and ordinary meaning of the phrase 'scientific use.' "[40]

Finally, each dissent disagreed sharply with the majority (and with Justice Arabian's separate concurring opinion) as to the proper balancing of the policy interests at stake, rejecting the notion that conversion liability would sanction a "litigation lottery." If only researchers engaged in fraud and deceit were at risk, then researchers with no economic interests at the time of consent (the usual case) would be protected. The same would be true of researchers using stored tissue samples who are not involved in the consent process at all. (Broussard, J.)[41] On the other hand, whether or not liability is limited to instances of fraud, the fact of potential liability would encourage diligent record keeping, thereby affording the tools to avoid litigation. (Mosk, J.)[42]

For Justice Mosk, the law must take seriously the precept that each of us has a protected property interest in controlling the disposition of our body, its parts, and its products. The doctrine of informed consent alone is insufficient protection, for even if faithfully observed, it is limited to the right to "just say no." Recognition of a property interest would foster an affirmative right of participation and promote partnerships between patients and researchers.[43] Finding, as well, that many patients would be unable to persuade judge and jury that had they known of the physician's commercial interest, they would not have given their consent, Justice Mosk dismissed the breach of fiduciary duty cause of action as a "paper tiger."[44] At bottom, the tone and tenor of the dissenters expressed a sense of outrage, absent in the opinion of the court, over the fraud perpetrated on Moore and the unjust enrichment that would inure to researchers should the law fail to craft a more patient-friendly remedy.

Reflections on Moore. If John Moore were to meet Dr. Golde today under similar circumstances, any research involving Moore's cells would be governed by the Common Rule and subject to IRB review. At a minimum, Moore would have to receive the core disclosures mandated by the federal policy, including being told of the nature and purpose of the contemplated research, its potential benefits, and reasonably foreseeable risks. Whether failure to disclose financial incentives violates the federal policy is less clear, as this is not included among the expressly mandated disclosures.

There is, however, a good argument that since Golde set his sights on the potential for monetary gain rather early, he had an obligation to include this in an explanation of the purposes of the research, at least at some fairly early stage in the research. Moreover, the duty to disclose financial conflicts of interest, if not to avoid them altogether, finds significant support elsewhere in today's law. Physician self-referral is banned or restricted in numerous states[45] (as it was in California at the time of *Moore*) and under federal Medicare law.[46] Financial incentives imposed on physicians by managed care organizations are either banned or must be disclosed under the laws of more than half the states.[47] While this body of law generally contemplates a clinical setting in which diagnosis or treatment is the primary purpose of the physician–patient encounter, it is part of an overall legal climate that counsels either avoidance or disclosure of physician financial incentives.[48]

Far less clear—and far more controversial—is *whether a patient or research participant has any property rights* in removed tissues and cells. To what extent may research participants assert, "my cells, my property" or "my genes, my property"? The question highlights a related, but little discussed issue. Under federal policy, informed consent may not include "any exculpatory language through which the subject or the representative is made to waive or appear to waive any of the subject's legal rights, or releases or appears to release the investigator, the sponsor, the institution or its agents from liability for negligence."[49] When Golde sent Moore consent papers urging that he relinquish any and all rights in any cell line or any other potential product, was this a violation of the federal policy? If so, are investigators prohibited from offering or negotiating agreements under terms that involve waiver of participants' future property-based claims to a share of the profits or of specific rights, such as to sue for conversion? Should any such waivers be considered void and unenforceable? We argue later (Chapter 10) that federal policy should recognize that sample sources have *limited property interests* in removed tissues and cells and in personal genetic information. It follows that the consent process should allow for waivers of at least some sorts of future legal claims that might be brought against investigators or research institutions.

At least two other cases have also involved sample sources' asserted property rights based on tangible contributions of biological materials. In 1981 Hideaki Hagiwara, M.D., suggested that researchers at the University of California working to develop hybridoma cell lines to fight cancer use lymph cells from his own mother, who was suffering from cervical cancer. An immortal cell line was fused with the Hagiwara cells, creating a cell line that secreted cancer-fighting antibodies for which the researchers were granted a patent. A subsequent dispute between the Hagiwara family and the researchers over a share of the profits was settled prior to a court decision. Under the terms of the settlement, the university retained the patent and the Hagiwaras were granted exclusive license to market the patent in Asia, with an agreement to pay the University of California royalties on any commercial product sales.[50]

While this book was in press a decision was rendered in the Canavan disease dispute described at the end of this chapter. Here, families who had donated tissue

and information, together with the Canavan Foundation and two other private organizations, claimed that researchers had improperly applied for a patent on the gene
sequence for this disease and had, based on the patent they obtained, sought to limit
testing for Canavan through restrictive licensing agreements. The court's ruling
dismissed five of the six legal claims, including those based on lack of informed
consent and conversion of property (here the Florida court followed *Moore* on the
conversion issue). However, the court held that the families and the organizations
had stated a valid legal claim for unjust enrichment. The essence of this equitable
claim (not dependent on property rights) was that since their contributions to and
ongoing involvement in the research had benefited the researchers, it would be
unfair for the researchers (and the institution) to profit from extension of the research and its fruits beyond the terms on which participants' consent was based,
and therefore compensation should be provided to the families.[51]

Moore's posit of a fundamental tension between conversion law and biotech-
nological progress—the "litigation lottery" theme that resonates throughout the
stored tissue debate—warrants further explication. The essence of a conversion
claim is that if someone else intentionally exercises dominion or control over my
property in a manner inconsistent with my rights and deprives me of my property,
then I am entitled to compensation, unless the property is returned to me without
damage or loss of value.[52] Beyond these core elements, there can be considerable
variation from state to state in the doctrine's application. Most importantly here,
the law varies on the appropriate measure of damages, that is, on whether monetary damages for conversion are limited to the *fair market value* of the property
at the time of conversion (the general rule), or may also include the *value added
to the property* by the converter. A number of courts take the latter view, though
this remedy is sometimes awarded only where the converter has not acted in good
faith.[53] To illustrate two exceptions, someone who improperly converts stocks of
fluctuating value may be liable for their highest replacement value between the
initial taking and the time of restitution;[54] similarly, the converter of crops may be
liable for their increased market value up to the date of trial.[55]

Whether courts will, in the future, embrace the general rule or find analogy
to these latter sorts of circumstances persuasive holds enormous implications for
biomedical research. Under the general rule, damages available to sample sources
would be limited to the value of tissues at the time of removal (more than likely
a nominal amount). It is hard to see how legitimizing such claims would create
a duty to inquire into the "consensual pedigree" of each human cell sample,[56] or
spawn a "title insurance" market for cell lines.[57] These forebodings seem far more
apt if biomedical research were to be added to the list of exceptional circumstances
justifying substantially larger recovery. Among the significant hurdles for a sample
source arguing his or her case is that appropriation of removed tissues does not
ordinarily deprive one of a financial opportunity in the way that conversion of
crops, stocks, or other marketable items does, at least not in the current system.[58]

Of course, to succeed on a claim of conversion, a sample source must first establish that tissues and cells were his or her property post-removal, the key question on which Moore's claim failed to carry a majority of the justices. In biomedical research the issue is further complicated by the related question of whether investigators may "lay claim" to previously removed tissues that have been stored for possible future research on the ground that such tissues are, as argued by the majority in *Moore* (and by the Nuffield Council, apparently applying British law incorrectly), *abandoned property* in which the sample source has relinquished all rights. We turn to these and other matters below.

Ownership and Control of the Body and Its Parts

In some senses our bodies and body parts are obviously and intuitively our (unique) personal property. The legal significance of calling the body property is that doing so suggests the ascription of certain rights. It is often stated that the concept of property encompasses a "bundle of rights," including rights of possession, control, use, and transfer—usually by sale or gift—as well as power to exclude others from any of these rights.[59] To characterize something as personal property is to lay claim to all or part of this bundle. The term "ownership" is sometimes reserved for holding all the sticks in the bundle.[60]

Being vested with the full panoply of property rights (full ownership) does not mean, however, that the rights-holder's authority over the property is absolute. As shown by *Moore,* property rights are commonly limited by public policy considerations. To illustrate further, the owner of residential property ordinarily may not convert the land to commercial use without approval of the local zoning authority. Similarly, a restrictive covenant in a deed purporting to prevent an owner from selling the property to African Americans or other minorities is not enforceable.[61]

Property law can be understood as being comprised of a set of rights, rules, and remedies distinct in important ways from those governing personal rights or as a cluster of personal rights applied to things.[62] With respect to both rights in the body and in health information, the concepts of *personal rights* and *property rights* are often overlapping and confused, and it is useful to clarify some basic distinctions. Some of the sticks in this bundle—those involving possession, control, and exclusion of others—look much like personal rights of informed consent, privacy, and confidentiality. Whether understood in terms of autonomy or property, a person has a basic (and, most often, noncontroversial) right to authorize physical contact for diagnostic, therapeutic, or research purposes, or to decline unwanted intrusions upon bodily integrity. Similarly, a person's interests in controlling access to personal health information might be grounded in personal rights of confidentiality and privacy or in the idea that we own information about ourselves.

Alternatively, some of the ways we talk about privacy share important features of property discourse. In health care the concepts of informational, physical, and decisional privacy are most familiar. But our interests in personal health information, including one's genetic profile, sometimes also involve the concept of *proprietary privacy*.[63] The contention that special protections are needed to safeguard each person's "coded future diary," popularized by the authors of the model Genetic Privacy Act, invokes concerns about "the appropriation and ownership of interests in human personality."[64] The language suggests analogy to legal doctrines, developed elsewhere, holding that appropriation of a person's name or likeness—treating another's name or likeness like one's own property—without permission is an invasion of privacy. Both the common ground and the confusion between these two categories of rights are evident in state laws, reviewed in the next section, that label genetic information as personal property.

Within the framework of the debate over stored tissues, a critical distinguishing feature of the property paradigm concerns the concept of *transferability*. When and how may an individual transfer possession and ownership of his or her body parts? When and how may others acquire rights of ownership in parts of the body? Focusing on these questions, the discussion turns to whether removed tissues may be understood as having been abandoned by the sample source. We then ask, what does the law tell us about a person's right to transfer other parts of the body and biological materials—organs, blood, semen, eggs, and frozen embryos—and address another key property issue, setting forth the core features of the patent law as it may apply to genetics research.

In its oft-cited 1987 report, *New Developments in Biotechnology: Ownership of Human Tissues and Cells,* the federal Office of Technology Assessment identified eight broad sources of property-type rights relating to human biological materials and information derived from those materials. These include laws relating to (*1*) patents, (*2*) cadavers and autopsies, (*3*) organ transplantation, (*4*) blood and semen sales, (*5*) copyright, (*6*) trade secrets, (*7*) conversion and trespass to chattels, and (*8*) accession.[65] We address some, but not all, of these areas. Our focus is intentionally selective, directed to issues we believe to be of greatest importance and interest to those involved in the research enterprise, whether they be investigators, institutions, or potential research participants.

An Overview of State Legislation. As of this writing, a handful of state laws use the term "property" to characterize an individual's interests in genetic information. Colorado and Georgia state that "genetic information is the unique property of the individual."[66] Florida uses the phrase "exclusive property,"[67] while Louisiana uses the term solely in the insurance context, stating that genetic information is "the property of the insured or enrollee."[68] A few of these states define protected information as that which is derived from "DNA analysis" (e.g., Florida) or more generally "genetic testing" (Colorado, Georgia), while two (Louisiana, Oregon) include information derived from gene products, inherited characteristics, and family history. Colorado, Florida, and Louisiana make the term "property" part of the operative language of the law, but in Georgia "property" is found only in the legislative findings (technically, not part of the law, but an aid to its interpretation). In 1996 New Jersey's legislature passed a genetic privacy law with language making an individual's genetic information his or her property. However, following complaints from the state's biotechnology industry that any reference to "property" would have a chilling effect on research and development, the Governor vetoed the bill. New Jersey later enacted a far-reaching genetic privacy law, with no reference to "property."[69]

The primary purpose of these laws appears to be twofold: to promote privacy and to shield individuals from genetic discrimination. The term "property" is used in connection with professional duties of confidentiality, as if to reinforce the personal and confidential nature of genetic information. Several states, embracing some version of the approach found in the model Genetic Privacy Act, require specific consent and authorization for each disclosure, while also enumerating certain circumstances where disclosure is permitted without consent. These exceptions are usually for use in criminal proceedings, to determine paternity, and to identify a deceased individual, but may also include newborn screening programs.[70] Louisiana is alone in this group that expressly addresses the research setting, stating that consent is not needed for anonymous research if the identity of the subject will not be released.[71] Beyond the right to authorize or block release of personal information, none of these statutes establishes, denies, or refers to property-based rights of transfer in genetic information or biological materials.

Several states establish a cause of action and set forth specific remedies for violation of a person's rights in genetic information. For example, in both Colorado and Georgia, an insurance company that makes an unauthorized disclosure may be liable for actual damages or, if the harm that results includes loss or denial of health insurance, the insurer may be compelled to provide coverage on the same terms and conditions as the individual would have been able to obtain coverage absent the disclosure.[72] Under Florida law, a person who makes an unauthorized disclosure is guilty of a misdemeanor in the first degree.[73] In Louisiana, negligent collection, storage, analysis, or disclosure may result in liability for: (1) actual damages or $50,000, whichever is greater, or (2) "[t]reble damages, in any case where such a violation resulted in profit or monetary gain." Willful violation of consent requirements, or inducing another to collect, store, or analyze a DNA sample carries somewhat steeper penalties.[74] Whether these states intended these remedies to be exclusive, precluding, for example, claims for conversion where an aggrieved sample source might successfully lay claim to a share of the profits, is unclear. Often in law the failure to make specified remedies exclusive leaves the door open to other, even novel, legal claims and remedies. On the other hand, there is good reason to believe that the term "property" in this context is used to assert the importance of individual consent and privacy, not to ascribe a constellation of traditional property rights in biological materials.

The Oregon experience illustrates the controversy and confusion surrounding the "property" label, and confirms the understanding that these laws may be more about privacy than property. Oregon's 1995 genetic privacy law (the first such law to be enacted nationally) crafted a series of rules centered on the need for individual authorization for obtaining, releasing, and retaining genetic information or samples.[75] It directed destruction of samples upon request of the individual or an authorized representative and also specified that "an individual's genetic information and DNA sample are the property of the individual except when the information or sample is used in anonymous research."[76] The exception for anonymous research was emphasized in a separate provision: "An individual does not interfere with, infringe upon, misappropriate or otherwise damage an individual's property by obtaining, testing, retaining, disclosing or providing an individual's genetic information or DNA sample solely for anonymous research."[77] Collectively, these provisions seem to suggest that it would be a violation of property rights when identifiable or linkable genetic information or material is obtained, used, shared, or misappropriated without consent of the individual. On another reading the 1995 Oregon law might be understood in more familiar terms of personal rights of consent, privacy, and control.

Critics of the law contended that the property language would inhibit genetic research and create confusion over the rights of researchers and others in the biotechnology industry. In response, Oregon established a Genetics Research Advisory Committee (GRAC), charged with the task of recommending a solution to the property debate. After a year's deliberation, the GRAC concluded that the property clause was not essential to the intended purpose of its enactment, that is,"to provide a way for individuals and their families to retain some control over their genetic information." It also found that the property clause had never been used to enforce rights in genetic information or material and might be difficult to put into practice. The GRAC therefore recommended that this provision be deleted from the law and replaced with a more explicit privacy right, including a list of specific penalties, both civil and criminal, for illegally obtaining, disclosing, or retaining genetic information or materials. In 2001, Oregon enacted these and other recommended changes to its genetic privacy law.[78]

Like Oregon's first attempt to address the question, the few states to characterize a person's genetic information (or tissue sample) as his or her property likely did so for the same reason—to strengthen individual rights of privacy and control. They likely had notions of proprietary privacy in mind rather than a traditional property model. Property language may open the door to recognition of a panoply of property-based rights and remedies, but no known cases interpreting these statutes have yet put this possibility to the test. Regardless, as we have seen, property rights in bodily tissues and personal genetic information do not depend on explicit statutory recognition. At present the law is largely silent (it neither authorizes nor blocks) on the rights of individuals to sell their biological material or the genetic information that it generates, and the rights and remedies of those who may feel their tissues have been wrongly appropriated by others.

The next section explores another related question—whether patients who give tissue samples in connection with their clinical care have thereby relinquished all rights to control future use of these samples. In other words, may researchers treat these samples as if they have been abandoned? We then turn to the question of a commercial market for tissues.

Abandonment of Tissue Samples. In accordance with national standards issued by the College of American Pathologists and local state law, pathologists (and other physicians) routinely retain a portion of clinically derived tissues, test reports, tissue-banking records, and other patient information for a substantial period of time, sometimes decades. The primary purpose of retention practices is clinical follow-up, but they also ensure that tissue and information may later be available for other purposes, including research. In fact, this is the most common source of human research materials.[79]

Institutions and researchers often (but not always) rely on general consent forms that include a provision for consent to later research use. For example, a surgical consent form might state that "[a]ny tissues surgically removed may be disposed by the Hospital in accordance with accustomed practice, including use in research studies." This form also allows the patient to write in exceptions to this broad permission.[80] But many other tissues, routinely stored without any form of consent and treated *as if* they have been abandoned by the patient, may later be used for research. (Whether this type of general consent, when obtained, is sufficient is a question we address in Chapter 9.)

The legal basis for this traditional practice is unclear. The common law doctrine of abandonment states that abandoned property is property in which the owner has "voluntarily relinquished all rights, title, claim and possession," with the intention of terminating ownership and "of not reclaiming any future rights." Ownership rights are not thereby transferred to any other person. Abandoned property may be claimed by someone else, who may assert rights of ownership in it, such as by taking and holding possession of the item.[81]

Whether the frequent practice of tissue storage fits these parameters raises an interesting challenge. Following the diagnostic or therapeutic use of a tissue sample, it is fair to say that most of us have voluntarily relinquished, and have intended to terminate, ownership in that portion of our blood or other tissues without intending later to assert any of our constellation of property rights. But this is done with the expectation (intention?) that the removed material becomes medical waste to be disposed of when it is no longer useful for our care. Arguably, this widely shared understanding and expectation that tissue will be discarded and destroyed is the basis for the intent to abandon. Were it otherwise, we would expect to be asked for our consent, for an affirmative relinquishment of our rights in removed tissues and cells.

By the same token, clinicians and investigators may feel that because removed, post-diagnostic blood and other tissue otherwise constitute "medical waste," they may be *regarded as abandoned* and later appropriated for research. Virtually every state has some type of law or regulation concerning the disposition of medical waste in hospitals and other health care facilities. However, these laws seem to offer little support for appropriation of abandoned tissues. Medical waste laws typically cover disposal of sharps, infectious agents, blood, blood products, and pathological waste, and less uniformly, surgical and laboratory waste. Beyond these core concerns, operative definitions of "medical waste" can vary considerably.[82] But whatever their scope, the animating purpose of these laws is to safeguard public health. Medical waste laws do not address whether various forms of waste may be used for research, nor do they look to the patient's consent (intent) to determine disposition.

Abandonment of human biological materials has on rare occasion found its way into an American courtroom. In one Kentucky case, *Browning v. Norton-Children's Hospital,* the patient underwent emergency surgery to amputate his right leg above the knee in treatment of a serious blood condition. When he discovered that his amputated leg had been cremated, he became distraught. Asserting a "great fear of fire," he sued the surgeon and the hospital for mental anguish. Finding that "when one consents to and authorizes an operation while a patient in a hospital (absent any specific reservation, demand, or objection to some normal procedure), he . . . thereby accepts all the rules, regulations, and the modus operandi of that hospital," the court rejected the patient's contentions. (The court also found that in the absence of specific inquiry from the patient over a four-week period, the hospital could not be expected to retain the leg indefinitely.)[83]

Analogous situations have on occasion arisen in the criminal context. One case has held that hair samples obtained by the FBI from a haircut given to a prison inmate were abandoned and could be appropriated and analyzed by the Bureau.[84] In another case, *Venner v. Maryland,*[85] the defendant eliminated numerous balloons containing hashish oil during emergency treatment for a drug overdose. Ruling on motions to suppress this evidence of drug possession, the court held that Venner's stool was abandoned property that could be seized and used at trial by the prosecution. The ruling affirmed a prior judgment by the Court of Special Appeals that offers a more expansive statement of the question. There the court opined that a person has a property right in

wastes or other materials which were once a part of or contained within his body, but which normally are discarded after their separation from the body. . . . [But] when a person does nothing and says nothing to indicate an intent to assert his right of ownership, possession or control . . . [and] places, or permits others to place waste material from his body into the stream of ultimate disposition as waste, he has abandoned whatever legal right he theretofore had to protect it from prying eyes or acquisitive hands.[86]

This statement appears to lend important support to investigators' contentions that removed tissues that otherwise would become medical waste have been abandoned by the patient. The precedent should be interpreted cautiously, however; among other considerations, the individual and societal interests implicated by the Fourth Amendment right against unlawful search and seizure are quite different from those at stake in the daily retention and storage of blood and other tissues in the clinical setting. More important for our purposes is the centrality of expectations and intentions in the abandonment doctrine. Insofar as patients ordinarily expect biopsy samples, tumors, skin and so forth to be discarded as waste when no longer needed for diagnosis and treatment, *some form of consent* (general or specific) *seems required* for future appropriation for research, a position we develop later on.

Transfer of Human Body Parts and Biological Materials—Gift or Sale? Like human participants research generally, research with human tissues has for decades embraced a donation model for transfer of materials from individuals to researchers. Consent (when obtained) is not given in exchange for purchase of one's tissue samples. If consent has a price, it takes the form of modest compensation offered for the inconveniences and costs of participation (time, travel, transportation, discomfort). While it is commonly hoped that the compensation provides an incentive to enroll in a study, this is not understood as a transaction between buyer and seller, nor is there negotiation over the amount. This practice has relied heavily on altruistic and shared commitment to the enormous potential of biomedical research to improve the health and well-being of the community, usually, without the prospect of direct benefit for participants and, certainly, without consideration of market forces or negotiated contracts.

Viewed more broadly, our current system leaves the door open to commodification of the body and its parts in a variety of ways. In fact, Lori Andrews and Dorothy Nelkin have documented a diverse market for human tissue in a variety of settings.[87] Much of this commerce is permitted to occur in the absence of legal regulation of the manner in which tissues may legitimately be transferred. As noted in the previous chapter, federal policy is essentially silent on the commodification of the raw materials of human participants research.

This section looks by analogy to several areas where the law has addressed (or begun to address) whether individuals and society may treat human body parts and materials as property, and if so, what rights of alienability (methods of transfer) the law recognizes. Admittedly selective, the examples of the donation model for solid organ transplantation with its express ban on organ sales, the free market approach to sales of blood and gametes, and the ambivalence surrounding rights in frozen embryos, together offer a spectrum of useful analogies for consideration of whether commercialization of human tissues in research should be permitted, regulated, or considered what philosopher Michael Walzer calls "blocked exchanges"—those modes of transfer that are either legally banned (placed beyond the marketplace) or expressly restricted.[88]

Organs as Gifts. That transfers of transplantable organs should be understood as donations, not commercial transactions, seems an established societal norm. The basic concept is embodied in the language we use. We speak of organ donors and recipients, not sellers and purchasers; we refer to giving and receiving "the gift of life."

All 50 states and the District of Columbia have adopted some version of the UAGA, first promulgated by the National Conference of Commissioners on Uniform State Laws in 1968.[89] Under the UAGA, adult individuals have authority to consent to or refuse retrieval of organs, tissues, or other parts of the body for use for transplantation, medical education, or research. Family members may also give consent (in the order of priority given by statute), "in the absence of actual notice of contrary indications" of the decedent's wishes.[90] The basic framework of the UAGA was reinforced by the 1984 National Organ Transplant Act (NOTA), which states that transplantable organs may not be sold and imposes criminal penalties for attempts to commodify organs (reasonable payments are permitted for a range of expenses, including removal, transportation, and storage of organs and travel, housing, and lost wages incurred by the donor).[91]

A few years later, in an attempt to increase the scarce supply of viable organs, the UAGA was revised to embrace "required request laws" designed to ensure specific inquiry about intent to donate and to ease the burdens of the decision. The 1987 revision, adopted by more than 20 states and in federal law for all Medicare- and Medicaid-eligible hospitals, further establishes the voluntary gift model for organ procurement.[92]

The voluntary donation model rests on, among other factors, the social value of altruism, concerns that an organ market would lead to exploitation and coercion of the poor, concerns that such a market would give unfair access to organs based on ability to pay, and on the idea that the human body has special moral standing deserving of respect and dignity that can only be recognized by placing organ transplants beyond the reach of the market. Each of these views has repeatedly been challenged in the ongoing search for new approaches to closing the gap between supply and demand in transplantation. In recent years a growing chorus of voices has called for lifting the ban on commercialism. Some advocate simply lifting the prohibition; others advance the benefits of a regulated commercial market, including proposals for a government role in mediating organ sales, and allowing some form of organ sales but continuing to ban the private purchase of organs.[93]

Small steps in the direction of creating financial incentives to donate have been taken in a handful of states that offer a "death benefit" to assist families in paying funeral costs.[94] In 2002 the American Medical Association House of Delegates endorsed a proposal from its Council on Ethical and Judicial Affairs to offer a modest sum to the families of donors and to study whether this offer gave people more incentive to donate.[95] Neither these state initiatives nor the AMA proposal go so far as to advocate a market exchange for organs themselves (indeed, one would expect the price for life-saving organs to be much higher), an approach that would require explicit amendment of NOTA. At present, there appears to be little political support for a different approach to organ procurement advocated by some commentators, and in place in some countries[96]—a presumed-consent model that would vest in the state and community, through its medical personnel, a level of authority to retrieve organs without consent (and without a purchase price), so long as there is no objection from the decedent or family. Vesting ownership rights in the state or community would be a sea change from our firmly entrenched cultural commitment to individual autonomy and control, especially over one's own body.[97]

Significantly, legal bans on commercialization of the body are limited to transplantation. Neither the UAGA nor NOTA prohibit the sale of human tissues for research.[98] Thus, under current law, a sample source (or an authorized representative) could offer his or her organs or tissues to the highest bidder in the research community and an investigator could offer a sum of money for human tissue without fear of criminal prosecution. That neither federal nor state organ donation and procurement laws impose parallel rules and restrictions when human tissues and cells are to be used for research may suggest that the same factors that counsel a system of voluntary donation in organ transplantation lead to different conclusions when applied to research. It might also suggest that when the legal structure for the organ transplant system was developed, the possibility of a significant commercial market for the raw materials of human participant research was but a blip on the radar screen.

Blood, Semen, and Eggs for Sale. In marked contrast to the transfer of solid organs, neither federal nor state law prohibits transfer by sale of blood, semen, plasma, or other bodily fluids. A commercial market for each of these substances exists today. Each of us has not only a right of exclusive possession in our bodily fluids, but also the right to sell these substances for a profit.

The United States may be the only country that freely allows women to contract for the harvest and sale of their eggs to assist others to create a child. This practice is prohibited in many other countries; it is permitted in England only if the eggs sold are "leftover" from the woman's efforts to create her own child through in vitro fertilization.[99] In the United States, one need only check the local newspaper, especially in college towns, to see advertisements: "EGGS FOR SALE." One dramatic illustration of the absence of free market restrictions that captured national headlines in 1999–2000, was the creation of RonsAngels.com, a Web site auctioning eggs from fashion models to the highest bidder. (Sperm from fashion models was later added to the auction list.)

Though we are free to sell our blood (most often, of course, we choose to donate to blood banks or hospitals), the law does not straightforwardly see such transactions as sales of bodily commodities. Under state anatomical gift laws and state adoptions of the Uniform Commercial Code (UCC), a body of law that governs a variety of commercial transactions, paid transfers usually are characterized as transfers of services, not as the sale of goods. State law often reinforces the service model with respect to transactions in blood and blood products. For example, the California law states that "the procurement, processing, distribution, or use of whole blood, plasma, blood products, and blood derivatives for the purpose of injecting or transfusing the same . . . into the human body shall be construed to be . . . for all purposes whatsoever, the rendition of a service . . . and shall not be construed to be . . . a sale of such whole blood, plasma, blood products, or blood derivatives."[100] As observed by OTA, the primary rationale is to avoid application of certain doctrines of liability. If transfers of these sorts were understood as a sale of goods, they might be subject to product liability litigation or implied warranty claims under the UCC.[101] This understanding is reinforced in several cases involving transfusions of blood contaminated with HIV[102] or hepatitis,[103] where courts have consistently held that blood transfusions are services, not transactions for the sale of goods.

Disposition of Frozen Embryos. The 1990s saw the emergence of new controversies over rights to transfer and dispose of cryopreserved embryos (or, sometimes, "preembryos"). Insofar as these disputes have been about rights of control over a tangible thing (the frozen embryo), they resonate as disputes over property rights. On the other hand, courts have thus far been reluctant to characterize embryos as property and have looked to resolve these controversies on alternative grounds. Some of this reluctance can be attributed to the fact that these cases raise unique moral and policy issues regarding an embryo's status as "person" or "property."

Best known is the *Davis v. Davis* case, in which a Tennessee couple divorced, and then asked a court to decide whether seven frozen embryos created during their marriage should be released to the former wife for the purpose of implantation (her original position) or maintained in their cryopreserved state (his original position).[104] By the time the case reached the Tennessee Supreme Court, both partners had remarried, and both had changed their positions. The wife had decided she no longer wanted implantation for herself, but would like to donate the embryos to a childless couple; the husband opposed donation and insisted that the embryos be destroyed.[105]

The Tennessee Supreme Court concluded that "the preembryos are not, strictly speaking, either "persons" or "property," but occupy an interim category that entitles them to special respect because of their potential for human life."[106] Though each partner had certain ownership interests in the preembryos, neither had "a true property interest."[107] The court's ruling rested on analysis of constitutionally protected rights of privacy and reproductive freedom, not property (which the court characterized as "not an altogether helpful question").[108] Finding that the right to procreate entails, and deserves, the same respect as the right not to procreate, the court found the husband's interest in avoiding parenthood to outweigh the wife's altruistic intentions. It ordered that the fertility clinic be permitted to follow its normal procedures for disposition of "unused preembryos" (provided this did not violate the husband's rights not to become a father).[109]

Courts in New York, New Jersey, and Massachusetts have been asked to resolve similar disputes. In the New York case of *Kass v. Kass,*[110] prior to divorce, the couple had signed a consent form provided by the hospital expressly stating that in the event of dissolution of their marriage, any remaining frozen embryos would be donated to the IVF program. Finding no ambiguity in the couple's intent, the court ordered that custody of the embryos go to the IVF program, not to the wife for possible future attempts at pregnancy.

The Supreme Judicial Court of Massachusetts in *A.Z. v. B.Z.,* also concluded that a couple's prior agreement for future disposition should be enforced. The court, however, said that this couple's prior "agreement" was ambiguous, in part because it was embodied in a series of consent forms (sometimes completed only by the wife), not a formal contract. Echoing *Davis,* the court refused to compel the ex-husband to become a father against his will and suggested that even if the prior agreement to allow implantation and procreation were clear and valid, it would not be binding and enforceable if the man later changed his mind and refused his permission.[111] The New Jersey Supreme Court reached a similar result in *J.B. v. M.B.,* holding that, in the absence of an enforceable contract, the ex-husband did not have the right to direct that the remaining frozen preembryos be donated to another couple, a result that would compel the ex-wife to become a genetic parent against her will.[112]

In an unusual twist, a Virginia couple found themselves litigating their rights to their frozen embryo with the fertility center. In *York v. Jones*[113] the couple sought interinstitutional transfer of their remaining frozen embryo from the Jones Institute in Virginia to a fertility center near their new home in California. The agreement with the institute did not contemplate transfer of unused embryos to another facility. Due to the procedural posture of the case and an agreement to settle the matter, no decision was ultimately rendered, but the court's ruling suggests that the institute might well have had a duty to release the frozen embryo to the couple as bailors (holders in trust) of their personal property.[114] Pursuant to the terms of the settlement agreement, the institute did release the frozen embryo to the couple, who transported it by plane to California, where it was to be implanted in the hope of a successful pregnancy.[115]

Few in number, the frozen embryo cases do not represent a clear trend. Yet a consistent message is that each gamete contributor and the fertility clinic have property-like interests in cryopreserved embryos. The embryos are tangible things that can and should be the subject of an agreement setting forth the respective rights of the parties. However, the extent of property—as opposed to personal—rights in frozen embryos is unclear. Courts have not ruled, for example, on whether embryos can be sold like the gametes that created them. The prevailing model among fertility clinics for disposition of "leftover" embryos in the absence of prior agreement is one of adoption or donation, not commerce.

Gene Patenting

Important features of ownership of biological materials have been and will continue to be determined under the federal patent law, administered and enforced by the U.S. Patent and Trademark Office (PTO). This section describes the basic features of the law of patents and identifies some of the most salient issues in the area of "gene patenting."

Under U.S. patent law (we will not discuss international patent law), "[w]hoever invents or discovers any new and useful process, machine, manufacture, or composition of matter, or any new and useful improvement thereof, may obtain a patent [on the invention or discovery]."[116] The holder of a patent enjoys "the right to *exclude* others from making, using, offering for sale, or selling" the thing that is patented without the patent holder's permission. A patent holder thereby also acquires freedom from (direct) competition in the effort to make, use, or sell the patented invention, as well as the right to convey some but not all rights of ownership such as through a license or other forms of permission that might be arranged by contract.[117] Patent rights last for 20 years[118] and may sometimes be extended. For example, a company may be entitled to an extension when approval of a regulatory agency (perhaps the FDA) is pending for a number of years, resulting in substantial loss of market opportunities.[119]

These broad patent rights have their foundation in Article I, section 8, of the U.S. Constitution, which grants Congress broad power to "promote the Progress of Science and useful Arts, by securing for limited Times to Authors and Inventors the exclusive Right to their respective Writings and Discoveries." Consistent with this Constitutional mandate, the panoply of rights carved out by the patent law is designed to encourage individual and institutional pursuit of research and development, and to serve the public interest in new knowledge, new products and processes of manufacture, and economic and social progress. The public purpose of the patent law is also evident in the obligations of inventors to contribute to the "public storehouse" of knowledge by publicly disclosing the invention so that others "skilled in the art" may benefit from it,[120] a requirement that has been characterized as a "quid pro quo" for enjoyment of this cluster of rights.[121]

For something to be patentable, it must be novel, nonobvious, and have a utility, that is, it must do something. At first glance it may seem that one cannot, therefore, patent genes, since genes and DNA sequences that exist in nature can hardly be said to be novel. Indeed, as a general matter, the law does not allow patenting of "products of nature." For the same reasons, it may seem that one cannot patent things that depend on or are comprised of living matter, nor should one be able to patent the discovery of a gene in the form in which it already exists in the human body.

A brief overview of the history of DNA itself suggests some of the difficulty in applying these rules to scientific "discoveries." When DNA was first isolated in a pure form by Johann Meischer in the 1800s, it led to a number of seminal discoveries. Theodor Boveri first described the phenomena of chromosomes, the essential units of inheritance (also in the 1800s). The experiments of Fred Griffith, Oswald Avery, and Maclyn McCarty (1900s), and Colin MacLeod (1940s) demonstrated that DNA could confer genetic information. And, of course, in 1953, the classic descriptive work of James Watson and Francis Crick hypothesized a structure for DNA that was consistent with inherited principles and, for the first time, tied together structure and function. In the 1960s, the work of Gobind Khorana and Marshall Nirenberg identified the essential elements of the genetic code and how information from DNA was transcribed and translated into protein.[122] At any one of these steps (and there are other examples), one could argue that the essential finding or discovery might have contained patentable information and that it provided and conferred "utility." Yet each seems to be a discovery of something already existing in nature and therefore not patentable.

These criteria have not been impediments to patenting biotechnology inventions that use genetic material, largely because what is being patented involves something new and useful that is created by the researcher. The leading case interpreting application of the patent law to biotechnology is *Diamond v. Chakrabarty*,[123] decided by the U.S. Supreme Court in 1980. In *Chakrabarty*, a microbiologist employed by the General Electric company introduced genetic material from naturally occurring bacterial plasmids into a living microorganism to create a bacteria that would break down crude oil. He applied for a patent (assigned to General Electric) for "a human-made, genetically-engineered bacterium ... capable of breaking down multiple components of crude oil," a property not possessed by any naturally occurring bacteria. The bacterium was thought to be of potential value in cleaning up oil spills. Initially the patent officer rejected the claim for a patent on the bacterium itself, ruling that microorganisms are not patentable subject matter because they are both living things and products of nature, a decision upheld by the Patent Office Board of Appeals.[124] The Supreme Court disagreed, ruling that the researcher had created (manufactured) something from raw materials by giving these materials new forms and properties. He had "produced a new bacterium with markedly different characteristics from any found in nature and one having potential for significant utility. His discovery is not nature's handiwork, but his own; accordingly it is patentable subject matter...." Moreover, the terms "manufacture" and "composition of matter" are to be construed to include living things; hence it is no impediment to a patent application that the thing to be patented is a living organism.[125]

Subsequent legal developments, following a similar path,[126] fill out a legal landscape that invites what has been called the "genetic gold rush."[127] As of this writing, approximately 1,000 patents for human gene uses have been issued by the PTO. Thousands of other patent applications are currently pending.[128] The precise nature of these numerous patents, issued and pending, is too varied and complex to recite. A critical point, however, is that each application must satisfy the criteria of patentability set forth above. In particular, the patent applicant must demonstrate *human contribution* and *inventiveness, novelty, and utility.* Often this means, in the words of the *Chakrabarty* decision, giving raw genetic materials "new forms and properties."

The PTO has revised the criteria by which its examiners will evaluate the utility of the invention for which patent application is made. The revised criteria state that an invention has a well-established utility if its use is "specific, substantial, and credible."[129] The impact of these new rules remains to be seen; some believe they will make it more difficult to obtain gene patents, others that the PTO has simply restated already existing standards. Possibly, their greatest impact will be in pressing researchers to be more specific about what their inventions are likely to do, perhaps discouraging applications that make general claims such as "a 'gene' will be useful as a marker of disease or in diagnosing whatever disease may later be found to be associated with it."[130]

Much has been made about the idea of patenting another person's DNA. Alarming assertions that the patent code covers "your genes" and that "you've already been sold" have appeared in the press.[131] It has even been suggested that a person whose genome includes a patented gene could be guilty of patent infringement. Despite the hype, as should be clear from the foregoing description of gene patenting, extant law does not allow anyone else to patent *my* DNA, nor may anyone patent the human genome as it naturally occurs in the human species. Watson and Crick may have discovered the biological structure of DNA, but they did not patent it. Neither investigators in the NIH-sponsored Human Genome Project nor Craig Venter and Celera Genomics hold patents on the map of the human genome itself. Patents have been and will continue to be granted when researchers give raw genetic materials, such as those obtained from stored tissue samples, new forms and properties that do not naturally occur in nature, with specific, substantial, and credible utility. As summarized by the PTO, "A patent on a gene covers the isolated and purified gene but does not cover the gene as it occurs in nature. Thus, the concern that a person whose body "includes" a patented gene could infringe the patent is misfounded. The body does not contain the patented, isolated and purified gene because genes in the body are not in the patented, isolated and purified form."[132]

Finally, we disagree with the *Moore* majority's conclusion that a patent award cuts off all property rights of the sample source. Our conclusion is not based on an interpretation of the law of patents.[133] Rather, it is based on the view that *defining the property rights of the sample source is a logically prior,* and in many respects *distinct question* from whether a researcher satisfies the criteria of patentability. Investigators and IRBs should confront questions of ownership and subsequent rights of sample sources at the time samples are collected. Depending on the circumstances, the potential patentability of material, information, and products derived from a genetic research protocol may be an important piece of a larger set of disclosures about an investigator's commercial interests that should be disclosed in the informed consent process.

Privacy of Genetic and Other Health Information

The state of the law governing genetic privacy and the risks of genetic discrimination are relevant to biomedical research in at least three significant ways. First, though investigators are not obligated to quote chapter and verse about existing law, fulfilling the duty of confidentiality and making accurate representations about the bounds of this promise require a basic familiarity with the legal terrain. Second, the legal landscape necessarily informs IRB judgments whether the research protocol poses minimal risk and the shaping of informed consent requirements. Last, as observed elsewhere, concerns about privacy and discrimination may play a pivotal role in a potential participant's willingness to enroll in a research study.

Federal Law. A small but important body of case law has recognized a right of *informational* privacy under the U.S. Constitution. In *Whalen v. Roe* (1977),[134] the U.S. Supreme Court upheld a New York law requiring physicians to disclose to the state health department information about prescriptions for specified drugs with a high risk for abuse. The Court acknowledged that electronic storage of large amounts of health information by the government posed a threat to privacy, finding that rights against unwarranted disclosure "arguably has its roots in the Constitution."[135] Three years later, a federal appeals court articulated a balancing test to determine the scope of the Constitutional right of informational privacy.[136] A number of other courts have found such a right in either the federal or their state constitutions.[137] Collectively, these cases articulate an important constitutional grounding of the right of informational privacy, one that extends to electronic records and databases. The Constitutional right of informational privacy, however, is limited in at least three significant ways: (*1*) it protects individuals against governmental, but not private, disclosures; (*2*) cases have tended to limit the right to particular circumstances; and (*3*) courts have generally been deferential to the government's need to gather and use information for public health or other purposes.[138]

The primary source of specific protections against unauthorized disclosure of personal health information is statutory law. Several important federal laws are pieces of this patchwork. The Privacy Act of 1974[139] regulates transfers of personal information, including health data, by government entities and expressly prohibits disclosures of personal information from records kept by federal agencies or its contractors without prior written permission of the individual. The Freedom of Information Act[140] mandates that various government records be available to the public, but shields certain medical records from disclosure. All Medicare- and Medicaid-participating healthcare providers are required to maintain the confidentiality and privacy of patient records.[141] And, as discussed previously, federal regulations impose duties of confidentiality in research and authorize Certificates of Confidentiality that may shield research information from administrative and court-ordered disclosures.

These laws offer important protections, but they also have significant limitations. Several apply only to government or government-supported actions. Enacted at different times and for different purposes, they fail to establish strong and uniform privacy protections. Moreover, enforcement of these rights is sometimes problematic and relatively untested. As Larry Gostin and colleagues conclude, "Privacy protection is fragmented and inconsistent with major gaps in coverage.... [A] patchwork of federal and state laws and judicial theories prescribe narrow privacy protections for selected types of individual health information or information held by certain entities."[142] Currently, there is no law or combination of laws that guarantees health information privacy.[143]

The Health Insurance Portability and Accountability Act of 1996[144] holds the promise of more significant, uniform privacy protections. HIPAA is perhaps best known for its efforts to improve access to and portability of health insurance (hence the title of the act), but it also promulgates new privacy and security standards for use of and access to individual health information. A core focus of HIPAA is to standardize electronic storage and transmission of PHI, in particular, information created and transmitted in connection with financial transactions in health care. The law also applies to protected health information that is not kept or communicated electronically. Information is only protected if it is "Individually Identifiable Health Information," that is, information that identifies, or reasonably could be believed to identify, an individual and in any way concerns that individual's health status, health care, or payments for his or her health care, whether in electronic or other form.[145] "Covered Entities," defined as health plans, health care providers, and health care clearinghouses (health information data processors) that engage in claims-type electronic transactions are directed to adopt policies and practices to comply with the privacy standards. Other entities doing business with a covered entity that involves disclosure of PHI are required to enter into a written agreement to be bound by HIPAA's privacy and security protections.[146]

HIPAA itself does not set forth a comprehensive plan to ensure health information privacy. Rather, Congress was directed to enact comprehensive legislation to accomplish this task by August 21, 1999 (three years after HIPAA's enactment); alternatively, should Congress fail to act, HHS was mandated to adopt implementing regulations by February 21, 2000. When Congress failed to meet its self-imposed deadline, HHS stepped in, proposing regulations to fill the void in November 1999. Final rules (known as the Privacy Rule) were adopted August 14, 2002, and took effect April 14, 2003.[147]

Under the basic scheme of the Privacy Rule, consent for use and disclosure of PHI—in the form of a written authorization—is required, unless it is for "routine" health care purposes, defined as treatment, payment, and health care operations.[148] Use or disclosure of PHI is subject to a requirement that "reasonable efforts" be made to limit the exchange of PHI to the "minimum necessary to accomplish the intended purpose."[149] As noted in Chapter 6, PHI is broadly defined as information that identifies an individual or "with respect to which there is a reasonable basis to believe the information can be used to identify the individual," if it relates to an individual's past, present, or future physical or mental health, including individually identifiable genetic information, whether derived from testing or family history, or relates to the provision of health care or payment for health care services.[150] Note that the Privacy Rule does not supplant existing law or practice. Numerous state laws and hospital policies call for written consent to a variety of diagnostic and therapeutic interventions, in particular surgical or other invasive procedures. The Privacy Rule "allows consent requirements already in place to continue."[151]

The rules bring a broad mandate for health care providers, institutions, and, to some extent, health plans to give patients written notice of their privacy practices and of patients' privacy rights and prescribe a standard form for doing so. Among the specifically enumerated rights are the right to request restrictions on disclosure, to receive detailed notice and an accounting of disclosures that are made, and to amend one's personal health record. These "rights," however, are subject to various exceptions and seem to give the holder of the information substantial discretion whether to comply with a patient's request.[152] It remains to be seen whether they impose meaningful and enforceable obligations.

As previously noted, HIPAA directs IRBs to expressly consider research participants' privacy interests and the risks of unwanted, unauthorized access to personal health information, including genetic information, in oversight and (dis)approval of research. Thus, investigators and IRBs alike should familiarize themselves with the larger meaning of the Privacy Rule beyond its immediate application to research. HIPAA compliance programs at the institutional level should include a broad look at the Privacy Rule in the approach to compliance and education in the research environment.

HIPAA establishes a floor for protection of health information, not a ceiling. HIPAA's minimum uniform standards do not preempt other federal or state laws, or professional standards, that may impose more stringent obligations to obtain consent or protect privacy than are mandated by HIPAA, as long as they do not conflict with HIPAA protections. Privacy standards "shall not supersede a contrary provision of state law, if the provision of state law imposes requirements, standards, or implementation specifications that are more strict than [those of the Privacy Rule]."[153] Thus, a more complete picture of privacy rights and protections must include state law.

Health Information Privacy in the Laboratory of the States. While several courts have recognized a right of informational privacy under their states' constitutions,[154] as with federal law the most important sources of privacy rights and protections are typically found in state statutes. According to a comprehensive, 50-state survey conducted by the Georgetown University-based Health Privacy Project, laws relating in some fashion to health information privacy are numerous and varied. Typically *state privacy laws* (sometimes termed *confidentiality laws*) are directed either to particular entities (the government, hospitals, physicians, insurance companies) or seek to regulate disclosure of information about particular health conditions (mental illness, cancer, HIV/AIDS). "[E]nacted at different points in time, over many years, to address a variety of uses and public health concerns," few laws can be said to provide a comprehensive privacy scheme.[155]

We narrow our focus to the approximately 25 states with statutes governing access, use, and disclosure of *genetic* information. The common theme of these laws is to protect privacy by requiring an individual's express authorization (consent) to obtain, use, or share identifiable genetic information. As summarized in Table 7.1, numerous states require consent to disclosure of genetic information; some (e.g., Florida, Georgia, Massachusetts, New York) also restrict access, mandating written consent for genetic testing. Some have chosen not to legislate consent to testing (California, Delaware, Maryland); only a handful have enacted a law in this area that does not require specific consent for disclosure of genetic information (Michigan, Nebraska, South Dakota). Slightly more than half of these state laws attempt to give teeth to privacy rights, imposing specific penalties for privacy violations. All carve out exceptions to the consent requirement, typically when the testing or information is for a criminal investigation, determination of paternity, pursuant to court order, or part of a newborn screening program. Some states (e.g., New Jersey) expressly exempt anonymous research, or research that is "not identified with the person or person's family" (New Mexico).

New York's privacy protections are among the strongest. New York mandates that "no person shall perform a genetic test . . . without the prior written informed consent of [the] individual;" specifies eight categories of disclosures to be included in the consent form, including the identities of those to whom test results "may be disclosed"; states that "[a]ll records, findings and results of any genetic test performed on any person shall be deemed confidential and shall not be disclosed without the written informed consent of the [individual];" and imposes penalties for violations.[156] A similar approach can be found in Massachusetts, New Jersey, and some other states.

Table 7.1 State genetic privacy statutes[157]

STATE	CONSENT FOR TESTING REQUIRED	CONSENT FOR DISCLOSURE REQUIRED	SPECIFIC PENALTIES FOR PRIVACY VIOLATIONS
Arizona	Yes	Yes	No
California	No	Yes	Yes
Colorado	No	Yes	Yes
Delaware	No	Yes	Yes
Florida	Yes	Yes	Yes
Georgia	Yes	Yes	Yes
Hawaii	No	Yes	No
Illinois	Yes	Yes	Yes
Louisiana	No	Yes	Yes
Maryland	No	Yes	No
Massachusetts	Yes	Yes	Yes
Michigan	Yes	No	No
Missouri	No	Yes	Yes
Nebraska	Yes	No	No
Nevada	No	Yes	Yes
New Hampshire	No	Yes	No
New Jersey	Yes	Yes	Yes
New Mexico	Yes	Yes	Yes
New York	Yes	Yes	Yes
Oregon	No	Yes	Yes
Rhode Island	No	Yes	No
South Carolina	Yes	Yes	Yes
South Dakota	Yes	No	No
Texas	No	Yes	No
Utah	Yes	Yes	Yes
Vermont	Yes	Yes	Yes
Virginia	No	Yes	No

These laws embrace an important commitment to genetic privacy and the right of individuals to control access to personal genetic information. In contrast to many state privacy laws on the books, one salutary feature of genetic privacy laws is that they typically apply to private individuals and businesses, not just to governmental entities. Still, these laws have important limitations. The nature and scope of rules governing access and disclosure vary considerably among the states. Many of these laws are directed only to insurance companies and health plans (e.g., Arizona, California, Maryland); some also apply to employers. Thus, while restricting access to information offers a measure of privacy, some states have focused more narrowly on shielding their citizens against discrimination. (Genetic nondiscrimination laws are discussed separately below.) In addition, some laws mandate consent for redisclosure of genetic information (Illinois); some limit retention of information without consent (New Jersey, New Mexico); many are silent on these matters. While many use broad definitions of genetic testing and genetic information to define the scope of what is protected, some states limit privacy protections to presymptomatic predictive testing and make an exception for testing and information related to diagnosis or treatment of an existing condition (Michigan). Family history is conspicuously absent in many states as a class of protected information.

To summarize, federal health privacy law is *a patchwork of incomplete protections*. State laws governing health information privacy sometimes provide stronger protections but are "uneven terrain," offering citizens of some states greater privacy than others. Although many existing protections for health information generally should apply as well to genetic information, almost half of states have also carved out specific rules for genetic information, adding our genes to the list of "conditions" deserving of special protection. These important pieces of the fabric of the law also leave numerous holes, not the least of which is that fewer than half of states have addressed the question. The fragmented nature of health information privacy law evidences the need for *a comprehensive, national approach that includes genetic privacy*.[158] Over the past several years, Congress has considered a number of more narrow bills to provide national privacy protection for genetic information (sometimes labeled "genetic exceptionalism"). In the fall of 2003, one bill has passed the Senate by an overwhelming 95–0 margin, but as of this writing none have been enacted.[159] That extant law does not guarantee that personal genetic information will be kept private and shared with others only with the consent of the individual heightens concerns about how those with access to genetic information (e.g., lab personnel, insurance companies, employers) will use it—and whether the law shields us against unfair, discriminatory uses.

Genetic Discrimination: Health Insurance

By far the most prevalent concerns about genetic discrimination involve areas of access to the important social goods of health insurance and employment. For the millions of Americans who get their health insurance through employer-sponsored group health plans, the two may be closely linked. We first review pertinent laws addressing discriminatory use of genetic information in health insurance and then turn to employment decisions.

As with privacy law, legal protections against discriminatory use of genetic information in health insurance are *fragmented and uneven*. The primary concern is with access to insurance, hence access to care, both personally and for families. This concern is sometimes expressed by patients in genetics clinics and clients in genetic counseling programs who choose to pay out-of-pocket for genetic tests and services, lest their health insurance companies learn about their genetic conditions and terminate coverage or raise premiums. Likewise, the concern about health insurance is sometimes voiced by research participants, who fear that information about their participation in a genetics study will get into their medical record and thereby become accessible to their health plan.

Federal Law. HIPAA establishes for the first time a national shield against some aspects of genetic discrimination. It prohibits use of genetic information to impose preexisting condition exclusions, except under narrow circumstances. To its credit, the law uses the broad term "genetic information," avoiding the pitfalls of more limited terms like "genetic testing" or "DNA testing." Under HIPAA, *asymptomatic genetic status* does not count as a "condition" that insurance companies may consider to impose coverage limitations, regardless of the manner in which genetic information is obtained.[160]

Still, the reach of the federal law is limited. An analysis undertaken by HHS in 1997, shortly after HIPAA's enactment, identifies a number of shortcomings. HIPAA applies only to group insurance plans, offering no protection to many family and small businesses or to purchasers of individual plans. Though only approximately 5% of the population buys health insurance in the individual market, this gap also affects those of us participating in employer-sponsored group plans who may move to the individual market with a change of job or retirement. HIPAA prohibits differential treatment within a group, but does not prohibit increased premiums for all members of the group based on the genetic characteristics of a small number of group members. Thus, group health plans may not exclude particular members of the group (company employees) on the basis of their genes, but all participants may be asked to subsidize the increased health risks of those with genetic predispositions. Finally, HIPAA does not prohibit companies from asking insurance applicants to disclose personal genetic information and family history or requiring genetic testing as a condition of insurability. Nor does it prevent insurance company access to genetic information; in most cases disclosure to one's health plan will be with consent of the individual in order to obtain coverage and payment to the provider. These shortcomings led HHS to recommend additional, more comprehensive legislation.[161]

Insurance Regulation under State Law. For the most part, health insurance regulation is a matter of state law. More than 30 states have enacted some form of legislation that prohibits or restricts health insurance discrimination on the basis of genetic status. (States typically have not regulated use of genetic information in life and disability insurance underwriting.) These laws vary considerably from state to state, affording important protections to some citizens in some parts of the country, but leaving significant loopholes that disadvantage residents elsewhere.

Most states ban the use of genetic information to establish rules for eligibility (such as preexisting condition exclusions). Most also restrict risk classification (rate setting) based on genetic test results, but there are numerous exceptions. A number of states (e.g., California, Connecticut, Virginia) extend these protections to genetic information obtained from genetic tests of individuals and family members, as well as other information about inherited characteristics. Others apply more narrowly to genetic testing of the individual (Alabama, Arizona). Most states appear to permit insurance companies to obtain and use genetic information in applicant questionnaires. Many of these laws apply to both group and individual policies; some (Iowa, Texas) only apply to one or the other insurance market. Few prohibit premium adjustments based on genetic status.

As we saw in the discussion of privacy, few states expressly restrict sharing of genetic information with others, such as insurance companies, the Medical Information Bureau, or employers. A number of states require informed consent for genetic testing, but some seem to allow companies to deny coverage if consent is withheld. Thus, like HIPAA, many states currently leave the door open to what amounts to coerced consent to disclosure of genetic information, that is, applicants are not required to disclose personal and family history nor to submit to genetic testing, but they may be unable to obtain health insurance if they do not.[162]

It is too early to tell whether state laws against genetic discrimination will make a meaningful difference. As noted in Chapter 2, some question whether genetic discrimination is a real problem that occurs with any frequency. It has been suggested, for example, that these laws may do little to prevent or to punish genetic discrimination. But they may serve an important deterrent function by making the practice not only unlawful but socially illegitimate.[163]

Genetic Discrimination: Genes in the Workplace

Federal Law. The most important potential source of federal protection against genetic discrimination for individuals in the workplace is the Americans with Disabilities Act (ADA). Title VII of the Civil Rights Act may offer another, limited source of legal rights for those who can establish that the nature of the discrimination is correlated with discriminatory treatment based on race, national origin, religion, or gender.[164] For example, one case, *Norman-Bloodsaw v. Lawrence Berkeley Laboratory,* holds that an employer's routine practice of testing its employees for syphilis, pregnancy, and (using genetic testing) for sickle-cell trait, a condition that disproportionately affects African Americans, may violate Title VII[165] (see a description of this case at the end of the chapter). Federal employees are shielded against discriminatory treatment based on genetic information pursuant to an Executive Order signed by President Clinton in February, 2000.[166]

Enacted in 1990 (the same year the Human Genome Project was launched), the ADA extends basic civil rights protections to persons with disabilities. Title I of the Act, which governs employment, prohibits employers from discriminating against qualified disabled persons on the basis of their disability. It imposes affirmative obligations to make "reasonable accommodations" to assist otherwise qualified applicants or employees to perform essential job functions, as long as requisite accommodations would not impose "undue hardship" on the employer (that is, "significant difficulty or expense").[167] The ADA applies to all employers, with the exception of private businesses with less than fifteen employees.[168]

Employers can gain access to genetic information if they choose to do so. The ADA prohibits mandatory medical screening (including examinations and inquiries) of all job applicants designed to determine whether applicants have a disability, or the nature or severity of disability. (Other types of inquiries are permitted if related to applicants' job qualifications, for example, the ability to use a computer or lift heavy objects, as are questions concerning infectious and communicable diseases, and drug and alcohol use.) But the ADA permits health examinations and inquiries of prospective employees if a conditional offer of employment has been made (preplacement exams), provided all prospective employees are treated the same without singling out individuals or groups with disabilities. For current employees, further medical examinations, including periodic exams, may be required, if "job-related and consistent with business necessity" (postplacement exams).[169]

The law is silent on the permissibility of genetic testing, but since a genetic test is a medical test administered by trained professionals, it seems clear that genetic tests and inquiries are permitted by the ADA under the same terms and conditions as other health inquiries and examinations. Where specific questions or tests are not imposed, genetic information may sometimes be revealed by medical records or family history. The ADA imposes duties of confidentiality and requires maintenance of separate files for medical information—rules that may provide some privacy protection outside the workplace—but this does not prevent employers from using this information in employment decisions.[170] Arguably, the preplacement process puts individuals at greatest risk. Once employment has been offered, medical examinations may be required—without limitations on the types of tests that may be performed—and individuals may be required to release their medical records. Refusal to comply may mean losing the job opportunity.[171]

Whether the ADA adequately protects individuals against genetic discrimination in employment looms as a large, unresolved question. Scholarly review of the legislative history has found scant evidence that Congress expressly intended for the ADA to apply to genetic information.[172] During legislative debates, several members of Congress asserted that one reason to vote for the law was that it would protect carriers of genetic conditions who were regarded as disabled. However, as Mark Rothstein concludes, on the whole, "Congress enacted the ADA without any serious consideration about the law's effect on individuals with various genetic conditions."[173]

To come within the protective reach of the law, an individual with a positive genetic test must fit within one of the three prongs of the definition of "disability." Individuals are disabled and entitled to protection if they (1) have "a physical or mental impairment that substantially limits one or more major life activities," (2) have a "record of such impairment," or (3) are "regarded as having such an impairment."[174] Clearly, the ADA applies to situations where a person has an illness or disability with a genetic component. Here, either of the first two definitions might apply; the genetic factor is essentially irrelevant once disability is manifest. The critical question is whether the "regarded as" clause applies to persons with *asymptomatic* genetic conditions under circumstances where (prospective) employers make adverse personnel decisions by treating someone as if he or she is currently disabled or will become disabled in the future. This would be discrimination on the basis of predicted future disability—the same issue that arises with insurance discrimination on the basis of genetic status.

The Equal Employment Opportunity Commission (EEOC), the agency responsible for administration, interpretation, and enforcement of the ADA, has twice issued policy guidance (1995 and 1998) contending that asymptomatic individuals with a gene predisposing to disease or illness are protected against discrimination under the "regarded as" clause.[175] (These statements reverse the position taken by the EEOC shortly after ADA enactment.)[176] As policy guidance, not embodied in statute or regulation, the EEOC position is not binding on a court, though it may be adopted as persuasive authority.

In 2001 the EEOC put its interpretation of the ADA to the test for the first time in a court action challenging genetic testing conducted by the Burlington Northern Santa Fe Railroad Company to determine employees' susceptibility to carpal tunnel syndrome. The lawsuit was brought in response to six formal employee complaints, including one that the railroad employees who made worker's compensation claims for carpal tunnel injuries were required to give blood samples that were subjected to genetic testing for predisposition to this syndrome, without their voluntary and informed consent and under threat of disciplinary action (including possible termination) for noncompliance.[177] The litigation was settled before trial. Under the terms of the settlement, the railroad agreed to pay $2.2 million in damages to 36 of its employees and to end its practice of blood sample collection for genetic testing.[178]

Burlington Northern makes an important statement about the EEOC's desire to extend the ADA's umbrella to genetic discrimination. Nonetheless, settlement of this case prior to trial does little to resolve uncertainty surrounding the issue. Pending resolution of this issue by the U.S. Supreme Court, or congressional amendment of the ADA (a path suggested by some commentators),[179] neither patients nor research participants can be assured of protection against genetic discrimination in the workplace under federal law.[180]

Even were definitive extension of the ADA's shield to instances of genetic discrimination imminent, other questions about when genetic discrimination *may be justified* remain. The ADA carves out a zone of justified discrimination in the workplace under the "direct threat" exception. Decisions not to hire or adverse job actions are permissible if based on "a significant risk of substantial harm" to the individual's health and safety or the health and safety of others, such as co-workers or the public, where the threat "cannot be eliminated or reduced by reasonable accommodation."[181] The Supreme Court recently ruled that an oil company could withdraw a conditional offer of employment to an applicant with a liver abnormality, based on the judgment of the company's physician that the individual's liver condition would be aggravated by continued exposure to toxins in the workplace.[182] This decision suggests that the ADA permits similar practices based on the results of genetic tests.

To illustrate, hypothetically, a chemical company might be within its rights to refuse to hire an applicant with the gene for glucose-6 phosphate dehydrogenase (G-6-PD) deficiency, a sex-linked, X-chromosome disorder that increases the risk of acute hemolysis from chemical exposures (harm to self).[183] Or an airline might be within its rights to dismiss a pilot diagnosed with the gene for sudden cardiac arrest (harm to others). Each such case (and many more possibilities likely will emerge with advances in predictive genetic testing) should be examined based on all the facts and circumstances, and would need to meet a heavy burden of proof establishing that the genetic test constitutes the "best available" objective evidence and supports the required finding of a "significant risk of substantial harm" likely to occur "imminently."[184]

Workplace Discrimination under State Law. Early state laws in this area singled out specific genetic traits or disorders for special protection. Florida and North Carolina are among the states that prohibit workplace discrimination against employees or job applicants with sickle-cell trait.[185] New York protects those with genetic markers for sickle-cell trait, Tay-Sachs disease, and beta-thalassemia against discrimination.[186] New Jersey adds hemoglobin C and cystic fibrosis to this list.[187]

Mostly in the 1990s, states began to enact more comprehensive legislation expressly intended to prohibit all forms of genetic discrimination in employment.[188] Today, more than half the states have such laws on the books. (Some, like New Jersey, have kept trait-specific laws on the books, while enacting more comprehensive protections.) In addition, many states prohibit genetic testing; virtually all do so in an effort to regulate how genetic information might be used in employment decisions. A number of states do both, as illustrated by Table 7.2, which summarizes the state of the law.

For workers in these states, these important protections fill a current void in ADA coverage. But like nondiscrimination in insurance laws, these laws need to be examined closely to assess both their strengths and limitations. Most of these laws should protect asymptomatic individuals against adverse employment decisions based on predicted future illness or disability. New York expressly prohibits discrimination based on "genetic predisposition or carrier status."[189] Iowa, Texas, Wisconsin, and several other states extend prohibitions against discrimination to labor organizations, employment agencies and licensing agencies.[190] Minnesota may have the tightest restrictions on employers' access to genetic information, stating that employers have lawful access only to "job-related" medical information.[191]

Table 7.2 Access to and use of genetic information in employment

STATE	BANS REQUIRED TESTING	BANS USE OF INFORMATION GENERALLY	OCCUPATIONAL QUALIFICATIONS/ OTHER EXCEPTIONS
Arizona	No	Yes	Yes
California	No	Yes	Yes
Connecticut	No	Yes	Yes
Delaware	Yes	Yes	Yes
Florida	Yes	Yes	Yes
Hawaii	No	Yes	Yes
Illinois	No	Yes	Yes
Indiana	Yes	Yes	Yes
Iowa	Yes	Yes	Yes
Kansas	Yes	Yes	No
Louisiana	No	Yes	Yes
Maine	No	Yes	Yes
Michigan	Yes	Yes	Yes
Missouri	No	Yes	Yes
Nebraska	Yes	Yes	Yes
Nevada	Yes	Yes	No
New Hampshire	Yes	Yes	Yes
New Jersey	No	Yes	No
New York	Yes	Yes	Yes
North Carolina	No	Yes	Yes
Ohio	Yes	Yes	Yes
Oklahoma	Yes	Yes	No
Oregon	Yes	Yes	Yes
Rhode Island	Yes	Yes	No
Tennessee	No	Yes	Yes
Texas	No	Yes	Yes
Utah	Yes	Yes	No
Vermont	No	Yes	Yes
Virginia	No	Yes	Yes
Wisconsin	Yes	Yes	Yes

Most states use a broad definition of genetic testing for abnormalities or deficiencies that includes "tests of genes, gene products, or chromosomes."[192] Yet some states appear to permit (because they do not prohibit) use of genetic information that comes to the employer by means other than direct testing (e.g., in medical records). Like the ADA, a number of state laws that ban use of genetic information make an exception if related to "occupational qualifications" (Connecticut, Maine, Ohio); others (Iowa, Wisconsin) expressly permit testing for susceptibility to workplace toxins. By contrast, the New Jersey law, hailed as one of the strongest, most comprehensive commitments to genetic privacy, appears to prohibit employers from taking these risks into account when making hiring and employment decisions.

In sum, employment discrimination law is more uniform—and more consistently strong—in its protections of individual rights than are privacy and insurance discrimination laws across the states. There are, however, important gaps in coverage, and a cloud of uncertainty concerning the protective reach of the ADA.

As much as the law has evolved in the quarter century since John Moore first met David Golde, the law, like the larger ethical and policy discourse, reveals many unanswered and unsettled questions. One consistent theme has been the extent to which *individuals should, through the mechanism of informed consent, control access to and use* of their bodily parts and tissues, and access, use, and disclosure of health information, including genetic information that our bodies reveal about us. Returning to the research setting, the next chapter offers another, policy-oriented perspective on these many questions, that of the National Bioethics Advisory Commission.

Cases and Vignettes

A legal dispute developed over the control of a gene for a rare disease that affects some Ashkenazi Jewish children. Prior to the legal battle, the case involved a father of two children suffering from Canavan disease—a fatal illness whose symptoms began three months after birth—and a scientist working at Miami Children's Hospital (MCH). Daniel Greenberg, the father, contacted the investigator, Reuben Matalon, and persuaded him to begin developing molecular probes that might locate the gene that causes Canavan disease. In this collaborative arrangement, Greenberg helped set up a registry of families affected by this disease and helped recruit tissue donors. The Canavan parents contributed $100,000 as partial funding for the research study. Matalon, in turn, succeeded in 1993 in finding the Canavan gene on chromosome 17, turned over his intellectual property rights to MCH, and later moved to a new position in another state. MCH obtained a patent on the gene sequence in 1997, began licensing a diagnostic test for the disease, and restricted access to the test. Feeling betrayed by MCH's commercial use of the Canavan gene, Greenberg and some other Canavan parents joined the Canavan Foundation and two other nonprofit groups in a federal lawsuit—the first time tissue donors have taken researchers (or an institution) to court for control of a gene.[193]

In 1998 the U.S. Court of Appeals for the 9th Circuit decided for the seven former and current employees who initiated legal action against the Lawrence Berkeley National Laboratory (LBNL). It was the first successful class-action lawsuit claiming discrimination and invasion of privacy related to genetic and other medical testing. The plaintiffs claimed that LBNL, by using stored blood samples to test some of its workers for pregnancy, sexually transmitted diseases, and sickle-cell trait without their consent, was guilty of discrimination (sexual, racial, and genetic) and invasion of privacy. As the legal opinion noted, "the conditions tested for were aspects of one's health in which one enjoys the highest expectations of privacy." LBNL denied the charges, claiming that the tests were part of comprehensive medical screening to which the employees had consented earlier. After 18 months of mediation, LBNL agreed in 2000 to a provisional $2.2 million class-action settlement, including $25,000 to each of the named plaintiffs and $2,000-$10,000 to other former and current employees.[194]

In 2001 hundreds of family members related to patients with Alzheimer disease sued Texas Tech University and the administrators connected with the medical school's Alzheimer DNA Bank. The suit claimed that the DNA Bank possessed approximately 10,000 blood samples from 2,200 families; it also had 150 brains, with 137 of the brains showing scientific signs of Alzheimer disease. Research at the DNA Bank had been suspended a year earlier because a number of required consent forms had been misplaced. University officials claimed that without the proper consent documents on file, research could not proceed, and the samples must be destroyed. The plaintiffs, many of whom had donated brains of their dead relatives to the DNA Bank and had backed the research with financial support, wanted the research to continue. Rather than permitting the blood samples and brains to be destroyed, they hoped to force the university to transfer the stored tissue samples to another university that will continue Alzheimer research.[195]

Notes

1. *Moore v. Regents of the University of California,* 51 Cal. 3d 120, 271 Cal. Rptr. 146, 793 P.2d 479, 501 (1990) (Broussard, J., concurring and dissenting), *cert. denied,* 499 U.S. 936 (1991).
2. U.S. Department of Health and Human Services, Report of the Secretary to the President, *Health Insurance in the Age of Genetics* (Washington, D.C.: HHS, 1997), p. 3.
3. Further discussion of many of the legal issues raised by genetic research can be found in the various references cited in this chapter. For a broader overview of legal issues in genetics, see Mark A. Rothstein, Maxwell J. Mehlman, and Lori B. Andrews, *Genetics: Ethics, Law and Policy* (Minneapolis: West, 2002); Bartha M. Knoppers, Timothy Caulfield, and Douglas Kinsella, eds., *Legal Rights and Human Genetic Material* (Toronto: Emond Montgomery Publications, 1996); and Bartha M. Knoppers, Claude Laberge, and Marie Hirtle, eds. *Human DNA: Law and Policy—International and Comparative Perspectives* (The Hague: Kluwer Law International, 1997).
4. See, for example, Richard Gold, *Body Parts: Property Rights and the Ownership of Human Biological Materials* (Washington, D.C.: Georgetown University Press, 1996); Sharon Nan Perley, "From Control Over One's Body to Control Over One's Body Parts: Extending the Doctrine of Informed Consent," *New York Univ Law Rev* 67 (1992): 335–65; and Bernard M. Dickens, "Living Tissue and Organ Donors and Property Law: More on Moore," *J Contemp Health Law Policy* 8 (1992): 73–93.
5. 51 Cal. 3d 120, 271 Cal. Rptr. 146, 793 P.2d 479 (1990).
6. Beth Burrows, "Second Thoughts about U.S. Patent #4,438,032," *Genewatch* 10 (1996): 4.
7. *Moore,* 793 P.2d at 481.
8. *Ibid.*
9. Burrows, pp. 3–4.
10. *Moore,* 793 P.2d at 481.
11. *Ibid.* at 482, note 2.
12. *Ibid.* at 481–82. The patent is reproduced as Appendix A to the intermediate appellate court opinion, *Moore v. Regents of the University of California,* 249 Cal. Rptr. 494 (Ct. App. 2d Dist. 1988).
13. *Moore,* 793 P.2d at 481–83.

14. The consent form is reprinted in "Patient's Informed Consent—John Moore," *Biotechnology Law Report* 7 (1988): 425.
15. Burrows, pp. 4–5.
16. *Ibid.*, p. 5.
17. *Ibid.*
18. *Moore,* 793 P.2d at 482–83.
19. *Cobbs v. Grant,* 8 Cal. 3d 229, 104 Cal. Rptr. 505, 502 P.2d 1 (1972).
20. *Moore,* 793 P.2d at 483.
21. *Ibid.*
22. *Ibid.* at 484 and accompanying note 5.
23. *Magan Medical Clinic v. California State Board of Medical Examiners,* 57 Cal. Rptr. 256, 262 (Cal. App. 1967) (quoted in *Moore,* 793 P.2d at 483).
24. *Moore,* 793 P.2d at 483.
25. *Ibid.*
26. *Ibid.* at 487.
27. *Ibid.* at 488–89.
28. *Ibid.* at 489–90 and accompanying notes.
29. *Ibid.* at 492–93.
30. *Ibid.* at 493.
31. *Ibid.* at 495–96.
32. *Ibid.* at 497.
33. *Ibid.*
34. *Ibid.* at 496.
35. *Ibid.* at 499.
36. *Ibid.* at 515.
37. *Ibid.* at 503.
38. *Ibid.* at 511–12.
39. *Ibid.* at 505–06, n. 5; see 517–18.
40. *Ibid.* at 508.
41. *Ibid.* at 504–05.
42. *Ibid.* at 515.
43. *Ibid.* at 520.
44. *Ibid.*
45. See generally Robert W. McAdams and Mary L. Gallagher, *State and Federal Prohibitions on Physician Referrals: A Guide to Compliance* (Gaithersburg, Md.: Aspen Publishers, Inc., 1998).
46. 42 U.S.C. § 1395nn (2001).
47. Tracy Miller, "Managed Care Regulation: In the Laboratory of the States," *JAMA* 278 (1997): 1102–09.
48. But see *Greenberg v. Miami Children's Hosp. Research Institute,* 264 F. Supp. 2d 1064, 1070 (S.D. Fla. 2003) (declining to extend duty to disclose economic interests to researchers).
49. 45 C.F.R. § 46.116 (2001).
50. For discussion of the Hagiwara case, see Ivor Royston, "Cell Lines From Human Patients: Who Owns Them? A Case Report," *Clin Res* 33 (1985): 442–43; Leon E. Rosenberg, "Using Patient Materials for Product Development: A Dean's Perspective," *Clin Res* 33 (1985): 452–54; and U.S. Congress, Office of Technology Assessment, *New Developments in Biotechnology: Ownership of Human Tissues and Cells—Special Report,* OTA-BA-337 (Washington, D.C.: USGPO, 1987), pp. 4, 26. [hereafter OTA Report.]

51. *Greenberg,* 264 F. Supp. 2d at 1072–73.
52. Dan B. Dobbs, *The Law of Torts* (St. Paul, Minn.: West Group, 2000), pp. 125–26; Restatement (Second) of Torts § 22A (1965).
53. Restatement (Second) of Torts § 927 (1979).
54. *Ibid.*
55. OTA Report, pp. 79–82 (discussing cases).
56. *Moore,* 793 P.2d at 479.
57. This suggestion comes from *Miles, Inc. v. Scripps Clinic and Research Foundation,* 810 F. Supp. 1091, 1097–98 (S.D. Cal. 1993) (discussing *Moore*).
58. For an analysis of how conversion law might apply to biomedical research, see OTA Report, pp. 79–82, 84–86.
59. To be more precise, in American law there are three ways we commonly transfer property to another: (1) sale; (2) gift; and (3) gift after death such as by testamentary will. It is also possible to transfer or alter particular rights in property by contract or the creation of trust arrangements. Property also passes by operation of law, such as by intestate succession in the absence of a testamentary will, or in disposition of a bankruptcy. See generally R. G. Hammond, *Personal Property: Commentary and Materials* (Auckland: Oxford University Press, 1992), Ch. 7.
60. Stephen R. Munzer, *A Theory of Property* (Cambridge, U.K.: Cambridge University Press, 1990), pp. 22–27.
61. *Shelly v. Kraemer,* 334 U.S. 1 (1948); *Mayers v. Ridley,* 465 F.2d 630 (D.C. Cir. 1972).
62. Munzer, especially Chs. 2 and 3; Joseph Singer, *Introduction to Property* (Gaithersburg, Md.: Aspen, 2001), esp. Ch. 1.
63. Anita L. Allen, "Genetic Privacy: Emerging Concepts and Values," in Mark A. Rothstein, ed., *Genetic Secrets: Protecting Privacy and Confidentiality in the Genetic Era* (New Haven: Yale University Press, 1997), pp. 49–50.
64. George J. Annas, "Privacy Rules for DNA Databanks: Protecting Coded 'future diaries,' " *JAMA* 270 (1993): 2346–50.
65. OTA Report, p. 70.
66. Colo. Rev. Stat. § 10-3-1104.7(1)(a) (1999); Ga. Code Ann. § 33-54-1(1) (Michie 1996).
67. Fla. Stat. Ann. § 760.40(2)(a) (West 1997).
68. La. Rev. Stat. Ann. § 22:213.7 (West Supp. 2002).
69. N.J. Stat. Ann. §§ 10:5-44–5-49 (West Supp. 2002).
70. La. Rev. Stat. Ann. § 22:213.7(D) (West Supp. 2002).
71. *Ibid.*
72. Colo. Rev. Stat. § 10-3-1104.7(12) (1999); Ga. Code Ann. § 33-54-8 (Michie 1996).
73. Fla. Stat. Ann. § 760.40(2)(b) (West 1997).
74. La. Rev. Stat. Ann. § 213.7(F). Ordinary course of business dealings in connection with life, disability, income, and long-term care insurance are exempted from these penalties.
75. The law stated: "A person may not retain another individual's genetic information or DNA sample without first obtaining authorization from the individual or the individual's representative" unless specified exceptional circumstances are present. Among the exceptions were retention for purposes of enforcing the criminal law; pursuant to court order; under state health division rules for identification or testing for the benefit of living relatives of deceased individuals; and under rules for newborn screening. Or. Rev. Stat. § 659.715(3) (1995). Oregon's repeal and revision of this law, Or. Rev. Stat. §§ 192. 531 et seq. (2001), retains similar language.

76. *Ibid.* The earlier law provided that "[t]he DNA sample of an individual from which genetic information has been obtained shall be destroyed promptly upon the specific request of that individual or the individual's representative," subject to certain exceptions. *Ibid.*, § 659.715(4), repealed 2001. Here again, the 2001 law retained similar language to its predecessor. Other states have embraced a similar approach without importing the language of property.

77. *Ibid.*

78. Or. Rev. Stat. §§ 192. 531 et seq. (2001). Also see the Report of the Genetic Research Advisory Committee, "Assuring Genetic Privacy in Oregon," November 15, 2000, pp. 8–9. Available through the Geneforum Web site: www.geneforum.org/learnmore/gp/or_gpa.cfm (visited May 2002).

79. National Bioethics Advisory Commission, *Research Involving Human Biological Materials: Ethical Issues and Policy Guidance* (Rockville, Md.: National Bioethics Advisory Commission, 1999), p. 2.

80. This form, "Consent for Operation or Procedure," is used at the University of Iowa Hospitals and Clinics.

81. *American Jurisprudence* 2d, vol. 1, "Abandoned, Lost, and Unclaimed Property," §1 (1994). Numerous other sources also stress the centrality of a person's intention to terminate ownership rights and not to transfer ownership to another.

82. Lisa A. Jensen, "Medical Waste Regulation in the United States," *Natural Resources & Environment* 9 (1994): 21–46.

83. *Browning v. Norton-Children's Hospital,* 504 S.W.2d 713 (Ky. 1974).

84. *United States v. Cox,* 428 F.2d 683 (7th Cir. 1970).

85. 367 A.2d 949 (Ct. App. Md. 1977).

86. *Venner v. Maryland,* 354 A.2d 483, 498–99 (Ct. Spec. App. 1976).

87. Lori Andrews and Dorothy Nelkin, *Body Bazaar: The Market for Human Tissue in the Biotechnology Age* (New York: Crown Publishers, 2001). See also Andrew Kimbrell, *The Human Body Shop: The Engineering and Marketing of Life* (San Francisco: Harper Collins Publishing, 1993).

88. Michael Walzer, *Spheres of Justice: A Defense of Pluralism and Equality* (New York: Basic Books, 1983).

89. Alexander M. Capron, "Reexamining Organ Transplantation," *JAMA* 285 (2001): 334–36.

90. This language, quoted from *N.Y. Pub. Health Law* § 4301 (McKinney 2002), mirrors that enacted across the country.

91. 42 U.S.C. § 274e (2000). Numerous states have similar provisions.

92. For a concise summary of the evolution of law governing organ donation, see Capron, note 89.

93. For discussion of various proposals for reform, including a commercial market, see Monique C. Gorsline and Rachelle L.K. Johnson, "The United States System of Organ Donation, The International Solution, and the Cadaveric Organ Donor Act: 'And the Winner Is . . .' " *J Corp L* (1995): 6–50. For a range of views on the issue, both pro and con, see the essays in Part 3 of Arthur L. Caplan and Daniel H. Coelho, eds., *The Ethics of Organ Transplants: The Current Debate* (New York: Prometheus Books, 1998). The issue of commercialization of body parts is discussed further in Chapter 10.

94. See, e.g., 20 Pa. Cons. Stat. Ann. § 8622 (West Supp. 2001).

95. Report of the Council on Ethical and Judicial Affairs, American Medical Association, "Cadaveric Organ Donation: Encouraging the Study of Motivation," CEJA Report 1-A-02, adopted at the 2002 Annual Meeting of the AMA House of Delegates; Andis

Robeznieks, "Feds have final say on organ donor initiatives," *Am Med News* (July 22, 2002).

96. See Gorsline and Johnson, pp. 20–25.

97. For an informative and useful discussion of various conceptual approaches to transfer of organs for transplantation, see James F. Childress, *Practical Reasoning in Bioethics* (Bloomington: Indiana University Press, 1997), Chap. 14.

98. OTA Report, p. 76.

99. Rebecca Mead, "Eggs For Sale," *The New Yorker*, August 9, 1999, pp. 57–65.

100. Cal Health and Safety Code § 1606 (West 1990). See Gorsline and Johnson, pp. 11–12 and accompanying notes (noting that some courts have found the sale of blood to be the sale of a product for purposes of imposing products liability).

101. OTA Report, pp. 76–78.

102. For example, *Silva v. Southwest Florida Blood Bank,* 601 So.2d 1184 (Fla. 1992); *Bradway v. American National Red Cross,* 263 Ga. 19, 426 S.E.2d 849 (1993).

103. For example, *Zichichi v. Middlesex Memorial Hospital,* 204 Conn. 399, 528 A.2d 805 (1987); *Kidder v. Savoy Medical Center,* 673 So.2d 210 (La. Ct. App. 1996).

104. *Davis v. Davis,* 842 S.W.2d 588 (Tenn. 1992), *cert. denied sub nom., Stowe v. Davis,* 507 U.S. 911 (1993).

105. *Ibid.* at 597.

106. *Ibid.*

107. *Ibid.* The trial court had found that the frozen embryos were "persons" with a right to life and that their future should be determined by application of a "best interests of the child" standard. *Davis v. Davis,* No. E-14496, 1989 WL 140495 (Tenn. Cir. Ct., Sept. 21, 1989).

108. 842 S.W.2d at 598.

109. *Ibid.* at 603–605.

110. 91 N.Y.2d 554, 673 N.Y.S.2d 350, 696 N.E.2d 174 (1998).

111. 431 Mass. 150, 725 N.E.2d 1051 (2000).

112. 170 N.J. 9, 783 A.2d 707 (2001).

113. 717 F. Supp. 421 (E.D. Va. 1989).

114. *Ibid.* at 425.

115. Starr Spencer, "Pair's hopes tied to embryo/Couple's custody battle over, now it's up to doctors," *Los Angeles Daily News,* September 27, 1989.

116. 35 U.S.C. § 101 (2001).

117. 35 U.S.C. § 271(a), 154(a)(1) (2001).

118. 35 U.S.C. § 154(2) (2001). The 20-year rule applies to most, but not all patents. "Design" patents are valid for a period of 14 years. 35 U.S.C. § 173 (2001).

119. 35 U.S.C. § 156 (2001).

120. *Ibid.,* § 112; *Application of Argoudelis,* 434 F.2d 1390, 1394–95 (C.C.P.A. 1970) (Baldwin, J., concurring).

121. *U.S. v. Dubilier Condenser Corp.,* 289 U.S. 178, 186–87 (1933). Stating that a patent is sometimes described as having a monopoly, *Dubilier* rejects this characterization, observing that the term *monopoly* usually refers to exclusive control over the "buying, selling, working, or using a thing which the public freely enjoyed prior to the grant." By contrast, the patent holder (inventor) creates something new that did not exist before in the public domain. In addition, if patent rights are akin to grant of a monopoly, patent law makes it a time-limited monopoly.

122. For some of the major scientists in the history of DNA, see this Web site: http://www. accessexcellence.org/AE/AEPC/WWC/1994/geneticsln.html.

123. 447 U.S. 303 (1980).

124. *Ibid.* at 306. The patent board found that the new bacteria were not products of nature because they were not naturally occurring, but agreed that as a living organism the bacteria was not patentable.

125. *Ibid.* at 308, 310 ff.

126. For a discussion of *Chakrabarty* and other legal authorities pertinent to patent protection for DNA sequences, see Rebecca S. Eisenberg, "Patenting the Human Genome," *Emory L J* 39 (1999): 721–45. Applying these same principles in a patent infringement action, the U.S. Supreme Court recently held that newly developed plant breeds are patentable subject matter. *J.E.M. AG Supply, Inc. v. Pioneer Hi-Bred International, Inc.*, 534 U.S. 124 (2001), *rehearing denied,* 535 U.S. 1013 (2002).

127. Andrews and Nelkin, *The Body Bazaar,* Ch. 3.

128. David Malakoff and Robert F. Service, "Genomania Meets the Bottom Line," *Science* 291 (2001): 1193–1203.

129. U.S. PTO, Dept. of Commerce, *Manual of Patent Examining Procedure,* 8th ed. (Aug. 2001), 2107(II)(B)(3), available at http://www.uspto.gov/web/offices/pac/mpep/mpep_e8_2100.pdf. This section of the manual also states that to pass muster under the "useful invention" criterion as having a well-established utility, the subject matter of the patent application must be such that "a person of ordinary skill in the art would immediately appreciate why the invention is useful based on the characteristics of the invention (e.g., properties or applications of a product or process)."

130. *Ibid.*

131. Wil S. Hylton, "Who Owns This Body?" *Esquire,* June 2001, p. 102.

132. 66(4) Fed. Reg. 1093 (2001).

133. It has been held that gene patents do not automatically cut off claims for unjust enrichment. *Greenberg,* 264 F. Supp. 2d at 1072 (citing *Chou v. Univ. of Chicago,* 254 F.3d 1347, 1363 (Fed. Cir. 2001)).

134. 426 U.S. 589.

135. *Ibid.* at 605.

136. *U.S. v. Westinghouse,* 638 F.2d 570 (3d Cir. 1980).

137. Lawrence O. Gostin, "Health Information Privacy," *Cornell L Rev* 80 (1995): 495–498 (discussing cases).

138. *Ibid.,* pp. 495–98.

139. 5 U.S.C. § 552 (1988).

140. 5 U.S.C. § 552 (1988).

141. 42 C.F.R. §§ 401, 482 (2001).

142. James G. Hodge, Lawrence O. Gostin, and Peter D. Jacobson, "Legal Issues Concerning Electronic Health Information: Privacy, Quality, and Liability," *JAMA* 282 (1999): 1467–68.

143. Others have reached the same conclusion. See, for example, American Health Lawyers Association, *Privacy of Health Information* (Washington, D.C.: AHLA, 2001), report; and John R. Christiansen, monograph, *Electronic Health Information: Privacy and Security Compliance Under HIPAA* (Washington, D.C.: AHLA, 2000).

144. Health Insurance Portability and Accountability Act (HIPAA), Pub. L. No. 104–191, 110 Stat. 2033 (1996) (codified in various sections of titles 18, 26, 29 and 42 of the United States Code).

145. 45 C.F.R. § 164.501 (2002); *Assoc. of American Physicians & Surgeons, Inc., v. U.S. Dept. of Health and Human Services,* 224 F. Supp. 2d 1115 (S.D. Tex. 2002).

146. Christiansen, *Electronic Health Information,* esp. ch. 2.

147. 45 C.F.R. § 164.501 et seq. (2002). The regulations discussed here supplanted those adopted as "final" by the Clinton administration on December 28, 2000. The cornerstone of the Clinton rules was a prohibition against disclosure of an individual's protected health information without prior written consent or authorization of that person, subject to certain exceptions or as required under other law. 65 Fed. Reg. 82462 (Dec. 28, 2000); codified at 45 C.F.R. Parts 160 and 164. Primarily due to this consent requirement, the Clinton administration rules were hailed as strong privacy protections. They also generated considerable debate and criticism. For discussion of the meaning of these rules for research, see Jennifer Kulynych and David Korn, "The Effect of the New Federal Medical-Privacy Rule on Research," NEJM 346 (Jan. 17, 2002): 201–04; George J. Annas, "Medical Privacy and Medical Research—Judging the New Federal Regulations," NEJM 346 (Jan. 17, 2002): 216–20. Following initial endorsement of the Clinton plan, the Bush administration proposed various modifications to the privacy rules; most importantly, to make it optional to obtain an individual's written consent prior to release of health information obtained in the course of treatment, payment or health care operations. The new proposed privacy rules, 67 Fed. Reg. 14775 (March 27, 2002), also stirred considerable controversy and generated substantial public comment prior to their August 2002 adoption.

148. 45 C.F.R. §§ 164.502, 506. Press release, HHS News, "HHS Issues First Major Protections for Patient Privacy," August 9, 2002, available at http://www.hhs.gov/news/press/2002pres/20020809.html; 45 C.F.R. § 164.502 (2002); Joanne L. Hustead and Janlori Goldman, "Genetics and Privacy," Am J Law Med 28 (2002): 289 (quoting the December 28, 2000, final rules).

149. 45 C.F.R. § 164.502(b).

150. Ibid., § 164.501.

151. See HHS Fact Sheet, "Modifications to the Standards for Privacy of Individually Identifiable Health Information—Final Rule," August 9, 2002, p.2, available at http://www.hhs.gov/news/press/2002pres/20020809.html (visited August 15, 2002).

152. 45 C.F.R. § 164.520.

153. 42 U.S.C. § 1320d-2 (Supp. 2002). See Christiansen, pp. 8–11.

154. Richard C. Turkington and Anita L. Allen, Privacy Law: Cases and Materials (Minneapolis: West, 1999), p. 125.

155. Joy Pritts, Janlori Goldman, Zoe Hudson, et al., "The State of Health Privacy: An Uneven Terrain (A Comprehensive Survey of State Health Privacy Statutes)," Practicing Law Institute, Patents, Copyrights, Trademarks, and Literary Property Course Handbook Series 607 (2000), pp. 630–31. For a national review of laws governing health care record confidentiality, see Lisa Dahm, 50-State Survey on Patient Health Care Record Confidentiality (Washington, D.C.: American Health Lawyers Association, 1999), monograph.

156. N.Y. Civil Rights Law § 79-1 (McKinney 2002).

157. This table is adopted in part from the Web site of the National Conference of State Legislatures, www.ncsl.org/programs/health/genetics/prt.htm (visited August 15, 2002).

158. Hodge, Gostin, and Jacobson, pp. 1469–70.

159. See "Genetic Information Nondiscrimination Act of 2003," S. 1053, 108th Cong. (2003).

160. 29 U.S.C. § 1182(a)(1)(F) (2001).

161. Department of Health and Human Services, Report of the Secretary to the President, Health Insurance in the Age of Genetics (Washington, D.C., 1997).

162. For an analytical table of state nondiscrimination in insurance laws, see the Web site of the National Conference of State Legislatures, www.ncsl.org/programs/health/ genetics/ndishlth.htm (visited August 15, 2002).

163. William Nowlan, "A Rational View of Insurance and Genetic Discrimination," *Science* 297 (July 12, 2002): 195–96; Mark A. Hall and Stephen S. Rich, "Laws Restricting Health Insurers' Use of Genetic Information: Impact on Genetic Discrimination," *Am J Hum Genet* 66 (2000): 293–307. Arguably, state laws against genetic discrimination face potential legal challenge under the Employee Retirement Income Security Act (ERISA), the federal law designed to ensure uniform national standards that safeguard employee benefits, including pension plans and health insurance for all employees of self-insured employers (approximately 125 million Americans). This is accomplished by imposition of federal standards and the preemption of state laws inconsistent with these standards in a way that impairs employee benefits (ERISA preemption), 29 U.S.C. § 1021 et seq. (1999). See testimony of Meredith Miller, Deputy Assistant Secretary, Pension and Welfare Benefits Administration, *Hearings Before the Senate Committee on Labor and Human Resources,* 105th Congress, 2d sess. (1998). A significant line of cases, including *Metropolitan Life Ins. Co. v. Massachusetts,* 471 U.S. 724 (1985), supports the view that if interpreted as mandated benefit laws, state genetic nondiscrimination laws would likely be upheld as permissible regulation of the business of insurance, a function traditionally left to the states and therefore not subject to federal preemption.

164. 42 U.S.C. § 2000e (1994).

165. 135 F.3d 1260 (9th Cir. 1998).

166. Exec. Order No., 13,145, "To Prohibit Discrimination in Federal Employment Based on Genetic Information," appears in 65 Fed. Reg. 6,875 (2000).

167. 42 U.S.C., §§ 12112(a), 12111(8), 12111(10) (2000).

168. 42 U.S.C. § 12111(5)(A).

169. *Ibid.,* §§ 12112(d)(2)(a), 12113(d), 12114.

170. *Ibid.,* § 12112(d)(3)(B).

171. Mark A. Rothstein, "Genetic Discrimination in Employment and the Americans with Disabilities Act," *Houston L Rev* 29 (1992): 52–61.

172. Rothstein; Larry Gostin, "Genetic Discrimination: The Use of Genetically Based Diagnostic and Prognostic Tests by Employers and Insurers," in Robert F. Weir, Susan Lawrence, and Evan Fales, eds., *Genes and Human Self-Knowledge: Historical and Philosophical Reflections on Modern Genetics* (Iowa City: University of Iowa Press, 1994), pp. 122–63.

173. Rothstein, pp. 49–50; see also Gostin, "Genetic Discrimination," pp. 134–35.

174. 42 U.S.C. § 12102(2).

175. *EEOC Compliance Manual,* vol. 2, no. 915.002 (March 14, 1995); EEOC, "Genetic Information and the Workplace," www.dol.gov/dol/_sec/public/media/reports/ genetics.htm (Jan. 20, 1998). See also Peter David Blanck and Mollie Weighner Marti, "Genetic Discrimination and the Employment Provisions of the Americans with Disabilities Act: Emerging Legal, Empirical, and Policy Implications," *Behav Sci Law* 14 (1996): 411–32 (discussing the 1995 statement).

176. Rothstein, "Genetic Discrimination," pp. 45–47 (discussing the EEOC's 1991 position); Frances H. Miller and Philip A. Huvos, "Genetic Blueprints, Employer Cost-Cutting, and the Americans with Disabilities Act," *Admin L Rev* 46 (1994): 373–74 (same).

177. *Equal Employment Opportunity Commission v. Burlington Northern Santa Fe Railroad,* No. C01-4013-MWB (N. D. Iowa 2001).

178. Press release, "EEOC Settles ADA Suit Against BNSF For Genetic Bias," available at http://www.eeoc.gov/press/4-18-01.html; David Hechler, "Railroad to Pay $2.2 Million Over Genetic Testing: Landmark Settlement Under the ADA," *The National Law Journal* 24 (May 13, 2002), p. A22.

179. Gostin, "Genetic Discrimination," pp. 147–49.

180. In addition to the sources already cited, for further discussion of the ADA and arguments for its extension to genetic discrimination, see Robert S. Olick, "Genes in the Workplace: New Frontiers for ADA Law, Policy and Research," in Peter David Blanck, ed., *Employment, Disability, and the Americans with Disabilities Act* (Chicago: Northwestern University Press, 2000), pp. 285–314. See also Paul Steven Miller, "Is There a Pink Slip in My Genes?: Genetic Discrimination in the Workplace," *Journal of Health Care Law and Policy* 3 (2000): 225–65 (reviewing both federal and state law).

181. 42 U.S.C. § 12113(a) (2001); 29 C.F.R. § 1630.2(r) (2001).

182. *Chevron U.S.A. Inc. v. Echazabal,* 536 U.S. 73 (2002). The precise statutory language of the ADA states that employers "may include a requirement that an individual shall not pose a direct threat to the health and safety of other individuals in the workplace." 42 U.S.C. § 12113(b) (2001). The EEOC expanded this standard to include risks of workplace harm to the individual. *Echazabal* clearly affirms the EEOC's authority to interpret the direct threat provision in this way.

183. See Marc Lappe, "Ethical Issues in Testing for Differential Sensitivity to Occupational Hazards," *J Occup Med* 25 (1983): 798.

184. See 29 C.F.R. § 1630.2 (1997); House Education and Labor Committee, H.R. Rep. No. 485, 101st Cong., 2d Sess., 51, reprinted in 1990 U.S.C.C.A.N. 303, 356.

185. Fla. Stat. Ann. § 448.076 (West 2002); N.C. Gen. Stat. § 95-28.1 (2002).

186. N.Y. Civil Rights Law § 48-a (McKinney 1999).

187. N.J. Stat. Ann. §§ 10:5-5, 10:5-12 (West Supp 2002).

188. Paul Steven Miller, "Genetic Discrimination in the Workplace," *American Journal of Law, Medicine and Ethics* 26 (1998): 189–97. For further discussion of various issues surrounding workplace and other forms of genetic discrimination, including a survey of state laws, see Ellen Wright Clayton, "Ethical, Legal and Social Implications of Genomic Medicine," *N Engl J Med* 349 (2003): 562–69.

189. N.Y. Executive Law § 296 (Consol. 2001).

190. Iowa Code Ann. § 729.6 (West 1999); Tex. Labor Code Ann. § 21.402 (Vernon Supp. 2002); Wis. Stat. Ann. § 111.372 (West 1999).

191. Mark A. Rothstein, "Protecting Genetic Privacy by Permitting Employer Access Only to Job-Related Employee Medical Information: Analysis of a Unique Minnesota Law," *Am J Law Med* 24 (1998): 399–416.

192. Iowa Code Ann. § 729.6(1)(c) (West 1999). The language in many other states is similar.

193. Eliot Marshall, "Families Sue Hospital, Scientist For Control of Canavan Gene," *Science* 290 (2000): 1062; *Greenberg,* 264 F. Supp. 2d 1064.

194. Sally Lehrman, "Medical tests cost Lawrence Berkeley $2.2 million," *Nature* 405 (2000): 110; *Norman-Bloodsaw v. Lawrence Berkeley Laboratory,* 135 F.3d 1260 (9th Cir. 1998).

195. Linda Kane, "Judge refuses to bump families from DNA lawsuit," *Lubbock Avalanche-Journal,* June 5, 2001, p. A1.

8

The NBAC Report: Recommendations and Limitations

Fundamentally, the interests of subjects and those of researchers are not in conflict. Rather, appropriate protection of subjects provides the reassurance that is needed if individuals are to continue to make their tissue, blood, or DNA available for research. Indeed, public confidence in the ethics and integrity of the research process translates into popular support for research in general.
National Bioethics Advisory Commission, 1999[1]

Respect for subjects' rights and welfare in such circumstances [when the normal consent requirement to participate in research has been waived] will usually dictate that they be informed after-the-fact of the research in which they have been involved as naïve or unwitting subjects and perhaps offered the opportunity to withdraw their information from the investigator's data. In general, however, NBAC concludes that this fourth criterion for waiver of consent is not relevant to research using human biological materials and, in fact, might be harmful if it forced investigators to recontact individuals who might not have been aware that their materials were being used in research.
National Bioethics Advisory Commission[2]

Chapter 5 discussed a number of international documents, including comprehensive reports and recommendations developed by multidisciplinary committees in the Netherlands, England, and Canada. Here we discuss a report on research with stored tissues by the National Bioethics Advisory Commission (NBAC), a multidisciplinary committee established by executive order of President Clinton in October 1995. This chapter describes the goals of the NBAC report, analyzes its recommendations, assesses its strengths and weaknesses, and compares some of its recommendations and themes with those of the non-U.S. committees. We do not always agree with the NBAC report, but we applaud its important contribution to the ongoing debate about research with stored tissues.

NBAC's Mandate and Goals

During the last quarter of the twentieth century, the United States was well served by two national, multidisciplinary bioethics commissions with different mandates, methods, and accomplishments. The National Commission for the Protection of Human Subjects of Biomedical and Behavioral Research (1974–78) addressed significant ethical problems that had developed in biomedical research by the early 1970s and made recommendations to the federal government that, once established as policy, came to represent much of the nation's understanding of ethical research done with human participants. Soon thereafter, the President's Commission for the Study of Ethical Problems in Medicine and Biomedical and Behavioral Research (1980–83) addressed a different set of ethical problems in clinical medicine and biomedical research and published a series of influential reports on several topics, including improving access to health care, updating the definition of death, genetic screening and counseling, and deciding to forgo life-sustaining treatment. Both of these commissions were widely respected and influential long after their official tenure ended.

In the years following the President's Commission, several attempts were made to establish another multidisciplinary bioethics committee at the federal level to address a number of bioethical problems that emerged during the late 1980s and early 1990s. One such effort—the Biomedical Ethics Advisory Committee (1988–89)—failed, largely because of political problems in Congress related to the debate over the morality and legality of abortion. Other, more focused committees—the Fetal Tissue Transplantation Research Panel (1988), the Human Embryo Research Panel (1994), and the Advisory Committee on Human Radiation Experiments (1994–95)—were funded and later issued reports with sometimes controversial recommendations.[3]

On the heels of the Human Radiation Experiments Committee's work, and responding to one of its recommendations, President Clinton's executive order established NBAC with a far-reaching mandate:

a. NBAC shall provide advice and make recommendations to the National Science and Technology Council and to other appropriate government entities regarding: (1) the appropriateness of departmental, agency, or other governmental programs, policies, assignments, missions, guidelines, and regulations as they relate to bioethical issues arising from research on human biology and behavior; and (2) applications, including the clinical applications, of that research.

b. NBAC shall identify broad principles to govern the ethical conduct of research, citing specific projects only as illustrations for such principles.

c. NBAC shall not be responsible for the review and approval of specific projects.

d. In addition to responding to requests for advice and recommendations from the National Science and Technology Council, NBAC may accept suggestions of issues for consideration from both the Congress and the public. NBAC may also identify other bioethical issues for the purpose of providing advice and recommendations, subject to the approval of the National Science and Technology Council.[4]

Harold Shapiro, president of Princeton University, was selected as the NBAC chair. When he and the original NBAC members met with President Clinton in July 1997 for the official beginning of NBAC's work, the president emphasized, among other points, an increasing concern that the genetic information contained in stored human tissues might be misused to discriminate against individuals and families.

By the time NBAC published its report on research with human biological materials in 1999, the committee had already published other reports on cloning human beings and on research with persons having mental disorders. In addition, the membership of the committee had undergone some changes. The 16 NBAC members responsible for the report on research with human biological materials included four physicians (one of them a geneticist) in academic medical centers, another geneticist, a physician-attorney in private practice, a retired dean of nursing, an academic psychologist, two health-law professors, three lay persons (leaders of a biotechnology firm, a private bioethics consortium, and a national organization for the mentally ill), and three academic bioethicists.[5]

These commission members chose to address the issue of research with stored tissues because, as they put it, the issue stands at "the confluence of two important developments." On the one hand, there is "the remarkably enhanced ability of biomedical researchers to study human biological materials . . . to increase knowledge about human diseases; and to develop better means to prevent, diagnose, and treat those diseases." On the other, there is an increasing concern about the ability of biomedical investigators to "reveal clinical and sometimes personal information about individuals" through their research with tissue samples and the related concern that "the use of genetic and other medical information found in [tissues] might infringe upon an individual's privacy, and if misused could result in discrimination."[6]

After months of data collection, public hearings, several commissioned papers (including one by RFW), and numerous committee discussions, the NBAC members agreed on four basic premises they would use in writing their final report and making their recommendations. First, "research use of human biological materials is essential to the advancement of science and human health." Second, "the people who provide human biological materials for research should be protected and respected." Third, the rapid achievements in genetics research and the widespread application of "a molecular-based approach to understanding human disease" have raised issues of concern related to "autonomy and medical privacy." Fourth, "there is disagreement within the scientific community about the nature of risks to individuals and about the . . . types of protections that are needed to ensure that biological samples can be used in research with minimal risks to those whose materials are used." In addition, NBAC organized its final report around five other important considerations:

1. Whether the biological materials are already collected and stored, or will be collected for prospective research studies
2. Whether the tissues are obtained in a clinical setting or a research setting
3. Whether a research sample can be linked to the person from whom it came
4. Whether the risks posed by the research affect individuals or communities
5. The types of protections that might be used to protect sample sources against harms, such as invasion of privacy or discrimination[7]

The majority of NBAC members decided, after considerable discussion, to use the Common Rule as the framework for their analysis and recommendations, both because American biomedical scientists are familiar with these regulations and because NBAC's charge included reviewing the adequacy of the federal system of protections for human participants in research studies. They therefore set out to answer two central questions:

1. "How well does the existing Federal Policy for the Protection of Human Subjects . . . meet the objective of protecting human subjects from harm in research involving human biological materials?"
2. "[Does the Common Rule] provide clear direction to research sponsors, investigators, IRBs, and others regarding the conduct of research using these materials in an ethical manner?"[8]

They concluded early in their deliberations that the Common Rule "was not entirely responsive" to these questions. Going further, they agreed that the present regulatory language is "inadequate," provides "ambiguous guidance," and requires some "modification." Nevertheless, they agreed to make the following statement the cornerstone of their analysis, recommendations, and overall position: "Properly interpreted and modestly modified, present federal regulations can protect subjects' rights and interests and at the same time permit well-designed research to go forward using materials already in storage as well as those newly collected by investigators and others."[9]

NBAC's major goal became to provide the National Science and Technology Council and other federal agencies with a series of recommendations that would, if followed, provide clearer federal rules for research with human participants and, more important, produce long-needed revisions to the Common Rule. To achieve that overall goal, they listed several secondary goals or objectives they hoped to accomplish along the way:

- To address "perceived difficulties in the interpretation of federal regulations"
- To ensure that research with human biological materials continues "to benefit from appropriate oversight and IRB review, the additional burdens of which are kept to a minimum"
- To provide investigators and IRBs "with clear guidance regarding the use of human biological materials in research, particularly with regard to informed consent"
- To provide "a coherent public policy for research in this area"
- To provide "the public (including potential research subjects) with increased confidence in research that makes use of human biological materials"[10]

The NBAC Analysis and Recommendations

The NBAC report begins with a helpful—and much needed—description of collected data regarding the types of human tissues currently in storage in this country, the various locations in which the tissues are stored, the multiple ways in which the tissues are stored, and the purposes for which they are stored. The collection of this data by Elisa Eiseman and her colleagues at the RAND Institute, as well as their estimates of the total number of tissues in storage in tissue banks, ranging in size from the Armed Forces Institute of Pathology to state newborn screening laboratories to university-based research laboratories, provided NBAC with a solid empirical "floor." Using the Eiseman data available at the time the report was published, NBAC estimated that over 282 million tissue specimens are now in storage in the United States. This figure, large as it is, turned out to be somewhat low; as indicated in Chapter 2, subsequent published data by Eiseman and Haga identified 307 million tissue specimens, plus innumerable tissue samples outside repositories, and the number grows by approximately 20 million specimens annually.[11]

The NBAC report also provides a helpful analysis of the multiple beneficial ways in which stored human tissues are used for research purposes. With descriptive information about the value of human tissue research in pathology, cancer studies, genetics, epidemiological studies, and infectious disease investigations, the report leaves no doubt that NBAC members greatly (and correctly) value the work done by biomedical investigators and hope their report encourages that work to continue, perhaps with greater public confidence and support. To support the descriptive information about biomedical research, the report includes a number of historical examples and recent cases (including, briefly, the NHANES and Iceland cases discussed in Chapter 1) that highlight the extraordinary value of research done with stored tissues.

The central feature of NBAC's report is its conclusion that current federal regulations governing research with human tissues can provide, if modified along the lines that NBAC recommends, adequate protection for human participants in biomedical research studies and appropriate guidance both for the scientists who do the work and the IRB members who provide oversight for the studies. According to the commission, the Common Rule is not broken, but only in need of minor repair. NBAC's prescription is intended to provide the repair, while maintaining strong commitment to the potential benefits of biomedical research and increasing popular support for research. According to NBAC, adoption of its recommendations as federal policy would effectively quiet the controversy about human tissue research.

What kind of current guidance does the Common Rule provide, and in what ways does it need to be fixed? NBAC's analysis proceeds with a series of questions:

1. Does the biomedical use of stored human specimens constitute research? The question is important because, after all, federal regulations governing biomedical research do not apply "to exclusively clinical interventions, even if they are experimental procedures." If the use of tissues occurs solely as a part of clinical diagnosis and treatment interventions, federal regulations do not apply. If, by contrast, a pathology laboratory (or other investigators) "saves tissue that was left over from a clinical intervention in order to conduct further, research-oriented testing, that research would be subject to the federal regulations."[12] NBAC fails to address, however, the fairly common problem of post-diagnostic research without appropriate consent, a point to which we will return later.

2. Is the research done with human biological materials subject to the federal regulations? Yes, clearly so, if the research is funded by any of the 17 federal agencies that subscribe to the Common Rule or is carried out at an institution that has agreed by means of signing a Multiple Project Assurance document to be governed by the Common Rule. But the regulations do not apply to research with human tissues conducted with private funds or at an institution free of affiliation with the Common Rule (or regulation by the FDA).

3. Does the research involve a "human subject"? (As indicated earlier, we prefer the term "participant," but understand the traditional use of this language and the importance of this question.)

   The NBAC members point out that the regulations define a "human subject" as being both alive and "identifiable." They also observe that OPRR (now OHRP) interprets this policy in human tissue research to include coded tissue samples as well as identified samples. Members apparently have no reservations regarding this common interpretation, even though they note that genetics and other biomedical research using archived tissues from deceased individuals can, in some circumstances, "pose risks for living relatives of the deceased." More specifically, they point out that some genetics research done with these tissues can result in psychosocial harm to a dead individual's identifiable, living descendents (e.g., troubling new self-knowledge, possible discrimination with employment or health insurance). Yet, reflecting a serious flaw in the report, NBAC does not suggest that this possible harm needs to be remedied in any way, such as by recommending that good-faith efforts be made to contact living descendents to give them an opportunity to consent or that IRBs be required to review this kind of research studies. Instead, in a sort of dismissive manner, the report simply states, "Of course, ethical concerns may pertain to the use of such tissues that are beyond the scope of current laws or regulations."[13]

4. Is the research eligible for an exemption from the federal regulations? As we discussed in Chapter 6, the federal rules provide two conditions under which research with human tissues from living individuals may be exempt from IRB review and informed consent requirements: stored samples have to be anonymous or anonymized ("unidentified" and "unlinked," to use NBAC's terms) and they have to be "existing and publicly available." The NBAC report appropriately notes that two problems with these exemption conditions are the difficulty of making sure that anonymized samples are truly unlinked and unlinkable to any identifiable persons and the ambiguity in interpreting the "publicly available" requirement. NBAC concludes, correctly in our view, that "publicly available" samples should be interpreted to mean samples that are available to the general public, not merely to scientists in a specified field. They also correctly interpret the "existing" condition to mean tissue samples that are "on the shelf" at the time research on them is initiated, regardless of whether the tissues were previously collected for other research or for nonresearch purposes.

5. What are the IRB requirements for research requiring review? NBAC points out that "two basic protections" exist for participants in research studies: informed consent by the participants themselves, and IRB review by a multidisciplinary committee with the responsibility of local oversight for such studies. The report also states, as we previously discussed, that the informed consent requirement can be waived under four criteria: (1) the research involves no more than "minimal risk" to the participants, (2) the participants' "rights and welfare" will not be adversely affected, (3) the research cannot be done without a waiver of the informed consent requirement, and (4) the participants will be given, "whenever appropriate," pertinent follow-up information.

NBAC's comments on these requirements seem to move in two different directions. On the one hand, they indicate that the regulations need to be strengthened by moving beyond "the strict focus" of the regulations on the individual research participant to include, in some instances, the interests of third parties such as groups of which an individual is a part. On the other, they state that the regulations need to be modified to include more attention to "the practicability of obtaining consent," a modification that would weaken the consent requirement and make waivers of this requirement easier to get.

Certainly, policy and practice need to be realistic about the difficulties sometimes created by the current informed consent requirement, but making it easier for investigators to obtain waivers goes too far in weakening informed consent, especially with prospective research studies. The NBAC report also offers inadequate guidance for analyzing when investigators' claims about the "impracticability" of getting informed consent is an authentic assessment of reality or simply an attempt to avoid the burdens of giving people informed choices about how their stored tissues are going to be used in research.

Before setting forth their recommendations for updating and modifying the Common Rule, NBAC briefly discussed some ethical perspectives on human tissue research. The chapter on ethics is organized around three principles of biomedical ethics—beneficence, respect for persons, and justice—formulated by the National Commission in its influential *Belmont Report* (1979). NBAC uses these principles as a general framework for discussing several of the ethical issues involved in research with stored tissues: the benefits, harms, and wrongs (for individuals *and* groups) that can be produced by such research; the ways of respecting the persons who are the sources of the tissues; and the justice-related concerns about this research (i.e., whether individuals have a property right to tissues removed from their bodies, whether the commercial gains sometimes possible through stored-tissue research will result in a commodification of the body). They also provide a brief analysis of privacy and confidentiality, genetic discrimination, stigmatization, objectionable research, post-mortem uses of biological materials, and other controversial matters in this ongoing debate.

NBAC's collective ethical perspective, stated in Chapter 4 of the report, is that any ethically sound policy about human tissue research has to have "a defensible balance" between "the ethical reasons that support greater control" over the research use of tissues and greater protection of persons who provide those tissues, and "the ethical reasons that support greater access" to tissue samples by scientific investigators.[14] Yet, in trying to achieve *this* essential balance, they fail to achieve *another,* namely, between the federal regulations and the various ethical perspectives that comprise the ongoing debate about human tissue research, including the perspectives of various professional organizations, of ethics and policy statements on this issue produced outside the United States, and of individual scientists, health-law attorneys, and bioethicists in this country who have articulated numerous ethical concerns regarding the appropriate boundaries for research using stored tissues.[15] While NBAC clearly reviewed a wide range of perspectives, heard extensive testimony, and commissioned numerous papers and reports, only some of these other perspectives get serious attention in the report. The ethical perspective that clearly dominates is that of the federal regulations, which are repeatedly discussed. After a brief introduction of the *Belmont* ethical principles, for example, the chapter on ethical perspectives "also draws [primarily] upon the ethical guidance provided by federal regulations designed to protect human research subjects."[16]

The 23 NBAC recommendations are grouped into eight areas. Recommendations one through five address the adequacy of existing federal policies as they apply to research studies with human tissue samples. Again, NBAC finds the regulations fundamentally sound; the committee's task is to recommend "ways to strengthen and clarify the regulations." Whatever recommendations they make should keep "additional burdens" to scientific investigators and IRB members "to a minimum." To help achieve the goal of greater regulatory clarity, the first five recommendations are introduced with a helpful categorization of human biological materials, a categorization that first distinguishes between *tissue specimens* that are stored in repositories (such as pathology laboratories) and *tissue samples* that are in the possession of individual investigators. Next, the categorization uses descriptive labels for the identity status of stored specimens or samples (the terms differ somewhat from the ones used in this book). The label "unidentified" is suggested as a replacement for the more common "anonymous," and the label "unlinked" as a replacement for the "anonymized" reference familiar to geneticists and other scientists. As to the status of other stored tissues, NBAC uses the conventional "identified" samples, but prefers "coded" samples to synonyms such as "linked" or "identifiable."[17]

NBAC's interest in strengthening and clarifying the current federal regulations is clear in their first five recommendations. Recommendation one suggests that research with unidentified (anonymous) samples be clearly understood to be exempt from the Common Rule, whereas research with unlinked (anonymized) samples would be subject to the Common Rule (but may be eligible for exemption). Research with coded or identified samples is also subject to the regulations without, in most instances, being eligible for exemption. The next four recommendations attempt to simplify the work of scientific investigators and IRB members by suggesting that investigator-created unlinked samples usually be exempt from IRB review, that all "minimal-risk" research with tissues be eligible for expedited IRB review, and that IRBs require investigators to include in their protocols specific descriptions of their plans to minimize risk to research participants who provide identified or coded tissue samples.

Recommendations six through nine deal with matters pertaining to informed consent. The report correctly notes some of the current problems related to informed consent, including the inadequacies of most hospital and surgical consent documents regarding future research with stored specimens (such forms "rarely . . . provide an adequate basis for inferring consent to future research"). Most existing specimens in clinically related repositories have, therefore, "been collected without disclosure" to patients about future research possibilities or any psychosocial risks they may face in connection with that research, especially genetics research. NBAC suggests that "additional studies are needed" to improve and strengthen the process of informed consent for prospective research studies with tissues obtained in clinical settings.

Specific recommendations about informed consent aim to clarify the role of the informed consent requirement in regard to both existing tissue collections and to future research projects. Recommendation nine stands out from the others and clearly caused considerable disagreement among NBAC members. It calls for the development of consent documents that might include providing potential research participants (in clinical or research settings) with a number of options: (*1*) refusing to consent to have their tissues used for research, (*2*) permitting their tissues to be used only if they are unidentified or unlinked, or (*3*) placing limits on the kind of research that will be permitted to be done with their coded or identified tissues. That the committee could not reach full agreement about this recommendation (three commissioners partially dissented in the published report) reflects some of NBAC's struggles with the informed consent requirement.

Recommendations 10–13 continue with the theme of informed consent, focusing on the waiver criteria currently required under the federal regulations. Given the frequent questions about these criteria from scientific investigators and IRB members, NBAC specifically addresses each one: the concept of minimal risk, the rights and welfare of research participants, the "practicability" of consent, and the debriefing of research participants after their participation in a study. In each instance NBAC makes recommendations that, if followed, would make waivers easier to get, weaken the informed consent requirement for human tissue research, and disregard some oft-noted concerns. They label concerns about psychosocial harms as only "speculative at present," recommend that IRBs *presume* the "impracticability" of getting consent for research with coded or identified samples in repositories, support the common practice of anonymizing identifiable tissue samples without consent from the sample source (they aptly label this action "rendering existing identifiable samples unidentifiable *to avoid the need for consent*"), and, surprisingly, recommend that the fourth criterion for waiver, the debriefing requirement, be ignored by investigators and IRBs because it "usually does not apply to research using human biological materials."[18]

Recommendations 14–16 deal with the controversial issue of whether investigators should report research results to individuals who have participated in a specific study. Advocates of reporting maintain that research participants have a right to know the results of a study; critics argue that revealing preliminary, unconfirmed data to participants can cause them harm and may cause them to make decisions based on incomplete and possibly inaccurate information. NBAC helpfully recommends that IRBs develop specific guidelines for investigators regarding the disclosure of research results, advise investigators to develop individual policies for possible disclosure of research results consistent with IRB guidelines, and urge that appropriate medical advice or referral be provided to participants whenever clinically significant research results are disclosed to them as participants in a study.

The NBAC report does not address the related, but separate question of whether investigators have a duty to try to contact previous participants in a specific study, perhaps years after that study was completed, with follow-up information about related scientific studies that would be relevant to them.

Recommendations 17–18 are, perhaps, the most important recommendations in the report. They call for the regulations to be amended to include considerations of potential harm (and benefit) to persons other than individual research participants. NBAC observes that "the exclusive focus of the regulations on the individual research subject is arbitrary from an ethical standpoint" because others can be harmed as a consequence of a research study.[19] In particular, NBAC discusses the risks of stigmatization and discrimination against group members as a result of some studies (without giving examples) as well as the potential risks and benefits to relatives of individual participants in some studies.

In general, these two recommendations are excellent. NBAC calls on investigators to anticipate the possibility that a tissue-based study might be "harmful to groups associated with the individual," that investigators work in advance with representatives of relevant groups "to minimize such harm," and that IRBs not grant exemptions from committee review for studies using unlinked (anonymized) samples if the research "poses a significant risk of group harms." They also recommend that the risk of harm to any specific group be disclosed as a part of "any required informed consent process."[20] Yet they choose to narrow the scope of these important recommendations by limiting consideration of possible harm to relatives to studies involving tissues from living persons, thus ignoring possible harm (or benefit) to living relatives through retrospective research on the tissues of deceased individuals.

Recommendations 19–23 complete what NBAC describes as "a model framework for considering research in which the human subject is defined through his or her biological material."[21] NBAC calls for two changes in the publication of research results: (1) more attention by investigators to the possibility of causing harm to individuals *and* families through the publication of identifiable information about them, and (2) a new journal policy whereby scientific journal editors would require certification of investigators' compliance with the Common Rule as a condition for publishing their research results. The report concludes by calling for more professional education about the ethical issues in research, more NIH funding to help investigators comply with NBAC's recommendations, and greater access for investigators to patient medical records since human tissue research often involves work in research settings *and* clinical settings. The last recommendation, in fact, is emphasized in Harold Shapiro's cover letter to President Clinton: "NBAC concluded that not only is it critical that human biological materials continue to be available to the biomedical research community, but, increasingly, it is essential for investigators to collect human biological materials from individuals who are also willing to share important ongoing clinical information about themselves."[22]

Assessment

Like other bioethics commissions, NBAC faced considerable challenges in its quest for internal consensus in a diverse, multidisciplinary group, discussing complex information and debating a controversial issue in a public forum. To its credit, the NBAC report has numerous strengths. Four important features of the report stand out as significant contributions. First, the report includes specific data, such as the Eiseman calculations about stored samples and the Wells/Karr analysis of public opinion published in volume II, and specific case examples that ground subsequent policy recommendations. Unlike some reports by national bioethics committees, this report provides real-life numbers and examples that helpfully buttress and strengthen the more theoretical and interpretive portions of the report. For example, the committee's descriptions of the identity labels they use for tissues ("unidentified," "unlinked," etc.) are supported by illustrative cases that add substantial clarity to the distinctions being made. Readers are also given several published case examples (e.g., research involving atherosclerosis, the hormone diethylstilbestrol, smoking and lung cancer) that clearly illustrate the tremendous value of human tissue research.

Second, the report clearly reflects the committee's dominant interest in bringing greater clarity to federal regulations by means of their interpretive comments and recommendations about how the Common Rule can be improved for the joint benefit of scientific investigators and local IRB members who review their protocols. Of particular help in achieving their goal of addressing "perceived difficulties in the interpretation of [the] federal regulations" is their analysis and interpretation of several important concepts: "human subject," "minimal risk," "practicability," "privacy," "respect," and "harm." Committee members correctly recognized that the debate about human tissue research has sometimes tended to flounder over the meaning of these concepts, and they succeeded in providing some needed conceptual clarification.

Third, NBAC's emphasis on considerations of group harm brings important attention to this under-discussed subject. We agree that the exclusive focus on "the individual research subject" in the regulations needs to be changed to address the multiple kinds of population- and group-based research commonly carried out by geneticists, epidemiologists, and other biomedical scientists. Such research not only takes place with identifiable groups in this country but, as we have seen, increasingly occurs in other parts of the world as well. It would have been helpful, however, if the NBAC members had not only called for the federal regulations to be revised to include considerations of group benefit and harm (and given some examples to illustrate this concern), but had also provided an analysis of some of the possible benefits and practical difficulties that occur when scientific investigators try to adapt the process of informed consent to include an appropriate form of "group consent."[23]

Finally, this NBAC report picks up a central theme of one of their earlier reports and appropriately applies it to the issue of informed consent in the context of prospective research with stored tissues. In that earlier report NBAC focused on research involving persons with mental disorders.[24] The committee considered whether such persons, while having decision-making capacity, should be permitted to give "prospective authorization" to their participation in research done at a later time, even if by that time, they might have lost their capacity to consent. NBAC recognized that individuals could give prospective authorization to "a particular class of research" if its possible benefits, known risks, and realistic alternatives had been discussed with them. In the tissue research report, they apply the same reasoning to the possibility that some persons, appropriately informed about particular categories of research with stored tissues, may be interested in and capable of giving prospective authorization to participate in that future research through their banked samples. NBAC states, correctly in our view, that such prospective consent to research is "consistent with respecting persons" and the preferences they express. Moreover, NBAC concludes that such future-oriented consent to participate in human tissue research is not only possible, but less problematic than some kinds of biomedical research because "the research will be conducted not on their bodies but on biological materials they provided" in the context of being informed about the psychosocial risks they are taking.[25] We return to this possibility in Chapter 11, recommending the use of research advance directives for thoughtful individuals who want to exercise choice now regarding how their tissues may later be used in research studies.

Other features of the NBAC report are problematic. Our three major concerns about the report—its methodology, its proposed weakening of the informed consent requirement, and the basic imbalance of some of its recommendations—are shared by some of those who sent NBAC public comments about the penultimate draft of the report.[26] First, while we applaud NBAC's collection of much helpful data about stored tissues, provision of numerous examples documenting the tremendous benefits of human tissue research, and active solicitation of public opinion on several controversial topics, we do not agree with the central feature of their methodology. As indicated earlier, NBAC made an early and formulational commitment to working within the framework of the federal regulations. As a result, the report inadequately considers other ethical perspectives that should have been given greater weight in their analysis and recommendations.

Of course, the Common Rule had to be emphasized, for the reasons given: American biomedical scientists are familiar with the regulations, and part of NBAC's charge was to review the adequacy of the regulations in protecting human participants in research studies. But the published report is, unfortunately, unbalanced because their review process and analytical methodology were too narrowly constrained by considerations of current federal regulations, OPRR (now OHRP) interpretations, and federal and state laws to the point that other important ethical perspectives did not sufficiently influence the committee's recommendations. For example, they used the three ethical principles of the *Belmont Report* as an analytical framework for Chapter 4, their main chapter on ethics, but these ethical principles seem to have little influence on the content of Chapter 5, the chapter containing their own recommendations. If NBAC had stayed with some of their earlier expressed views about respecting persons and justice-related concerns in human tissue research, some recommendations in the final chapter would be substantially different. Likewise, if NBAC had done more with some of the traditional, core features of research ethics (e.g., the voluntariness of participation in research, the right to make informed choices, the right to withdraw from a research study), the report's methodology would have had a better balance between ethics-based reasoning and regulatory issues.

Second, the report weakens the informed consent requirement, at least when important trade-offs are involved in the context of human tissue research. Informed consent is, of course, a recurring theme throughout the report. But when difficult calls have to be made and recommendations on controversial issues have to be put forward, the report consistently sides with the interests of biomedical investigators and the potential benefits of their research, frequently giving informed consent short shrift. With a few exceptions, the report repeatedly makes the same move: it uses language that suggests the importance of informed consent (e.g., "Seeking this consent demonstrates respect for the person's right to choose whether to cooperate with the scientific enterprise, and it permits individuals to protect themselves against unwanted or risky invasions of privacy."[27]), then makes comments and recommendations that, if enacted as federal policy, would undoubtedly *weaken the informed consent requirement*. Thus NBAC describes informed consent as "merely one aspect of human subjects protection" and "an adjunct to IRB review"; shows preference for a standard of general consent (rather than a "layered" or a "specific" standard of consent); provides a long case illustration suggesting that informed consent is not really important, but only a necessary regulatory hurdle; accepts the anonymization of tissue samples by investigators "to avoid the need for consent"; and recommends lowering the bar for waiver of consent by making the test of impracticability easier to pass.[28]

The one notable exception is, it turns out, not much of an exception after all. Recommendation 9, as mentioned earlier, calls for the development of consent documents that will "provide potential subjects with a sufficient number of options to help them understand clearly the nature of the decision they are about to make."[29] This strong recommendation is buttressed by subsequent commentary commending the National Action Plan for Breast Cancer and other advocacy groups for their efforts to develop "multi-layered consent forms that are both informative and practical."[30] Unfortunately, sandwiched between these statements are a soft suggestion about the options that consent documents "might" include, a suggestion that such forms could be "administratively burdensome," and a long, detailed, dissenting footnote (the only one in the report) that highlights important differences within NBAC. Collectively, this material dilutes the strength of the recommendation about consent documents.

Third, NBAC states more than once that it hopes to achieve "the right balance" or at least "a defensible balance" between two sets of competing values at stake in the debate about research with stored tissues. At one point the report describes the competing values as "greater control" (plus "stronger protections") for research participants over the research done with their stored tissues and "greater access" to those stored tissues by scientific investigators who want to study them for beneficial purposes, including "clinically beneficial research and/or clinical interventions."[31]

NBAC fails to achieve "the right balance," for three related reasons. First, as indicated by the first quotation at the beginning of this chapter, NBAC members sometimes minimize the competing interests of scientific investigators and participants in research studies. It is true that many people, including us, greatly value the work done in biomedical research and welcome each new report of another research discovery that may lead to better medical care and improved health. In this respect, the "interests of subjects and . . . researchers are not in conflict." But it is also true that individuals (and families) who participate in research studies do not usually choose to do so blindly or thoughtlessly, nor do they want to be used as only "means" to investigators' projected beneficial "ends" (the older literature on research ethics sometimes used to refer to human research participants as "guinea pigs"). In this respect, the interests of research participants sometimes are in conflict with the interests of researchers, which is one of the reasons that individuals occasionally exercise their right to withdraw from a research study.

When NBAC does mention these competing interests, it underplays the mutuality of interests in control between researchers and participants. Yes, undoubtedly, researchers are interested in gaining greater access to stored tissue samples, and appropriately informed participants in research studies may have some interest in controlling the types of research done with their tissues and may be thankful for the protection that well-constructed, informative consent documents provide them. We are also convinced that many patients in hospitals and clinics would be interested in exercising some control over the post-diagnostic research uses of their tissue samples and, we hope, would be appreciative of consent documents that try to protect their interests to some degree by informing them about the possibility of post-diagnostic research. We suggest, however, that the competing interests of researchers and participants in human tissue research are more correctly framed by saying that *persons in both groups are interested, in varying degrees, in control* over what is done with stored tissues. For investigators, the understandable interest in control not only involves greater access to stored tissues but also the freedom to work with stored tissues with as few bureaucratic hurdles (such as IRB review and OHRP requirements) as possible. For research participants, whether in research or clinical settings, the interest in control not only involves stronger protections but also being able *to exercise choice,* a central feature of the concept of informed consent.

Again, when faced with the challenge of balancing these competing interests, NBAC consistently favors the side of the investigators. As indicated earlier, the report is filled with good, generally correct, and important statements about researchers and the persons who provide them, knowingly or not, with tissues for their research. But when hard choices have to be made, NBAC *usually opts to go with researchers* and the extraordinary possibilities contained in the work they do in the lab and, one hopes, later in the clinic. Therefore, most of the secondary goals of the report are focused on scientific investigators and IRB members who review their research protocols, with NBAC recommendations backed up by the committee's expressed hope (with which we agree) that important research with stored tissues will continue to be done and any additional burdens will be "kept to a minimum."

NBAC's imbalanced emphasis is best illustrated by the commentary preceding Recommendation 13, a portion of which is quoted at the beginning of this chapter. Here the report attempts to justify dropping the debriefing requirement for a waiver of informed consent concerning human tissue research by saying that if investigators were required to recontact previous participants with additional information about a research study, those former participants *might be harmed* because they "*might not have been aware*" that their materials were being used in research."[32] This statement seems to support the familiar saying, "What they [former participants in human tissue research] don't know won't hurt them." This position is untenable, open to abuse in practice, and counterproductive to NBAC's own desirable goal of providing the public "with increased confidence" in human tissue research.

Finally, the NBAC report is silent or surprisingly incomplete on a number of cases and issues that have had prominent places in the debate about research with stored tissues. Regarding cases, NBAC gives a particularly brief account of *Moore,* provides only two paragraphs on the NHANES III study without even mentioning the ethics controversy at the CDC over informed consent, and describes the Icelandic controversy over the DeCODE database with only a passing reference to the ethical concerns over privacy, informed consent, and commercialization.[33] The report never specifically addresses the problem of secondary research, never says anything about the participation of children in research studies, mentions the practice of post-diagnostic research several times without any indication that it might raise ethical concerns, and provides only a very brief description of problems connected with patenting and the commercialization of human tissue research. As mentioned earlier, the report simply dismisses or ignores without argument concerns about objectionable research, ownership or property claims regarding tissues (taking no position on this hot-button issue), and a possible duty for investigators to recontact former research participants in some way with follow-up information that might be clinically significant.

The NBAC Report in an International Context

NBAC places its work in an international context, at least to a limited extent, by including a brief section on international perspectives regarding the use of human biological materials in research. In this section the report provides helpful information on published statements about human tissue research by the European Group on Ethics in Science and New Technologies, the HUGO ethics committee, the Canadian Tri-Council, and the WHO Human Genetics Program. They do not mention the reports by the Health Council of the Netherlands and the Nuffield Council on Bioethics.

Given the global nature of this issue, NBAC might have done more with this impressive body of thought than merely noting some of the common themes— respect for privacy, respect for autonomy "operationalized by a requirement of informed consent," and recommendations against commercialization of research— that appear in the midst of "a rich diversity of positions" in the international documents. If any common position emerges from these documents, it is, according to NBAC, that "a person's rights and interests are best protected if that person *has some form of control* over his or her removed biological material."[34]

We can briefly compare NBAC's work with published reports by national committees in the Netherlands, England, and Canada on the same subject, as well as the shorter policy statements from the HUGO ethics committee. The most notable difference is that after reporting that the international documents tend to agree on the importance of research participants having some measure of control over the research done with their stored tissues, NBAC does not place as much emphasis on this point as do most other national reports. Certainly, in comparison with the documents from the Netherlands and Canada, NBAC places less emphasis on either personal control or, more specifically, consent documents as ways of exercising control (we prefer to say, "choice"). Thus the theme that is repeated in the Netherlands report—"People are entitled to a say in what happens to their body"—is less prominent in NBAC's thinking, especially in terms of the common practice of doing research with DNA samples that have been anonymized without the knowledge and consent of the persons whose bodies were the source of the tissues.

The NBAC report does not share another theme common to all the international documents we have discussed, namely an emphasis, vague though it has to be, on what we have called the "special-ness" of human tissues and the individuals who provide them. The result is that although NBAC discusses the importance of respect for persons in one chapter, the report as a whole does not emphasize this theme. Moreover, the report does not place much emphasis on the dignity of human beings, as the other international documents do, nor does NBAC make any use of a paper it commissioned on religious perspectives, which could have been helpful in developing this theme.[35] Possibly for these reasons, as well as its goal of clarifying the policy implications of the Common Rule, the NBAC report does not express the same concerns as some international documents about secondary research with tissue samples (especially emphasized in the Netherlands report) or the commercial possibilities connected with human tissue research (given particular emphasis by the Nuffield Council).

By contrast, the NBAC report is more practical in certain ways than some of these international documents. It provides substantially more national data about stored tissue repositories than the other national documents do, makes better use of public opinion (even though the NBAC data on public opinion is quite limited), and certainly clarifies national regulations better than the reports produced in the Netherlands and England (the Canadian Tri-Council report is, by mandate and design, a much more comprehensive document than the NBAC report). In addition, NBAC's recommendations are much more specific and practical than those in most of the other reports.

We now turn to Part III of the book. We begin by discussing the importance of the informed consent process, and make some recommendations for updating the process of informed consent in the era of genomic medicine.

Cases and Vignettes

When a national committee began deliberations about research with stored tissues, a physician wondered aloud why anyone would seriously question the societal benefits of biomedical research and, given that perspective, why any intelligent persons would want to place ethical or legal restrictions on this research, even in an effort to strengthen the informed consent process. To support his position, he came to one of the committee meetings with copies of 20 biomedical publications that had been done in recent years with research using human tissues (normal tissues, malignant tissues, and cell lines) supplied to investigators by the National Cancer Institute's Cooperative Human Tissue Network. To him, the evidence was crystal clear: this important research using tissue samples and cell lines must continue with as few ethical and legal encumbrances as possible.[36]

An IRB at a children's hospital needed to develop institutional guidelines for the collection and use of tissue samples for research. The committee discussed federal regulations, read much of the literature about informed consent and research with stored samples, and struggled to put an array of proposed pediatric research studies in the correct review categories. Some of the proposed research would be retrospective in nature, using tissue samples that were already frozen or otherwise "on the shelf": anonymous frozen plasma samples that were collected on patients previously enrolled in an investigational drug trial for nongenetic purposes; identified gastrointestinal mucosal biopsies stored in a freezer from a previous, completely different research protocol; and identified osteosarcoma tumor tissue stored in pathology, now planned to be used for genetic marker studies. Other proposed studies would be prospective: the future collection of blood samples from normal controls; the future collection of urine from patients seen in the emergency room with fever; and the future extraction of DNA from blood specimens to be obtained from muscular dystrophy patients.

The IRB had to develop guidelines to help investigators understand which protocols did not require informed consent, which protocols might qualify for a waiver of informed consent, and which protocols required informed consent and complete IRB review.[37]

One issue of the monthly "Medical Ethics Advisor," published and distributed by American Health Consultants, discussed the NBAC report. After pointing out that "hospitals across the country may be·sitting on a research gold mine and not even know it," it continued, "Although most hospitals currently are not set up to allow researchers access to the tissue samples, the fact that they exist raises questions about whether these samples could be used in genetic research." Jeff Botkin, M.D., a physician-ethicist interviewed for the article, commented that NBAC recommended the practice of anonymizing samples without consent, thus eliminating the privacy risk to individual sample sources but leaving open the possibility of stigmatizing large population groups. Moreover, Botkin stated that NBAC was "split" on whether individuals can appropriately give general consent to letting their personal tissues and data be used for future, presently unknown, genetics studies. The article's conclusion: NBAC made many recommendations, but "bioethics policy is falling behind the pace of scientific advancement," in part because the federal OHRP "has not released any formal policies or standards to govern hospital ethics committees or IRBs."[38]

Notes

1. National Bioethics Advisory Commission, *Research Involving Human Biological Materials: Ethical Issues and Policy Guidance,* Vol. I: *Report and Recommendations of the National Bioethics Advisory Commission* (Rockville, Md.: National Bioethics Advisory Commission, 1999), pp. ii, 55.
2. *Ibid.*, p. 70.
3. Eric M. Meslin and Harold T. Shapiro, "Some Initial Reflections on NBAC," *Kennedy Inst Ethics J* 12 (2002): 95–102.
4. NBAC, Vol. I, inside front cover. Another multidisciplinary bioethics committee at the federal level is the NIH's Recombinant DNA Advisory Committee, which, unlike NBAC, continues to function. A more recent bioethics committee is the President's Council on Bioethics, established by George W. Bush in 2001. For a progress report on this committee, see Stephen Hall, "President's Bioethics Council Delivers," *Science* 297 (2002): 322–24.
5. NBAC, Vol. I, unnumbered page.
6. *Ibid.*, copy of Shapiro cover letter to President Clinton.
7. *Ibid.*, p. 9.
8. *Ibid.*, cover letter to President Clinton.
9. *Ibid.*, pp. ii, 55.
10. *Ibid.*, p. ii.
11. See Elisa Eiseman and Susanne B. Haga, *Handbook of Human Tissue Sources: A National Resource of Human Tissue Samples* (Rockville, Md.: RAND, 1999), p. 141.
12. NBAC, p. 27.
13. *Ibid.*, p. 29.
14. *Ibid.*, p. 51.
15. See Chapters 2, 5, and 9–10 in this book.
16. NBAC, p. 42.
17. *Ibid.*, pp. i, 58.

18. *Ibid.*, p. 70, emphasis added.
19. *Ibid.*, p. 72.
20. *Ibid.*, p. 73.
21. *Ibid.*, p. 75.
22. *Ibid.*, p. 75, and p. 2 of Shapiro cover letter.
23. See, for example, Eric T. Juengst, "Groups as Gatekeepers to Genomic Research: Conceptually Confusing, Morally Hazardous, and Practically Useless," *Kennedy Inst Ethics J* 8 (1998): 183–200.
24. See NBAC, *Research Involving Persons with Mental Disorders That May Affect Decisionmaking Capacity,* 2 vols. (Rockville, Md.: USGPO, 1998).
25. NBAC, *Research Involving Human Biological Materials,* Vol. I, pp. 48–49.
26. Eric Meslin graciously sent us copies of the written comments on NBAC's February 22, 1999, draft of the report.
27. NBAC, *Research Involving Human Biological Materials,* Vol. I, pp. v and 66.
28. See, for example, NBAC, Vol. I, pp. v, 66, 31–32, 68–71.
29. *Ibid.*, p. 64.
30. *Ibid.*, p. 66.
31. *Ibid.*, p. 51.
32. *Ibid.*, p. 70, emphasis added.
33. *Ibid.*, pp. 22–23.
34. *Ibid.*, p. 34, emphasis added.
35. See NBAC, Vol. I, Chapter 4. By contrast, one of the earlier NBAC reports made substantial use of religious perspectives. See Chapter 3 in NBAC, *Cloning Human Beings* (Rockville, Md.: National Bioethics Advisory Commission, 1997).
36. This event occurred at one of the National Bioethics Advisory Commission meetings (open to the public) in Bethesda, Maryland in 1998.
37. Susan Kornetsky et al., "Guidelines for the Collection and Use of Biological Specimens for Research Purposes," Committee on Clinical Investigation, Children's Hospital, Boston, unpublished manuscript.
38. "Stored tissue samples: Gold mine or land mine?" *Medical Ethics Advisor* 17 (2001): 40–43.

III

ETHICAL, PROFESSIONAL, AND LEGAL IMPLICATIONS

9

Updating Informed Consent in the Era of Genomic Medicine

> According to the law, the data in the IHD [Icelandic Healthcare Database] will be collected under the assumption of "presumed consent." ... Some argue that presumed consent is inconsistent with the right of individuals to decide for themselves and actually amounts to no consent at all. However, presumed consent is the standard used for research on health care data that is produced in the process of delivering medical services. It is not certain that we would have health care as we know it today if explicit consent had been a prerequisite for the use of medical data.
>
> Jeffrey Gulcher and Kari Stefansson, 2000, DeCODE, Inc.[1]

> Although it is their DNA and not their bodies that will be studied, individual consent must be obtained for the collection of DNA (because it is removed from the body), for storage (because the DNA belongs to the individual) and for analysis and the use of the information obtained by analysis (at least if this information can be linked to the individual person). ... [A] blanket consent to non-hypothesis-based "data dredging" in the genetic database would be unacceptably vague.
>
> George Annas, 2000
> Boston University Schools of Public Health and Law[2]

Informed consent is one of the recurring themes in this book. The reason is simple: informed consent represents a kind of contested territory where an ongoing international debate is being waged by several interested parties. The point of contention is the conditions under which research with stored tissue samples can and should be done. The views of many of these interested parties—patients, research participants, geneticists and other biomedical scientists, pathologists and other physicians, IRB members, entrepreneurial "gene hunters," indigenous populations, biotechnology companies, bioethicists, attorneys, and distinguished multidisciplinary panels in several countries—were presented earlier.

The result of this debate, after several years, is an ongoing disagreement between two opposing camps, with each camp having several permutations of its fundamental position—and, it seems, numerous representatives of that basic position in many countries. Groups, committees, and individuals aligned with one camp strongly advocate continuing traditional biomedical research practices during the era of genomic medicine with, perhaps, only a minimal strengthening of the informed consent process. Groups, committees, and individuals aligned with the other frequently call for research participants and patients to be given more information and choice about taking part in human tissue research without, perhaps, giving sufficient consideration to how such changes may impede important research with banked DNA samples.

Informed consent is certainly not the only ethical and legal issue involved in human tissue research; we discuss several of these issues in the next chapter. Informed consent is, however, the most dominant feature in this international debate because reasonable people in multiple professional fields and in many countries disagree about how the concept of informed consent should be used in settings involving research with stored DNA samples. Why is this the case, and what recommendations for change are reasonable, ethically defensible options?

To answer these questions, this chapter provides several reasons for updating the informed consent process so that consent can be more relevant to the kinds of human tissue research being done worldwide. It also indicates why the "reasonable person" standard for disclosure is the appropriate disclosure standard for investigators who do research with stored tissues, especially if that research is prospective in nature but also, to a lesser degree, if the planned research is retrospective research with archived samples. Along the way, we analyze several versions of consent and make recommendations regarding how patients and research participants can be empowered to make choices about the possible use of their tissues for research, especially when that research is on identified or linked samples containing personal and familial genetic information.

The Need to Update the Informed Consent Process

Informed consent has evolved over the decades until it has come to occupy a place of central importance in clinical medicine and biomedical research. In clinical medicine, informed consent has largely moved over the years from a concept relegated to courtroom proceedings, judicial decisions, and law journal commentaries to the point that practices related to informed consent are a routine, daily feature of clinical medicine in its various settings. Depending on the invasiveness, importance, frequency, and risk of harm associated with various medical procedures, the process of informed consent is commonly carried out in two ways: either (1) the explicit signing of a procedurally relevant consent document by an autonomous patient (or a nonautonomous patient's surrogate), or (2) a hospital/clinic policy stating that all adult patients are understood to have given consent (i.e., implied consent) to any fairly routine procedure simply by agreeing to be treated in the facility. A third way is used by physicians from technologically developed countries who do clinical work, often on a volunteer basis, with indigenous populations in other parts of the world. They adapt the conventional, individual-focused process of informed consent to meet the requirements of providing medical care in a specific third-world group setting.

In biomedical research, the process of informed consent is clearer, generally more formal, more predictable, and regularly reviewed by an IRB, at least in university settings. (The role that informed consent has, if any, with the numerous tissue samples obtained in the private sector by pharmaceutical and biotechnology companies is impossible to know.) Any scientific investigator planning to conduct a publicly funded research study is required by institutional agreements with funding agencies to have the study approved in advance by the investigator's local IRB, unless the study meets the criteria for exemption. In addition, even investigators doing unfunded research studies with human participants in university settings are obligated to comply with local IRB requirements, because most U.S. universities have given the federal government written assurances that all investigators working with human research participants will comply with federal regulations.

Alternatively, if the research study is to be done with an identifiable group or indigenous population in another country (or, in recent years, Native American groups in the United States), the research team is expected to work with appropriate IRB-type committees in those settings, whenever such a review mechanism is available. This external IRB-type approval, like the approval of a proposed study by an investigator's local IRB, includes discussions and revisions of a carefully formulated consent document and other investigator-generated information that may be pertinent to getting committee approval and, later, informed consent by potential participants in the research study.

In both clinical medicine and biomedical research, the elements of the informed consent process are these: (*1*) providing relevant information in appropriate ways (*2*) to patients and potential research participants possessing decision-making capacity (DMC) so that these persons are (*3*) enabled to understand the information and (*4*) make voluntary and (*5*) adequately informed decisions about consenting (or refusing to consent) to recommended medical procedures, or taking part (or declining to participate) in research studies. Depending on the situation, the medical procedures and research studies may involve obtaining one or more tissue samples from the patients' or research participants' bodies. This theoretical model of the informed consent process, however, sometimes runs into several practical, professional, personal, and institutional problems in both clinical and research settings, the analysis of which lies beyond the scope of this book.

A more limited analysis is pertinent to this book. Why does the process of informed consent in clinical medicine and biomedical research need to be updated in the era of genomic medicine? What is there about common practices worldwide of using the tools of molecular biology to do research with banked DNA samples that threatens the process of informed consent in unprecedented ways? How can the review of human tissue research by local IRBs be improved to enhance the possibility that potential research participants in research settings *and* clinical settings will be more adequately informed about planned research with their tissues?

Eight current problems need to be addressed. (*1*) Physicians, scientific investigators, IRB members, and the rest of us need to understand that informed consent is a process, not merely an event symbolized by the signing of a consent document. Sometimes, unfortunately, busy physicians give orders to another person on the health-care team, such as a nurse or medical student, to "consent the patient," suggesting with that statement that the only important thing about informed consent is getting the patient's signature on a required consent document. Sometimes, when questions come up about informed consent in meetings of investigators and their research teams, they are dismissed with comments suggesting that the main concern about informed consent for research is getting the wording of a consent document approved by the local IRB. Likewise, members of IRBs sometimes spend a disproportionate amount of time during their meetings with prospective grant recipients on a detailed analysis of the wording in consent documents, thereby reinforcing the widely held view that informed consent=consent document=single event.

That view needs to be replaced by an understanding of informed consent as an important process of communication and mutual decision making that may involve several conversations and use various forms of communication, thus allowing for subsequent thoughts and follow-up questions. From the perspective of physicians and investigators (and members of their teams), taking part in this process involves the disclosure of relevant information (e.g., the planned medical intervention or research study, its anticipated benefits, its risks, acceptable alternatives, etc.), the assessment of comprehension and decision-making capacity on the part of patients and prospective research participants, and the response to pertinent questions raised by those persons. From the perspective of patients and prospective participants in research studies, taking part in the process involves getting relevant information about the recommended medical procedure or planned research study, thinking about its possible benefits and known risks, asking questions (about the risks, acceptable alternatives, costs or compensation, etc.), and making a decision about whether to consent to having the recommended procedure done or participating in the planned research.

The conventional way this process of communication and decision making is formalized is, of course, through the use of consent documents, whether signed upon one's admission to a clinic or hospital, admission to a hospital critical care unit, at some point prior to undergoing a recommended procedure of some importance, or before actually beginning to participate in a research study (by filling out a survey, giving a family medical history, taking part in a clinical trial, and/or providing a blood sample or other tissue sample). Fortunately, health professionals have developed additional ways of supplementing consent documents. Especially since the information is often technical in nature, multiple ways are now used in clinical settings to clarify that information and enhance patients' comprehension of the specific words contained in consent documents: brochures with user-friendly language and pictures, visual aids, and videos. These supplemental communication tools are especially helpful in clinical settings that involve complicated, but repetitious procedures with large numbers of patients.

(2) More scientific investigators and research teams need to follow the model increasingly found in specialized clinical settings of using technology in creative ways to enhance the informed consent process. An increasing number of professionals in some clinical fields and subspecialty clinical areas are giving patients the choice of viewing interactive CD-ROM programs to improve the informed consent process for diagnostic tests and treatment options. The Foundation for Informed Decision Making at Dartmouth University, for example, has produced dozens of these interactive communication tools for numerous clinical areas (e.g., orthopaedic surgery, genetics) as a way of improving decision making by patients and saving time for health-care professionals.[3] The American College of Obstetrics and Gynecology has produced a series of interactive CD-ROM programs called PACE (Patient Advice and Consent Encounter) as a way of improving communication with patients.[4] The Patient Education Institute, a company with headquarters at the University of Iowa's research park, has produced over 150 CD-ROM and Web-based patient education programs that use multimedia software (including animation) to enhance the informed consent process in a variety of clinical settings.[5]

Similarly, some scientific investigators and research teams already use technology in creative ways to inform potential participants about specific areas of biomedical research. By contrast, other investigators and research teams, who regularly use state-of-the-art technology in their analysis of DNA samples, seem not to be doing as much in using technological communication tools with prospective research participants. These investigators and research teams could, as some labs are already doing, supplement written consent documents with brochures containing pictures of the laboratory setting, some of the lab equipment, and some of the lab personnel who will be carrying out the planned research study. The CDC, for example, provided prospective participants in the NHANES III study with a professionally produced brochure that combined their consent document with photos of physicians, nurses, and the mobile unit that would go to participants' homes to enable tissue collection, lab tests, and other data collection to be done at those sites. If such brochures are produced by investigative teams, however, we hope that the primary purpose for doing so is to enhance the decision-making process of prospective participants in a planned research study, and not simply to produce a recruiting tool.

There are other possibilities. For instance, videos could be produced that would give prospective participants in a genetics research study a better idea of the laboratory equipment, techniques, and processes that will be used to move from the collection of a blood sample from an individual participant to a later point in time at which lab personnel will have produced multiple types of information from that blood sample (information about possible inheritance patterns, DNA sequence information, gene identification, mutations, genetic similarity with relatives, etc.). Medicine labs, pediatrics labs, psychiatry labs, and other labs that do prospective research on tissues could produce similar videos that would provide helpful, discipline-specific information to individuals considering participation in a particular type of research study. Such information about the "lab world" is, of course, common stuff to people who develop a research study protocol and do the work to complete the research study. But it is very different from the world inhabited by most people, and a user-friendly video with helpful information that could be used over and over again with many people might result in more research participants, and certainly better informed research participants, than seems to be common at the present. Yet even the best videos still need to be supplemented by interactions with a member of a research team who can provide helpful answers to any number of serious questions raised by individuals who have viewed the videos.

In addition, more research-related Web sites could be developed and used creatively, not only for the purpose of attracting large numbers of prospective participants to a particular field of research (e.g., the genetic factors in Alzheimer disease, craniofacial disorders, panic disorder, various eye disorders) but also to provide general information about planned studies in those specialized fields. These Web sites could contain links to more information about more specific studies. This Web-based information would not take the place of much more specifically worded consent documents, but it could certainly introduce and supplement the use of consent documents. Such an approach is already being used by many research teams, including investigators affiliated with DNA Sciences, the company behind the widely publicized Gene Trust DNA bank that has recruited thousands of participants worldwide into their research on dozens of multigenic diseases.[6]

(3) Investigators and research teams are busy people who plan research studies, write consent documents related to the planned studies, prepare numerous pages of supporting information for IRBs, celebrate when research funding comes through, contact many persons who might be recruited for a research study, have conversations with prospective and actual research participants in the study, and carry the research study to completion. In the midst of this work, these professionals sometimes need to have a better understanding of the basic rationale that underlies the process of informed consent, whether the research being planned and done takes place with patients in clinical settings or with other persons in a multitude of research settings. Without such an understanding, the time and effort required to write consent documents and meet various IRB requirements can easily be considered as wasted time. Moreover, the efforts required to inform prospective research participants in language they can understand (i.e., consent documents written at a sixth-grade reading level) about the purpose, anticipated benefits, known risks,

and other relevant information about a planned research study can be regarded as a pointless "jumping through the IRB hoops," especially if scientists believe that prospective participants "can't understand" and are "not interested anyway."

What is the rationale that makes the process of informed consent for research studies important? Although volumes have been written on the topic, the rationale underlying informed consent is fairly straightforward. It has two necessary, complementary parts: to give autonomous individuals *a choice about how their bodies can be used* for medical and scientific purposes, and to protect research participants *from being harmed on balance* from their participation in research studies.[7] The first part of the rationale is necessary because no individual or group has a moral or legal right to use another individual's body in ways that go against his or her preferences and wishes, unless there are overriding public-health concerns. As self-determining individuals who regularly make decisions about how our bodies are used (and perhaps abused), we expect to make similar decisions whenever investigators try to enlist us to take part in a research study. Even if we agree—especially if we agree—with the scientific purpose of the study, we have the right as thinking, generally self-protective persons to exercise choice: to choose whether, when, and how we will permit our bodies to be used even for good scientific purposes.

The second part of the rationale is necessary because of the implications of a threefold truth: the relative ease with which humans harm each other, the almost limitless ways we have of harming others, and the expansive capacity we have to engage in self-delusion, whereby we are able to convince ourselves that we are helping others when we may be doing just the opposite.[8] In the context of scientific research using human participants, the possibility that all of us have of harming others is, unfortunately, sometimes actually done by researchers who have access to (possibly vulnerable) research participants and a mixture of motivating reasons for their work. Such possible motivations include, for example, not only the pursuit of scientific discovery, but getting additional grants, satisfying bosses, receiving promotion and tenure at academic institutions, and achieving fame and/or fortune.

The second part—protection of participants from harm—therefore has two components: permitting prospective research participants to make their own self-interested assessments regarding what would constitute an acceptable risk of harm to them, and requiring investigators to abide by protective policy rules for research (the federal regulations) and protective administrative mechanisms (IRBs) to help them avoid doing harm to others in the name of science. For egregious examples of physical and psychological harm done to others in the name of science, one has only to consult publications on the history of biomedical, behavioral, and other forms of scientific research.[9]

(4) Hospitals, clinics, and the physicians and nurses who work in these settings need to disclose a fairly widespread practice to patients, namely that post-diagnostic research is sometimes done on stored tissue samples in pathology,

genetics, and numerous other labs, and in some commercial labs receiving tissue samples from hospitals for diagnostic tests. Much of this post-diagnostic research is done on tissues sent to pathology labs by surgeons (including surgical specimens regarded as "extra" tissue or surgical "waste"). Some research is done on tissues of all kinds sent to pathology labs and other biomedical labs inside and outside hospitals by physicians providing diagnosis and treatment for patients in nonsurgical clinical settings. Some research is subsequently conducted by physician-investigators themselves on tissues (e.g., blood, urine, cheek cells, skin, amniotic fluid, muscle tissue, cerebrospinal fluid) obtained from patients for diagnostic purposes, but it remains available to the physician-investigators and some of their scientific colleagues after the diagnostic tests have been completed.[10] How much of this research is done with IRB approval and how much of it is done "under the IRB radar screen," as an NIH administrator commented to one of us, is an open question.

The John Moore case is, of course, the most publicized example of post-diagnostic research, with surgical samples of Moore's spleen and samples of his blood, urine, and bone marrow all ending up in Dr. Golde's lab. Elisa Eiseman and Susanne Haga have documented that most of the 307 million tissue specimens currently stored in tissue banks in the United States were originally collected for diagnostic and therapeutic purposes.[11] As noted in Chapter 3, the position paper by the Council of Regional Networks for Genetic Services (CORN) defends this common practice by saying that tissue samples obtained for diagnostic and therapeutic purposes may and should be used later for research in order to help the advance of medical science. They urge that all new tissue samples "be collected with the *dual intent* of providing immediate and/or future benefit for the source person *as well as* providing tissue for subsequent research in genetics or in other disciplines."[12] The AAMC recommends that this dual-intent practice be institutionalized by all hospitals and clinics by giving each patient "two unique identifiers, one for clinical use, the other for research," with linkage between the two numbers securely and confidentially maintained by an institutional databank.[13]

This AAMC recommendation could be helpful, depending on subsequent details, because it would represent a public move of candor and disclosure to patients about post-diagnostic research practices that are currently often hidden from (or at least not generally acknowledged to) patients, and because it could also improve health care. Even if the AAMC proposal does not become common practice, patients would be well served if the administrative personnel in hospitals and clinics regularly and clearly disclosed to them *at least the possibility* that any blood draw or other tissue sample obtained from them for diagnostic purposes might subsequently be used for research purposes as well and that they have a right to consent to that research. This disclosure by an institution could take several practical forms—through hospital and clinic admission forms, and/or via a video on biomedical research regularly shown on in-house TVs.

Patients would also be better informed if physicians and nurses (and phlebotomists) regularly disclosed the same possibility to them as a part of the process of informed consent. This disclosure through conversations with patients (or via printed statements or brochures) by physicians and nurses would be especially helpful if it also included the information that tissue samples obtained from patients might (*1*) continue to be identified with them as individuals, (*2*) be linked to them by a barcode or other institutional coding device, or (*3*) be anonymized after diagnostic tests had been completed.

One more item of information about post-diagnostic research would be helpful for hospitals, clinics, and health care professionals to disclose to patients: the possibility that some of this research might be done by genetics investigators (or others, such as investigators in infectious diseases), thereby perhaps *implicating other biological members of a patient's family* as well as providing intimately personal information about the patient. If such openness and regular disclosure about the possibility of post-diagnostic research were to become common, patients would be substantially better informed about human tissue research and enabled to make decisions about some of the important implications of providing blood and other tissue samples when asked to do so by physicians, nurses, and phlebotomists. Simply put, patients would be empowered to make choices that they do not currently even know they have, aided by important information they are not currently given.

Do patients want this information? We believe they do, based in part on some data we collected some years ago in a pilot study on patient attitudes toward biomedical research and, more specifically, regarding post-diagnostic research with stored tissues. As mentioned earlier, we had an IRB-approved survey instrument filled out by 93 adult outpatients in a family medicine clinic in Iowa City. Most of these patients indicated that they believed that biomedical research using stored tissue samples is "very important" (52%) or "somewhat important" (18%); and most (54%) thought it is a good idea for "people to support biomedical research by participating in research that does not pose unreasonable risks." Very few (3%) had ever had a physician tell them about the possibility of post-diagnosis research on their tissue samples, yet 69% of them thought "it is necessary for physicians to tell patients if research might be conducted on their tissue sample." Most would be "very bothered" (33%) or "somewhat bothered" (40%) if research were done "*without your consent* on tissue samples you provided for diagnostic tests."[14]

Would the kinds of disclosure regarding the possibility of post-diagnostic research we have suggested represent a significant impediment to biomedical research? We don't think so, because all the disclosure methods we have suggested could easily become regular practices and reasonably efficient parts of the communications process between health care institutions/health care providers and the patients they serve.

Would such disclosures of heretofore often hidden or unacknowledged research practices with tissue samples obtained in clinical settings make patients unduly concerned, less cooperative, or less inclined to consent to provide tissue samples? We doubt this would happen very often because the primary reason for patients' willingness to provide blood or other tissue samples upon request would remain fundamentally important to them, that is, they have an undiagnosed medical mystery that is most likely to be solved by means of a tissue-based "clue" that can only be helpful if it is used with an appropriate diagnostic test. Most patients will likely continue to consent to provide tissue samples for such tests, with some of them still not thinking very much about the subsequent possibility of research being done with the samples.

Regular disclosure of the possibility of post-diagnostic research is also likely to increase support among citizens for biomedical research, as well as building trust in the professionals to do the research. As discussed earlier, multidisciplinary panels in the Netherlands, Canada, and the United States have independently advocated such goals in the midst of the current controversy over research with stored tissue samples. Telling patients the truth about common research practices and giving them choices they do not currently have may be a way of achieving those goals.

(5) Another problem has to do with the consent documents that are a required feature of IRB-approved biomedical research, whether funded by the federal government or private companies. Given the commonness of research with stored tissues, consent documents need to do a better job of disclosing relevant information to prospective research participants about DNA banking. DNA banking, as indicated in Chapter 2, is a common practice involving two kinds of storage of DNA-related information for current research studies and possible future research: (a) stored biological materials, including tissue samples, extracted DNA, and/or transformed cell lines, and (b) genetic data derived from these biological materials, including stored DNA sequence data and other relevant information about the human being from whom the tissues came.

Consider the findings of an earlier research study. A few years ago one of us (RFW) was funded to direct several studies that examined some of the ethical, legal, and social implications of genetics research. One of those studies focused on how the informed consent process was actually being carried out among genetics investigators working with human participants in the United States, with particular attention given to the process of informed consent in the context of DNA banking practices. Requests for information and copies of consent documents went to 177 genetics investigators doing a wide range of genetics studies. Investigators in 47 states and the District of Columbia sent us 103 usable consent documents.

Only 23 documents explicitly asked prospective research participants for consent for DNA banking as part of larger research projects or contained more general language informing them that investigators wanted permission to store research participants' blood, other tissue samples, or transformed cell lines for subsequent research. These documents represented a variety of genetics studies: alcoholism, cystic fibrosis, Down syndrome, Huntington disease, the muscular dystrophies, schizophrenia, and so on. All of the other consent documents provided no explicit or general language that would have given prospective research participants even a vague notion that their blood or other tissues would be banked in genetics labs for long-term research studies, even though many of the responding investigators told us they had disclosed such plans in related documents given to their IRBs.[15]

When the investigators in this study analyzed the 23 consent documents that mentioned DNA banking, we found that only a few of them (three to nine documents, depending on the specific content being analyzed) disclosed even a portion of the information that would be relevant for a reasonably prudent, prospective participant in a research study to know about the DNA banking component of the study. None of the documents came very close to providing the several kinds of specific information that would seem to be required for a reasonable person to give *informed* consent to participating in a genetics study that would store blood or other tissue samples from that person for one or more genetics research studies spanning a number of years. The good news was, however, that the consent documents indicated that a few genetics investigators and research teams had decided to disclose at least some participant-relevant information about planned DNA banking in their consent forms.

In the years since that study (sometimes called the Iowa Study), it has become reasonably clear through anecdotal examples that other genetics investigators and other researchers using DNA banking practices have begun to include information about these practices in their consent documents. Unfortunately, it is also evident, through other anecdotal examples, that an unknown number of investigators and IRB members who review their research proposals continue to fail to provide relevant information to prospective research participants about some of the important aspects of long-term storage of any tissues they provide for planned (and likely) research studies, even when that information is shared by the investigators with the IRB members.

The upshot is that some progress is being made by some investigators and research teams in that they increasingly regard prospective research participants as reasonable, "want-to-know" persons; regularly consider the types of information about DNA banking and its implications that persons placed in the situation of being prospective research participants would probably want to know; and consistently write consent documents that provide that relevant information. Our hope is that additional progress along these lines will be made nationally and internationally.

But this trend, to the extent that it is a trend, needs to be quickened and expanded to include more research teams that use DNA banking practices as an indispensable part of their research protocols. Not to move in this direction—*the direction of greater disclosure and more adequately informed consent*—will be to continue the practices documented in the Iowa Study, namely, that many "consent" documents fail to disclose important, relevant information about DNA banking to prospective research participants and thereby prevent them from having reasonable choices and making informed decisions about providing tissue samples for research studies.

Consider one notable example. The Women's Health Initiative is one of the largest and most complex disease prevention studies ever conducted. This research study has 160,000 adult, female research participants who were recruited from 40 clinical centers across the country. The women participate in the study for 8–12 years. Each of them has gone through an exceptionally thorough, sequential, multicomponent process of informed consent involving verbal and written information, a video, and reading materials. Depending on where they fit into the study, however, each woman has signed one or more consent documents that includes, among many other pieces of information, *only a single sentence* telling them that their stored blood samples may be used for genetics tests. The documents fail to provide them with (*1*) additional information about how, where, or why their blood samples will be stored for research purposes or (*2*) any information about the kind of genetics testing that may be done, any possible benefits or risks in that research, or who may have access to the research results.[16]

(*6*) The procedures by which individuals can communicate their advance consent to participate in one or more research studies need to be expanded beyond consent documents. One way of expanding the options for communicating advance consent for an individual's possible participation in some future research studies using stored tissue samples would be through the development and use of research advance directives.

All adult American citizens have the moral and legal option of using advance directives to communicate their personal choices about decisions that might have to be made toward the end of their lives when they are unable to make health-care decisions for themselves, especially if the ends of their lives take place in a hospital or other health-care facility. They have the option of completing a treatment directive whereby they communicate their consent or refusal to consent in advance to the medical interventions that might be used to sustain their lives in the event of critical or terminal illness. They can also complete a proxy directive whereby they select one or more surrogate decision makers in the event they can no longer make health care decisions for themselves. If they choose, both types of advance directives can be used, perhaps in a combined form.[17]

Persons who have completed one or both of these end-of-life advance directives have engaged in prospective decision making, a type of decision making that all of us do from time to time as we make advance planning decisions in the present for projected circumstances we know could happen at some point in the future. We cannot be certain that these situations will occur (e.g., our death in a hospital critical care unit), and we certainly should know that the circumstances we project may differ in actuality in the future from the way we project them in the present. For that matter, we may seriously hope that the circumstances we project as a future possibility do not actually occur. We still engage in advance planning, nevertheless, as an exercise in prospective autonomy whereby we make choices and communicate consent in the present with the intention that, should the projected circumstances come to be and we are at that time unable to make the requisite health-care decision(s), the decisions we express now will be regarded as prospective authorization for decisions necessary at that later time. In this way we plan to enable our surrogates and responsible physicians to carry out our decisions in that possible future clinical situation.[18]

The same kind of prospective decision making and authorization—in the form of communicating advance consent—can and should take place for certain kinds of research, including human tissue research. As discussed in Chapter 8, NBAC used the concept of prospective authorization as an explanation of and justification for a new approach in research ethics, namely permitting scientific investigators to carry out research studies with individuals' bodies, minds, and stored tissues when the only evidence of informed consent by those individuals is in the form of future-oriented consent documents they signed months or years in advance of the actual study's being done. For NBAC, using such advance consent for future research studies is not a practice generally to be promoted or condoned because the research would be done with the bodies (and/or tissues) of individuals who, at the time of the research, would either be incapable of consenting to participate in the actual study (because by that time they would have a mental disorder causing them to lack DMC) or be uninformed about it (because they might have moved and would be difficult to contact).

NBAC thinks, nevertheless, that such a practice of prospective authorization for personal participation in specific classes or types of future research studies is justifiable in two types of research: research on some mental disorders involving individuals who previously consented to participate (while possessing DMC) but can no longer do so, and research on stored tissue samples involving tissues obtained from individuals who consented at the time of tissue acquisition by physicians or investigators to have the tissues used for particular types of future research studies. The justification of research in these two kinds of situations is based on NBAC's assumption that individuals providing such prospective authorization would have done so as a part of an adequately constructed process of informed consent.[19]

NBAC is correct in its conclusions about prospective consent for specified types or classes of future research on stored samples. We suggest, moreover, that the concept of prospective consent for particular kinds of research can also be expanded and made operational through the use of research advance directives, a point also made by the Canadian Tri-Council.[20] Several types of research advance directives should be developed and made available to patients and prospective research participants, thus supplementing the use of consent documents.

(7) IRBs need to update their committee membership, review procedures, and consent-related requirements for investigators in the light of widespread, quickly

evolving DNA banking practices in the biomedical sciences. The work done by administrators and members of IRBs is demanding, tedious, time-consuming, frequently the subject of criticism by scientific investigators, and insufficiently recognized and rewarded by departments and institutions. This work is also important, necessary to provide protections for research participants and investigators, and reflective of the values central to responsible research ethics, whether it is done by members of local IRBs, IRB-type committees at some federal agencies, research ethics committees in Canada, regional research review committees in Denmark, medical society-run research review committees in Slovakia, consultative committees in France, or a number of variations on this theme carried out in many countries in many parts of the world. India is the country most recently to establish a national network of IRBs.[21]

In the United States these research ethics committees are often understaffed, underfunded, and overwhelmed by the volume of work they are expected to do, including the review of research proposals in collaboration with research ethics committees in other countries. IRB members have a continually increasing number of research proposals to read, discuss, make decisions about (whether through an expedited review process or a full committee discussion), and continue to monitor at regular intervals.

This description of IRBs was confirmed by a report issued a few years ago by the U.S. Office of Inspector General. An earlier federal report had concluded that "the effectiveness of IRBs is in jeopardy" because they face major changes in the research environment, review too much and too quickly, have too little expertise, and provide too little training for committee members and investigators.[22] The OIG report concluded that "minimal progress" had been made in significantly changing IRBs. As discussed in Chapter 6, the OIG report led to a decision by the Department of Health and Human Services to establish the Office of Human Research Protections. HHS has also initiated educational programs to improve the training of investigators and IRB members regarding the informed consent process, the need for local monitoring of that process, and other ethical aspects of research done with human participants.[23]

Thus some important changes are taking place at both the national and local levels, including a widely used NIH Web-based course on the protection of human participants in research studies.[24] Pertinent to the topic of this book, however, are two additional changes that need to take place if the process of informed consent (and the review of that process by IRBs) is to be updated as it needs to be. First, we have commented earlier about the datedness and vagueness of some of the federal regulations as they apply to human tissue research. In this regard, we join forces with others who have pointed out that the regulations need serious revision and clarification for a new era of biomedical research.[25] Updating the regulations, however, will be difficult and slow in coming because the voices calling for reform (ours included) are not in unison regarding the specific revisions that need to be made, and any revision of the Common Rule requires agreement by all 17 federal agencies currently using these regulations.

Equally important, a second set of changes needs to be carried out at the local level to address some specific problems that limit the effectiveness of the IRB review process. At present, IRBs frequently lack expert committee members who themselves do research in molecular genetics or related fields. Moreover, they often have other committee members who do not understand DNA banking practices or how the informed consent process needs to be adapted to that research context, get significantly different interpretations among committee members regarding how the federal regulations apply to research using stored tissues, and make requirements of investigators (usually pertaining to the wording of consent documents) that when carried out provide insufficient protection for research participants once their tissue samples and DNA-based information are in storage.[26] The result is a review process for biomedical research that simply does not fit our time and the needs of investigators and research participants.[27]

Fortunately, alternative remedies are available. For large, complex research institutions, such as research-oriented universities, the problem can be handled through one administrative move: a requirement that the IRB always have a member who is an expert in molecular genetics or a related field. This expert in the research methods of molecular biology could, perhaps, be a geneticist no longer active in directing genetics studies. For IRBs in smaller institutions that have fewer— perhaps no—genetics experts available locally, but increasingly have to review research proposals that call for this kind of expertise, the problem is more difficult. A possible solution, however, would be the cooperation of several such institutions in the same geographical region in sharing a regional genetics expert as an IRB consultant, for a fee and on an "as needed" basis.

Even more sweeping changes for IRBs may be forthcoming. After the establishment of the OHRP, HHS commissioned the Institute of Medicine to perform a comprehensive assessment of the national system of IRBs. The IOM report was published in 2002. It made a number of recommendations, including a proposal that IRBs be reorganized into a system of three-tiered "research ethics review boards" that, whenever appropriate, would have regional responsibilities for reviewing multicenter research studies.[28]

(8) IRBs and other research ethics committees need to broaden their understanding of informed consent to include the important participation of identifiable communities and groups worldwide. As mentioned earlier, considerable genetics research and other types of research take place in remote corners of the world. Investigators, their research teams, and their financial sponsors (national research-funding agencies, biotechnology companies, etc.) are almost always located in technologically advanced countries, but the human participants (and their tissues) of central importance to these research studies are often found in isolated pockets of Africa or South America, on numerous islands throughout the world, or, in some

instances, "hidden" in geographically limited areas of the United States and other Western countries.

Because of this disparity between researchers and the persons on whom the research is being done, research studies in earlier years sometimes ignored the interests, cultural traditions, religious beliefs, and other values of the people being studied. In some cases these research participants were undoubtedly harmed and possibly wronged because of the greed, racism, ethical insensitivity, and cultural imperialism of the persons doing the research. In other cases the investigators, engaged in collecting tissue samples and various types of data on individuals, families, and groups, did so with a reasonably clear understanding of the traditional values of the people with whom they were working and the significant differences between those values and the values of the scientifically trained, usually Western-oriented investigators. Nevertheless, because of the frequency with which some researchers ignored the traditions and values of indigenous peoples in geographical settings other than their own, many investigators who travel great distances to collect blood samples, urine samples, bone fragments, and other tissues have often been grouped under the same pejorative labels: "bleed and run" scientists, "gene hunters," and so on.

Partially because the NIH and other federal funding agencies have recently taken important steps to address this problem, the practices of investigators and IRBs have begun to change. Now U.S.-based investigators and IRBs are no longer required to have a Single Project Assurance (SPA) for research studies done internationally. Rather, American investigators are required to conduct their international research studies according to the model of a Federalwide Assurance, as discussed earlier. The use of FWAs signals a new, more cooperative approach to research done by American investigators in collaboration with one or more home-country (Brazil, India, etc.) scientists. Likewise, the FWA model for collaborative international research studies represents a new, possibly better, way of reviewing research studies, including a more appropriate approach to the process of meaningful informed consent in other parts of the world.

According to this new model, the home-country collaborator works with a research ethics committee or another IRB-type committee, if one already exists, or constitutes an IRB-type committee following U.S. research guidelines. The home-country IRB then conducts the review(s) of the research study, with written assurance that it is following U.S. research regulations interpreted in the context of local standards. With this assurance, the IRBs in each American investigator's home institution may accept the study review done across a national border.[29]

Whether this new model for international research studies will actually be an improvement, whether the committee review of various studies will be done with sufficient consistency and stringency from country to country (and IRB to IRB), and whether the new collaborative research and review process will bring about a long-overdue recognition of the values and traditions of other cultures by IRBs in the United States are all questions waiting to be answered. But we hope that this new approach to collaborative research studies and the review of such studies—with American investigators, home-country scientists, home-country research ethics committees, and U.S. IRBs—will work well. If so, this new approach will enhance and strengthen community participation in the informed consent process for research studies done in other countries. This cross-cultural approach to informed consent is important because, simply put, Western-style consent documents that focus on individual research participants have limited relevance in many other cultural settings.

The Reasonable Person Standard of Disclosure

What information should be disclosed to prospective participants so that they will know a research study involves DNA banking? More specifically, what information should be disclosed to prospective participants about a research team's DNA banking practices (and the investigators' policies related to DNA banking) so that they will have a sufficient understanding of the long-term implications of providing a blood or other tissue sample for a study?

Likewise, in both inpatient and outpatient clinical settings, what information should be disclosed to adult and adolescent patients (and to the parents or guardians of children) about the possibility of post-diagnostic research so that they will have a reasonable expectation of what may happen to the blood sample or other tissue sample once it leaves a patient's body? Common practices suggest that the tissue sample may be (*1*) *discarded* as biological waste after the diagnostic tests are completed; (*2*) *stored* for an indefinite period of time (for quality control reasons, or medico-legal reasons) in a pathology or other hospital laboratory; (*3*) used for post-diagnostic *research* by one or more investigators; (*4*) used for *educational* purposes in teaching hospitals; or, less commonly, (*5*) *sold* to one or more biotechnology firms. How much of this information should be disclosed to patients so that they will know these possibilities exist?

Since an important part of the informed consent process is adequate comprehension of information by prospective research participants and patients (whether the information is received verbally, in a consent document, by video, or via a computer program), what standard of disclosure is the appropriate one for physicians, clinician-investigators, and other biomedical investigators to use? In particular, if the process of informed consent needs to be updated for the current era, as we believe it does, what standard of disclosure is the appropriate one for investigators to use in the context of studies involving DNA banking?

For the past several decades numerous attorneys, judges, physicians, bioethicists, and legislators in the United States (and other countries) have had differing views regarding the appropriate disclosure requirements for appropriately informed consent in clinical settings. Four alternative standards have been proposed and extensively debated: the professional (or "physician discretion") standard, the reasonable person (or "objective") standard, the specific person (or "subjective") standard, and the legislative standard (based on whatever state law requires, including some "cookbook"-type lists of possible risks and harms). No clearly dominant disclosure model has emerged, at least in terms of state laws, because deciding on the appropriate disclosure standard in any case depends on several variables: the jurisdiction in which a clinical case occurs, the common-law and legislative history of a state, the characteristic features of significantly different clinical settings, the institutional policies of hospitals and clinics, the different training and practice styles among physicians, the information available about individual patients' views and preferences, the different expectations about disclosure from culturally and educationally diverse patients, and the advice given physicians about informed consent requirements by clinical ethicists and institutional attorneys. Nevertheless, the reasonable person standard is not only the accepted legal standard in many states, as mentioned in Chapter 7, but often seems to be the standard of disclosure regularly being used by clinicians even in states having another official standard of disclosure for physicians.

In a parallel development, numerous persons at the NIH (and research agencies in other countries), health-law attorneys, bioethicists, members of IRBs or research ethics committees, scientific investigators, and activist groups in several countries have discussed how the consent process applies to biomedical research. As indicated earlier, the discussion in this country has focused primarily on federal rules for research and, in particular, the details, merits, implications, and flaws of the Common Rule. Curiously, even though substantial attention has been given to the specified items that investigators are required to disclose about their planned research studies, little if any attention has been given to the standard of disclosure investigators are expected to follow with prospective research participants. Yet the views of many investigators and IRB members about the ethics of disclosure to prospective participants seem to be based on the federal regulations and suggest that the reasonable person standard of disclosure is the appropriate standard for disclosures about research studies.

One gap in these long-running discussions is the failure to address disclosure requirements for clinical settings that may be precursors for and intertwined with post-diagnostic research. The gap pertains to a lack of discussion about the standard of disclosure to which biomedical professionals should be held when they are in the *dual role of physician-investigators*. The literature on informed consent has not until recent years even recognized that concerns about disclosure and consent exist in situations involving clinically derived tissue samples that are banked and used for long-term research purposes, some of which may have very little connection with the medical condition(s) that initially were the cause for obtaining tissues from patients.[30]

The reasonable person standard, in our view, is the appropriate one to use in virtually all clinical and research settings. It has one distinct advantage over the other standards: it fits equally well as a standard for disclosure in clinical settings, research settings, or in settings that involve a blending of clinical/research roles (e.g., pathology labs, cytogenetics labs) on the part of the physicians and other health professionals. For that reason among others, we are convinced that *the reasonable person standard is the best standard of disclosure* for all professionals involved in doing human tissue research.

When compared with other possibilities for disclosure—as well as with current, frequent practices of minimal disclosure and nondisclosure—the reasonable person standard is clearly preferable. The first standard of disclosure mentioned earlier, the professional standard, is often favored by physicians, especially when they think about informed consent in the context of legal liability, such as the possibility of being a defendant in a trial having to do with a clinical case. Likewise, if scientific investigators think about the remote chance of becoming defendants in an analogous trial setting with questions about informed consent (as in *Moore*), they, too, would probably prefer to be held accountable according to the professional standard. In either instance, defendants would be expected to show that they had disclosed pertinent information to a patient or a research participant in a manner and at a level of specificity that is consistent with the customary practices of their professional peers in a certain medical specialty or area of research. In some cases of human tissue research, the professional standard would thus seem to allow an investigator to take an updated, though extreme, position of self-defense analogous to trial defenses used by some American surgeons in court a century ago (e.g., "I didn't even tell her that we were going to store her blood sample for years, anonymize it, and use it for research studies because I didn't think it was any of her business.") as long as he or she could find several other like-minded investigators in the same field who would agree with that minimalist level of disclosure. A less extreme, far more likely rationale for an investigator to use in defending the professional standard would be an updated version of the social contract theory, that is, because humanity stands to benefit from the potential scientific findings resulting from human tissue research, everyone has a shared responsibility to participate in at least some research studies, even if scientific professionals disclose only a minimal amount of information about them.

To use another example, the professional practice standard (if it were applied to organizations) would seem to require the disclosure of little or no information by hospital administrations to patients regarding the possibility of post-diagnostic research, even in teaching hospitals affiliated with academic medical centers where such research may be fairly commonplace. Of course, surgical consent forms often have a single, very general sentence about possible future research with tissue obtained during surgery, but outside of this exception, hospitals tend not to disclose anything about possible post-diagnostic research with clinically derived tissue samples.[31] At least one reason for this silence is simple: the Joint Commission on the Accreditation of Healthcare Organizations does not currently require hospitals to make such disclosures to patients as part of the admissions process (where it could and should be done) or at any other time.

The professional standard is inadequate, in most instances, because it sets the standard of disclosure too low for physician-investigators and other scientific investigators in the twenty-first century. This standard requires only that investigators communicate the amount and kind of information that is commonly disclosed by other genetics investigators, pathologists, epidemiologists, or investigators in other fields using DNA banking techniques in their research. If used in connection with research with stored tissues, this standard would seem to require the disclosure of little or no information to participants about DNA banking practices. This would be true even if investigators had already told an IRB they planned to use banked samples in their research and even if some, perhaps many, prospective research participants would be interested in having that information prior to giving consent to participate in the planned study. This option is not justifiable because it suggests an "investigator [or hospital] knows best" approach to disclosure, and ignores the legitimate interests that prospective research participants (including patients) may have regarding their tissue samples.

The specific person ("subjective") approach to disclosure recommended by some bioethicists is, by contrast, not adequate in most instances of human tissue research because it sets the standard of disclosure too high for many physician-investigators—and especially for other scientific researchers who do not have professional contact with patients. The specific person standard is arguably the preferable standard of disclosure for the informed consent process in a limited number of clinical settings, notably those clinical settings in which individual physicians get to know individual patients through repeated encounters and conversations over several years and thereby have some understanding of a patient's medical history, value system, family relations, preferences, anxieties, and hopes.

In most situations involving disclosure of information about planned human tissue research, however, the specific person standard of disclosure is not acceptable because of its impracticality. Most investigators using stored biological materials in their research studies (e.g., population-based epidemiological or genetics studies) have little, if any, information about the value systems, preferences, anxieties, hopes, or much of anything else of a personal nature regarding the individuals who may choose to participate in a research study. Often a blood sample obtained from any individual participant is only one of many blood samples obtained from hundreds or thousands of other participants, thereby precluding investigators from having any personal knowledge about any of the specific research participants. Even in tissue-based research studies (e.g., studies involving clinically derived samples) in which individual blood samples or other tissue samples remain identified or, more commonly, coded as they are studied in a laboratory setting, the chances are slim that the clinician-investigators and members of their laboratory teams have a clue about the preferences, anxieties, or hopes of any of the specific individuals from whom the tissues came.

There is, however, an exception, even if a statistically rare one: When investigators *do* know one or more specific patients or prospective research participants sufficiently well that they understand how the disclosure of information about a planned research study would be received by them, they should tailor the information (e.g., how much is communicated about DNA banking practices and research plans, and how it is communicated) to fit their life situations, educational levels, preferences, anxieties, and hopes. For example, an investigator might, in rare instances, know a specific patient or prospective research participant well enough to know that this person would regard some kinds of research objectionable (e.g., studies of a particular medical condition, studies focusing on the prevalence of a medical condition in a specific ethnic or racial group, behavioral genetics studies trying to find a "gay" gene or a "violence" gene). When this unusual situation occurs, it most likely occurs in a clinical setting in which a physician-investigator gains this level of personal knowledge about a patient through his or her role as a physician. As investigator, however, he or she should disclose information about a planned research study at a level of specificity that fits that patient's perspective.

The legislative standard is also problematic in the unlikely event that a state legislature would decide to formulate a law stipulating the content that investigators would be expected to disclose to prospective participants about research studies using DNA banking. As discussed in Chapter 7, at present, only Louisiana (and, previously, Oregon) has legislation that specifically addresses some of the issues related to research done with DNA samples.[32] But even the Louisiana law does not stipulate elements of disclosure pertaining to research practices with banked DNA samples.

Using the legislative standard to impose specific content for investigators to disclose would be problematic for at least two reasons. First, it could result in a patchwork combination of state laws that would impose different elements of disclosure on investigators working in different states. Thus, differences among state laws would only exacerbate the variability in disclosure requirements that already exists as local IRBs in different research institutions impose different requirements and restrictions on investigators doing basically the same kind of research. Second, using the legislative standard of disclosure for research studies using DNA banking and a variety of research techniques in molecular genetics would be difficult because of the frequency with which DNA samples, cell lines, and DNA data are shared by investigators in different states and countries. The challenges thus imposed on investigators and IRB members would be considerable as they try to do state-of-the-art research and review that research appropriately—and also comply with specifically worded state laws that do not change as rapidly as research practices do.

That leaves the reasonable person ("objective") standard of disclosure. This standard is not without problems, of course, but the problems connected with using it are far outweighed by its possible benefits. The chief problem is that the central concept—the "reasonable person"—is inherently vague and impossible to define in a way that satisfies everyone. Nevertheless, the concept has been a part of Anglo-American common law for over 200 years (originally, as the "reasonable man"). More importantly, this standard gains its strength from three features it possesses: (*1*) it personifies "common behavioral assumptions that members of society must make about their fellows in order to interact efficiently," (*2*) it serves as a prescriptive "standard that individuals must meet or risk liability," and (*3*) it reflects the right of self-determination held in common by all autonomous individuals, whether they are patients, participants in research, or individual citizens engaging in business transactions and other regular activities.[33]

The reasonable person standard is also often misinterpreted. It is not correctly interpreted as applying to any single individual, nor is it to be confused with someone's possession of the virtues of reasonableness, cooperativeness, or being a team player. Rather, when correctly interpreted, this standard is an objective reference to "a composite of reasonable persons."[34] Most importantly for research settings, this composite person *is in the situation* of a potential research participant. As a result, the reasonable person standard, whether used in the context of clinical care or the context of research, is sometimes referred to as the "reasonably prudent" person standard.

How does this apply to the process of informed consent in the variable context of human tissue research? Consider the Iowa Study discussed earlier. In that study we (RFW and Iowa colleagues) used the reasonable person standard of disclosure in our analysis of the 23 consent documents dealing with consent for DNA banking. More specifically, these ELSI investigators analyzed the documents from the perspective of a reasonable person whose consent is being sought by a genetics investigator for a research study that will include long-term storage of biological materials. Placed in this kind of situation, that of a prospective research participant, what kinds of concerns or questions would a reasonable person have before he or she agreed to provide a blood sample that might be kept for an unknown period of years in a genetics lab?

Alternatively, what information would a reasonably prudent person wish that she had been given during the process of informed consent regarding the control and ownership of biological materials when, perhaps by coincidence, she discovers years later that the tissue sample supplied to a genetics investigator had been transformed into a cell line? What would she wish had been disclosed as a future possibility upon discovering that the cell line was subsequently shared with numerous other investigators and, given the unique features of the cell line, produced commercial profits for the genetics investigators and the biotech company with which they work? Or what would she wish had been disclosed about secondary research studies in the unlikely event of later finding out that other investigators, working in collaboration with the original investigator, had used many anonymized blood samples (including, almost certainly, one or more samples obtained from her body) for a genetics study that she personally finds objectionable?

The results of the Iowa Study were published in 1995. At that time the ELSI investigators were convinced that a reasonable person placed in the situation of a prospective research participant in an American study using DNA banking would have at least seven identifiable interests and information concerns:

- The privacy and confidentiality of personal information
- The control and ownership of banked materials (and, hence, possible commercial benefits)
- The possibility of withdrawing biological materials from a research study
- The length of storage planned for tissues
- Participants' access to any personal, clinically relevant information derived from the samples
- Third-party access to the biological materials and data
- The possibility of secondary research with the banked materials[35]

Based on subsequent experience in using this theoretical model with a variety of groups in diverse educational settings, we now think that a reasonable person placed in this situation would likely have up to *eight identifiable interests and concerns* constituting a definable core of information that he or she would want disclosed before agreeing to participate in a study using DNA banking practices. In addition to the original seven items of information, we include one more at the beginning of the list: the identity status of the samples. This core of desired information might be expressed by a reasonable person placed in the situation of a prospective research participant in some or all of these alternatively worded questions:

- "Will my tissue sample [my DNA sample] be identified or traceable to me when it is being studied in the lab?"
- "What are the chances that information derived from my stored sample [my stored DNA] will get into the wrong hands?"
- "It is my tissue sample [my banked DNA], right?"
- "Can I withdraw my personal involvement [my banked sample] from this research study at any time?"
- "How long do you plan to keep my banked sample [my DNA]?"
- "If you find out something clinically important about me from my banked sample [my DNA], will you tell me?"

- "Will other people have access to my DNA sample and data [genetic information about me] in the future?"
- "Will you or other scientists use my stored tissue sample [my DNA] for secondary research studies with different purposes?"[36]

In most instances, the reasonable person standard is the appropriate standard of disclosure for investigators to use when DNA banking is planned. It is also the appropriate standard according to which investigators should be held accountable if participants in a research study subsequently raise questions about the information they were given about planned research with tissue samples they provided. Likewise, the reasonable person standard is the appropriate standard of disclosure for physician-investigators to use with patients, especially when a physician (in a diagnostic and therapeutic role) *knows* that he or she (in an investigative role) is planning later, perhaps in collaboration with other investigators, to use a patient's stored tissues for research purposes.

Two of the professional genetics groups discussed in Chapter 3 agree with this view. The American College of Medical Genetics specifically calls for clinicians to inform patients about any subsequent research plans; the Council of Regional Networks for Genetic Services document calls for clearly acknowledging the "dual intent" involved in collecting tissue samples in clinical genetics contexts.[37] By contrast, even though the College of American Pathologists' policy statement specifically discusses "concurrent collection" of tissue samples (the practice of carrying out research on pathologic diagnostic specimens after the completion of the work necessary for a patient's care), the authors assert without documentation that patients neither want nor need this information about post-diagnostic research.[38]

We return to this CAP position later. For the moment we highlight our differences with this status quo position on minimally informed consent, even when put forth by a prestigious medical society, by calling for a rigorous updating of the informed consent process built around the reasonable person standard. Simply put, the time has come to add both (*1*) *additional specificity* to the informed consent requirement (by applying the reasonable person standard to DNA banking and research) and (*2*) *more widespread applicability* of the informed consent requirement (by making appropriately informed consent the norm for both prospective and, whenever practicable, retrospective human tissue research).

If the reasonable person standard were to become the professional standard for all human tissue research, what difference would it make? At the very least, it would mean that some current practices of doing prospective and retrospective research studies apart from the knowledge and consent of the key parties involved (the individuals from whom the tissues came or, in some cases, the surviving relatives of those individuals) would have to change. For example, the reasonable person standard of disclosure would seem to require hospital administrators and physicians on hospital staffs to agree on institutional policies of disclosure whereby patients would be informed (e.g., in a consent form signed upon admission, via a video on in-house TV, on clearly displayed notices) that post-diagnostic research is at least a possibility for any blood sample or other tissue sample they provide to the health-care professionals at that institution. The institutional disclosure would not need to go into great detail, but would at least have to disclose to patients that any tissue samples obtained through blood draws, surgical procedures, and other invasive procedures performed in that institution would become the property of the institution (with limited property rights) and might be stored for several long-term research purposes—while also assuring patients that this research would be done only with appropriately informed consent. In this way, an institutional policy based on the reasonable person standard would provide patients with pertinent information that hospitals functioning under the professional standard would probably not disclose.

As to retrospective research done on pathologic or other archived samples, the reasonable person standard seems to require that someone on any research team planning to do retrospective research on archived samples identified or linked with a previously living human being be given the responsibility of making, at a minimum, a good-faith effort to contact one or more members of the surviving family (e.g., by letter, by newsletter) before research is done on those tissues. The results of the effort to contact a surviving family for consent would need to be reported to the local IRB, which would have the discretion of deciding when such efforts to contact were, in fact, impracticable. Absent any contact with the surviving family, the responsibility of deciding if the proposed retrospective tissue study is justifiable should rest with the IRB.

Varieties of Consent

One of the complicating factors in the interdisciplinary debate about human tissue research and informed consent is multiplicity, both in the research done with stored tissues and in the interpretations given to the term "consent." Earlier chapters have suggested that not everyone in this debate addressing the topic of informed consent in the context of human tissue research means the same thing by the term "consent." While it may be true, according to Shakespeare, that "that which we call a rose by any other name would smell as sweet," it is not true that any procedure or process to which someone attaches the term "consent" actually constitutes consent, especially not informed consent, if this terminology is to retain much of its core meaning.[39]

James Childress has described "the spectrum of varieties of consent" that appears in academic discourse and legal statutes for the conditions under which "human body parts" can be transferred and subsequently used for transplantation and/or biomedical research. He uses the inclusive language of human body parts as defined in the revised (1987) Uniform Anatomical Gift Act (a human body part is "an organ, tissue, eye, bone, artery, blood, fluid, or other portion of the human body"). Childress is, however, primarily interested in describing six ways in which solid organs are transferred and used for transplantation: (*1*) express donation, (*2*) presumed donation, (*3*) routine removal, (*4*) expropriation, (*5*) abandonment, and (*6*) sale/purchase.[40] We discussed views about the abandonment of tissues and some of the concerns about the commercialization of tissues in earlier chapters; we return to both themes in the next chapter.

For now, Childress's depiction of the varieties of consent is important. He observes that three alternative interpretations of "consent" are sometimes used to justify and legally support the acquisition of solid organs for transplantation purposes: (*1*) express consent (or donation), (*2*) implied or implicit consent, and (*3*) presumed consent. Express consent, whether given orally or in writing, is "the paradigm case of consent" for organ transplantation and numerous other practices carried out daily in clinical medicine and in biomedical research. Implied consent, by contrast, is not expressed either orally or in writing, but is inferred from other actions, "even though the consenter may not have understood or intended such an implication."[41] Still further in contrast, presumed consent is basically tacit consent, neither specifically expressed nor inferred from specific other actions, but a passive condition characterized by silence, omissions, or in general "by failures to indicate or signify dissent."[42]

Childress's threefold typology of consent is too limited for human tissue research, especially given the multiple interpretations that are given to "consent" or "informed consent" in the debate. His typology needs to be expanded to make it more relevant to the complexities increasingly surrounding decisions to participate via one's tissue samples in research studies using DNA banking and to make it more comprehensive by adding other important categories, including a descriptive category appropriate for some legal minors. Thus, a more complete typology of the varieties of consent (and substitutes for actual consent) consists of these alternatives: (*1*) express, appropriately specific consent; (*2*) express, general consent; (*3*) assent and consent in pediatric settings; (*4*) community consent; (*5*) surrogate consent; (*6*) implied consent; (*7*) presumed consent; and (*8*) no consent.

Express, Appropriately Specific Consent. This version of consent, as Childress observes, is the paradigm case of consent. It is the gold standard for the process of voluntary, informed consent that has been advocated and defended for decades in the United States by many health-law attorneys, judges, and bioethicists. The result is that this interpretation of what consent can and should be is widely regarded as the normative type of consent for most U.S. clinical settings, especially those involving invasive and risky procedures for patients, and for most biomedical research done in compliance with the federal regulations.

When used in the debate about research with banked tissues, this conceptual model of consent posits a decision-making process, as discussed earlier, that is carried out by an individual adult (or older adolescent) who has decision-making capacity and is provided with relevant and sufficiently specific information about a planned research study. With that appropriately disclosed information, he or she can deliberate about the general scientific purpose of the proposed study, its anticipated scientific benefits and actual or possible risks (including psychosocial risks to self and family), and some of the implications involved in the planned long-term banking of tissue samples. Given the number of variables involved in specific research studies using DNA banking, the appropriate information is often presented in a "layered" consent document having several sections or offering a prospective participant several choices. He or she can then make a voluntary decision, one hopes, regarding participation in the study via stored DNA samples and expressly communicate that decision to a member of the research team, usually in writing when the decision is affirmative. The nature of that decision depends, of course, on personal, familial, and social factors that influence a reasonable person's decision when placed in this situation.

A number of individuals, groups, and policy statements subscribe to this normative version of informed consent and maintain that this version of consent is the appropriate standard for much human tissue research, most notably when this research is prospective in nature and will use identified or coded samples. Chapter 3 contains a discussion of several examples: the model law called the Genetic Privacy Act, the 1995 American College of Medical Genetics policy paper, the 1995 NIH/CDC workshop statement, and the 1997 CORN position paper. These documents also indicate substantial agreement about the moral need to extend this model of informed consent, with appropriate modifications, into several other types of human tissue research: planned or anticipated post-diagnostic research with clinically derived samples, prospective research using anonymized samples, and retrospective research using archived samples (when the consent process is modified to include surviving family members). Moreover, each of the documents contains several recommendations for specific types of content that should be disclosed to prospective research participants in consent forms, with the CORN group advocating the development of consent forms that will provide patients/prospective research participants with "a menu of options" to which individuals can respond with yes/no answers (see Chapter 3 for details).[43] Other model consent forms in the literature also contain multiple options for persons considering participation in genetics studies.[44]

There are additional advocates. The Tri-Council of Canada strongly advocates this kind of comprehensive, appropriately specific consent for research studies, as does the NBAC report, at least occasionally. As pointed out earlier, however, NBAC is not consistent in advocating layered consent documents.[45] By contrast, the National Action Plan for Breast Cancer coalition has developed a very good, layered consent document, tested it nationally with focus groups, revised it, and advocated its use for years.[46]

Some of the strength and enduring appeal of this model of consent rests on its unparalleled ability, when compared with other alternatives, to pass three real-world "tests" for consent models. These are: (*1*) *The test of appropriate disclosure:* Would adherence to this model of consent provide individuals with sufficient information on which to base an appropriately informed decision about participating in research using stored tissues? (Yes.) (*2*) *The test of voluntary decision making:* Would use of this consent model encourage individual patients/prospective research participants to make voluntary decisions? (Yes, depending on situational factors.) (*3*) *The test of objection to the point of withdrawal:* Would use of this model encourage investigators to disclose to prospective participants in a consent document that if they agree to provide requested tissue samples, they have a right subsequently to disagree with the stated research goal or research team even to the point of withdrawing from the study by requesting that their stored samples and derivative data be destroyed? (Yes, depending on details, and certainly more than other consent options.)

This model of consent also has numerous critics, many of them investigators who do human tissue research. From their perspective, this full-service model of informed consent begs to be rejected or weakened substantially because it is either too theoretical, too detailed, inefficient, impracticable in the real world of human tissue research, unnecessary, unwanted by patients and research participants, expensive to administer, or, if imposed on biomedical investigators through legislation or regulatory policy, would greatly impede important research from being done as rapidly as it needs to be done.

Express, General Consent. A second interpretation of the type of consent needed for human tissue research is advocated by many investigators and some biomedical societies as an adequate, real-world alternative to the first model. Instead of an itemized listing of options (e.g., selected identity status for banked samples, preferred types of research in which to participate, types of research that might be objectionable), this model of consent provides patients and prospective research participants with minimal information. It indicates that research may be conducted with clinically derived samples, but gives little or no indication of what that research might be, who might be doing it, when it might be done, or how long it might continue.

For adult patients (or parents/guardians of pediatric patients), general consent usually takes one or two forms: (*1*) a sentence on a one-type-fits-all surgical consent form that says only that surgically removed tissues may be used later in unspecified research studies (with generic wording along these lines, "Any surgically removed tissues may be used by the hospital according to customary practices, including for education and research") or, less commonly, (*2*) a sentence buried in minutely detailed hospital admission forms telling patients that biomedical research is one of the regular types of work done by some of the staff members in that hospital. An individual's signature on these forms signifies only that he or she has been given the form and signed it in order to get the necessary or recommended surgery, or to be admitted to the hospital as a patient. Among the strongest advocates for this general consent model are some pathologists, some geneticists, and other investigators who work with archived samples (e.g., surgical specimens in pathology labs, placental tissues and cord blood samples from delivery rooms, neonatal blood samples on newborn screening cards).

For the proponents of general consent, this approach to informed consent is preferable to the first consent model precisely because it begins and ends with the disclosure of very little information to patients or their families. Not only is this bare-bones disclosure acceptable to and popular with many investigators who do this research, they sometimes maintain that this general consent model is also acceptable to most patients and to the majority of the general public. Why? The reasoning is straightforward: most patients do not mind being kept uninformed about research practices, do not want to know any of the specifics about the kinds of research done with clinical samples, and could not begin to understand the information sufficiently to make informed choices even if it were given to them. In addition, advocates of this position maintain that the future research purpose(s) for specific tissues is sometimes not yet known at the time tissues are collected. The bottom line: patients are not going to be harmed by this lack of information and choice, and keeping disclosure to the legally permitted minimum has the additional benefit of saving time and trouble for investigators, hospital administrators, and hospital law/risk management offices.

Several groups support the model of general consent as being sufficient for human tissue research. The most notable, clearly stated policy statement backing this model of consent is the College of American Pathologists' position paper discussed earlier (see Chapter 3). The paper, entitled "Uses of Human Tissue," originally circulated in unpublished form and later published, states that members of 17 pathology societies in this country support a model of general consent that would simply consist of a statement telling patients that their tissues may be used in research approved by IRBs and then giving them a choice with no additional information: "I __ CONSENT __ DECLINE TO CONSENT to the use of my tissues for research."[47] Other groups that support the model of express, general consent are the British Nuffield Council of Bioethics (in 1995) and the Association of American Medical Colleges (in 1997).

An alternative form of general consent is sometimes recommended for some areas of biomedical research. Rather than using consent forms with detailed information about specific research studies, and repeating the consent process for other research studies in the same general area of research, its advocates suggest that "generic consent" can be an acceptable and more efficient option.[48] Another version of general consent, but with greater disclosure about the planned research, generic consent is a kind of informed consent that might bridge the gap between the detailed consent forms required for IRB-approved research and the approaches to general consent that provide patients and research participants (in post-diagnostic research) with no details about the research that will be done. Consider these examples: Prospective research participants interested in helping genetics research teams discover the genetic causes of multiple medical conditions could sign a "generic consent" form for "genetics research," thereby permitting their tissues to be used in a variety of studies rather than limiting their participation (via banked samples) in genetics research to specific types of studies. Patients with cancer interested in helping cancer researchers identify more of the causes and pre-disposing factors for cancer, including the type of cancer they have, could sign a "generic consent" for cancer research in addition to, perhaps, a more specifically worded consent document appropriate for a research study on their particular form of cancer.

The benefits of general consent are threefold: saving research time, cutting down on administrative paperwork, and avoiding hassles (with IRBs, hospital attorneys, bioethicists, and patients and their families) about the details of planned research with stored samples. The immediate recipients of those benefits would be clinician-investigators and other investigators who want to conduct as much important biomedical research with stored tissues as they can, do it well, do it quickly, and get funding to continue doing it. The long-term recipients of benefits from this research, we all hope, are people worldwide.

The fundamental ethical problem with this model of consent is also clear. General consent (or blanket consent) leaves patients in the dark about the types of research that may be done with their clinically derived tissue samples, whether they as individuals may be identifiable through their samples, the scientific pur-poses of planned research studies, the psychosocial risks that may be involved for persons providing samples, the possible risks that may occur if family members are implicated in genetics research on the samples, and even the types of antici-pated societal benefits that may occur through this research. This model of general consent fails to fulfill either part of the rationale for informed consent because it neither encourages choice nor tries to protect patients from psychosocial harm(s) (e.g., in family relationships, through acts of discrimination, through unwanted participation in objectionable research) that they or their family members might subsequently experience because of the unrestricted research done on their tissues.

This general consent model also fails the three real-world tests mentioned ear-lier, that is, there is insufficient disclosure to patients, constrained voluntariness on the part of patients, and no possibility for questions or objections except by persons who refuse to consent, if they are given that option. Simply put, patients are caught in a combined power/knowledge imbalance with physicians and/or other institu-tional research advocates and expected to go along with the research enterprise. This "going along" by patients can, of course, be done out of ignorance that their tissues may be used for research, or it can be an inadequately informed way of giving a "blank check" to investigators and research institutions to do whatever kinds of research they want to do with clinically derived tissue samples, limited only by IRB constraints.

Assent and Consent in Pediatric Settings. The standard of informed, deliberative, and voluntary consent does not work in most pediatric settings for a simple reason: children are not small adults. Children have differing blood values compared with adults, differing dosage requirements for medications, numerous medical conditions unique to younger human beings, faster recovery rates to injuries, pediatric versions of numerous medical conditions common to adults, differing perspectives on life and death, and so on. Important for our topic, children and adolescents present unusual challenges in terms of what "consent" to treatment or research can mean in a nonadult population. As a result, the exclusively adult perspective in most of the literature on informed consent needs to be modified to fit the developmental stages common to children and adolescents, including how the concept of "informed consent" to participation in human tissue research studies can and should be adapted to fit legal minors.

Sometimes "proxy consent" is suggested as the appropriate model of consent for pediatric settings. The American Academy of Pediatrics (AAP) points out, however, that the concept of proxy consent is flawed in pediatric practice because the fundamental idea contained in the action of giving consent requires that one "expresses something for one's self: a person who consents responds [e.g., to a request] based on unique personal beliefs, values, and goals."[49] Therefore, the concept of proxy consent cannot apply to pediatric settings because most children and young adolescents have not developed cognitively to the point that they are capable decision makers on important health-care matters. Most autonomous adolescents (in contrast to some adults) have not communicated their decisions about personal health-care matters sufficiently to parents or other trusted adults to enable one of those persons to consent on the behalf of an adolescent should the need arise (e.g., to refuse life-sustaining treatment on behalf of a terminally ill legal minor who cannot communicate that decision personally).

Fortunately, there is consensus about an age-based, developmental sequence that is appropriate for handling important decision making for and by patients in pediatric settings. This threefold sequence is widely regarded as combining appropriate recognition of the variability of children's cognitive development, respect for children's increasing interest in making their own decisions, and realism about the fact that most children and young adolescents are nonautonomous when it comes to making important personal health-care decisions.

The sequence calls for decisions about a legal minor's medical care and treatment to be made in the following ways. Appropriate authorization to carry out recommended diagnostic procedures and treatment interventions (e.g., invasive diagnostic testing, immunizations, casting broken or abnormal bones, surgery) in the medical care of any infant or young child (below age 7) should be based on oral or written *informed permission* given by that child's parent(s) or legal representative. With older children and younger adolescents who have more cognitive development (ages 7–13), appropriate authorization for recommended medical care should be based on a combination of *informed permission* by parent(s) or legal representatives *and assent* by the patient, thus providing older children and young adolescents with frequently desired, greater involvement in making decisions about their own lives and health. With older adolescents (ages 14–17), AAP guidelines advise pediatricians that they should obtain the *informed consent* of the patient along with appropriate support by that adolescent's parent(s) or legal representative, without (in many legal jurisdictions) having to obtain permission by these adults.[50]

As an alternative to informed consent, the concept of "assent" has come to have an increasingly important place in much clinical pediatric practice. Putting this concept into practice with many pediatric patients means several things: helping them to achieve "a developmentally appropriate awareness" of their medical conditions, telling them what they can expect with diagnostic tests and medical treatments, making a clinical assessment of a "patient's understanding of the situation," being alert to the factors influencing a patient's thinking (including inappropriate parental pressure to accept testing or therapy), "soliciting an expression of the patient's willingness to accept the proposed care," and weighing a patient's views (including objections) seriously in deciding whether to carry out the recommended medical procedures.[51] Like other practice guidelines in medicine, these guidelines about giving children the option of assenting or objecting to proposed medical interventions are not and cannot always be carried out in practice. They do, however, highlight the importance of giving children "a say" in their medical treatment, even if they are not yet capable of understanding at an adult level and going through the more deliberative process of informed consent or informed refusal.

Parallel to these efforts to give children an increased "say" about proposed medical treatment have been other efforts by pediatric health professionals and other professionals to give older adolescents an increased role in the decisions made about their medical care. Backed by research studies in developmental psychology, an increasing number of pediatricians, nurses, clinical psychologists, bioethicists, and health-law attorneys conclude that most neurologically normal adolescents aged 14–17 possess DMC comparable to most adults.[52] For that reason, many professionals maintain that the same general assumption should apply to older adolescents in clinical settings as applies to adults in similar situations, namely that these patients have the capacity to make informed, deliberative, and voluntary decisions about recommended medical treatment—and that unless circumstances in individual cases indicate otherwise, these decisions should be respected and carried out by adults.

Similar developments have not taken place in the regulations governing pediatric research studies. Guidelines for research with children in the United States, as well as international guidelines for research with children, tend to require that investigators and members of IRBs (or REBs in many countries) focus on balancing the potential benefits and risk of harm to research participants, including children in research studies. U.S. regulations specify four categories of possible research with children that differ in terms of (*1*) the projected risk of harm to participants, (*2*) the projected direct benefit for individual participants, (*3*) the projected benefit for biomedical science and society, and (*4*) the required steps for investigators to get proposed research studies approved. The regulations require more rigorous documentation of parental permission and children's assent as the projected risks of harm increase beyond "a minimal risk."[53]

The regulations fail, unfortunately, to provide an adequate definition of either "assent" or "minimal risk." They do not even address the possibility of applying the requirements of the informed consent process to adolescents. One result of this omission is that consent documents for research including adolescent participants often display uncertainty regarding whether adolescents are to be regarded as children (with consent documents requiring parental signatures) or adults (with adolescents signing consent documents for themselves).[54]

Moreover, the federal regulations fail to provide any specific guidance for long-term, human tissue research using tissues obtained from children and adolescents. Investigators and IRB members are therefore not required even to think about the unusual circumstances that exist (*a*) when children are asked to assent to research studies that will be done on tissues obtained from their bodies, (*b*) when adolescents may want to have more information about a research study and a more deliberative role (the role of consenters) in deciding about the possible long-term use of their tissues in the study, or (*c*) when the risk of harm in participating with one's tissues in research involves at least some risk of subsequent psychosocial harm to self or close biological relatives.

The regulations do not require or even suggest that investigators and IRBs recognize the legal change that occurs when adolescents reach the age of legal maturity. This "aging up" step should be recognized in research settings in one of two ways: by IRBs requiring investigators who work with tissues from children and adolescents to commit themselves to destroying all stored, coded samples as soon as the sample sources turn 18, or to using adult consent forms to "reconsent" individuals when they become legal adults.

In other countries, only one of the documents discussed in Chapter 5 expresses particular concern for legal minors in the context of human tissue research. The Nuffield Council on Bioethics refrains from calling for the prohibition of tissue donation by legal minors, but puts forth three ethical criteria for such research: negligible risk of minimal harm, parental permission, and the "agreement [assent] of the children themselves."[55]

This model of assent and consent in pediatric settings also has critics, of course, with the criticisms taking one of two forms. One form of criticism focuses on attempts to give children and adolescents a larger role in decisions about their health care and participation in research studies, with claims that "kids don't need to know," "kids can't understand," and "kids make crazy decisions anyway." The other form of the criticism emphasizes the overriding importance of research that needs to be done, including research with tissues obtained from the bodies of children and adolescents. For these critics, whatever importance there may be in giving legal minors a more significant "say" about (*1*) how tissues from their bodies may be used in research and (*2*) the kinds of risks of psychosocial harms they may be willing to take to help in the discovery of scientific knowledge pales in contrast to the importance of the research itself. As a well-funded pediatric investigator emphasized to one of us after an educational session on informed consent, "but we *really need* to get those tissues for research!"

Community Approval. As mentioned earlier, in the latter part of the twentieth century an increasing number of DNA-sampling scientists, anthropologists as well as geneticists, traveled from technologically advanced societies to remote pockets of the planet to collect blood samples, bone fragments, and other DNA samples from members of indigenous communities. Many scientists seem to have been successful in retrieving valuable DNA samples, sending them home, putting them in long-term storage, establishing cell lines with some of them, and publishing important results from this global research.

The ethically and culturally insensitive practices of some of these scientists later came under severe criticism by representatives and defenders of indigenous people. In addition, some geneticists and other academicians began in the early 1990s to promote the Human Genome Diversity Project (HGDP) as a supplement to the international Human Genome Project. One of the important themes for advocates of the HGDP was the need to redefine the concept of informed consent so that it was not limited to consent given by individual research participants, but, more generally, would help protect the rights of research participants in the context of the traditions, values, and goals of their communities. As a consequence, considerable discussion took place internationally regarding community consent as a possibly important, new option among the varieties of consent.

A basic claim by HGDP advocates was that just as it is important to do international genetics studies to discover and correctly document the genetic diversity that exists in the world, so is it important that tissues obtained to produce that scientific information be collected in a manner that involves the participation of the affected communities through community consent.[56] The proponents of the HGDP, whose proposal was adopted by HUGO in the mid-1990s, produced a model ethical protocol that discussed the rights of indigenous research participants and the importance of community consent.[57]

Subsequently, however, the HGDP failed to get approval and funding in the U.S., and the concept of "community consent" has faced substantial criticism. Most notably, the National Research Council (NRC) published a detailed critique of the proposed HGDP, including the interpretations that had been advanced about community consent. As a preferable alternative to this concept, the NRC Committee on Human Genome Diversity recommended that local social groups be involved in the design and implementation of any local DNA-sampling plan.

In particular, the NRC committee called for scientific investigators to involve indigenous groups in two ways: site-specific *community consultation* (working with appropriate community representatives to design sampling strategies, collection methods, and reciprocity agreements) and *community approval* (working with the process that a particular group uses to make collective decisions on issues related to community identity and interests). Further, they recommended that this communicative and interactive process be as closely analogous to the process of informed consent for individuals as possible, with investigators disclosing information in an appropriate manner to the community about the expected duration of the research, anticipated benefits, foreseeable risks, confidentiality measures, voluntariness of participation, rights of refusal and subsequent withdrawal by individuals, and availability of any compensation.[58]

The concept of community consent is problematic for at least three reasons. First, there are numerous definitional problems in determining what counts as a community in specific instances and in different parts of the world, how community membership is defined, how decisions are made for and by the community, and so forth. Second, there is the problem of what legitimately counts as consent. As noted earlier, consent is a voluntary act that individuals do for themselves. Authentic consent is neither something that a group can do for individuals without their participation in that decision, nor is it something that group leaders can coerce members of the group to do, a fact that is severely tested whenever women and children are coerced to participate in research in male-dominated groups. Coerced consent should not be regarded as authentic consent! Third, there are numerous procedural and implementation challenges involved in making a community-backed process of consent actually work, including challenges of maintaining individuals' rights, protecting the confidentiality and privacy of research-based information, protecting relatives' rights (e.g., in pedigree studies), establishing agreements with investigators about access issues with banked DNA samples and data, working out other reciprocity or profit-sharing agreements, and so forth.[59]

Yet these problems are not insurmountable. Some large groups and subgroups within the larger groups do, occasionally, work out a process for community consultation and approval of research studies that seems to meet the needs of investigators, community leaders, and individual community members. A case in point is the detailed explanation of the role of community in research contained in the 1997

U.S. Indian Health Service "Guidelines for the Collection and Use of Research Specimens."[60]

Two recent efforts to address cultural diversity and community rights in international research studies are also promising. One of them, the use of FWAs mentioned earlier, is a new approach being taken by the NIH, IRBs in the United States, and U.S.-based investigators that may transform the working relationships between these scientists and indigenous communities everywhere. The other is a major initiative taken by CEPH, the Centre d'Etude du Polymorphisme Humain (Center for the Study of Human Polymorphisms) in Paris, based on its worldwide collection of tissue samples. CEPH has made a panel of approximately 1,000 DNA samples—obtained with community approval from indigenous populations in Africa, Asia, Europe, North America, and South America—available without charge to an international consortium of over 100 investigators. These samples are to be used to identify DNA sequence variance throughout the world, with the expectation that the scientific findings will be made available on a publicly accessible database.

Surrogate Consent. This model of consent is an unlikely possibility for most human tissue research. Nevertheless, having an ethical and legal mechanism whereby a trusted relative or friend can, when a previously autonomous person no longer possesses DMC, step forward to make a health-care decision on that person's behalf has substantial precedent in this country. Likewise, the surviving members of a family in the United States and in some other countries have property-like rights in how the dead body of a relative is handled or placed.

Thus the model of surrogate consent has possible, but limited, applicability to human tissue research. First, the federal regulations or state laws could be revised to permit a previously autonomous person's "legally authorized representative" to consent (or refuse to consent) in a clinical setting to the use of clinically derived tissues from the patient's body in post-diagnostic research studies, just as he or she has the right to consent (or refuse to consent) to medically recommended treatment of the patient. Second, the model of surrogate consent could be applicable to the consent (or refusal) by a previously designated relative to proposed retrospective research studies in a pathology lab with identified or linkable cadaveric tissues in the designator's dead body, if the family were to be contacted for consent. If, for example, the designated relative knows that the dead relative either supported or was opposed to the type of research being proposed, that knowledge would provide a sufficient moral (and possibly legal) basis on which to give (or refuse to give) surrogate consent for the use of these tissues for the planned research.

Implied Consent. The first three models of consent can be oral or written in clinical settings, depending on differences among specific clinical contexts. The fourth model, correctly understood as community consultation and approval, may be connected in some geographical locations with the provision of medical care to members of a community, but usually focuses primarily on investigator-initiated, community-supported research. The fifth model, surrogate consent, might be based on an oral statement, but the chosen surrogate would certainly have a stronger legal claim if the statement had been made in writing.

When any of these versions of consent is used as a personal authorization by patients or research participants for human tissue research, that authorization typically occurs in writing. For the first three models of consent, each widely used, two written forms are common: (*1*) admissions documents signed by incoming adult patients (or parents/guardians of pediatric patients) acknowledging and accepting a hospital's printed policies (including, perhaps, a general statement indicating that research may be done with clinically derived tissue samples), and (*2*) consent documents signed by research participants (or parents/guardians of children and younger adolescents) for specific research studies. How many patients and research participants actually read these documents before signing them is, of course, open to question. A less common and more variable practice is the written documentation of community consultation and approval for a research study provided by community leaders in a third-world setting.

By contrast, the models of consent yet to be discussed usually involve no written documentation of the particular model of consent being described. Implied consent, as Childress notes, is expressed neither orally nor in writing. This model of consent depends on *inferences drawn by a third party* from specific situations or other actions. Situational examples include the provision of medical and nursing care in emergency situations outside hospitals (e.g., an accident victim on a roadside, a person who collapses in a public place). In such situations, temporary medical or nursing care can be provided (and legally defended later, if necessary) on the basis of a societal assumption about implied consent, namely that when a "Good Samaritan" renders aid in such a situation, he or she is correctly acting on the inference that a reasonable person needing help in that situation would normally consent to having the help provided. Since the person in need cannot give oral or written consent at the time, the ethical and legal interpretation of the situation is that the person's consent to receive care is implied in the situation itself.

Implied consent is also regularly used as a rationale within hospitals to justify the provision of medical and nursing care to patients in certain clinical contexts (e.g., emergency rooms, critical care units) without specifically seeking their oral or written consent for every procedure done with them. Thus, emergency rooms and critical care/intensive care units usually have unit-based policies that define certain kinds of procedures as being "routine care" within the units. Part of the rationale for such policies is the claim that a patient's physical presence in the unit (even if the patient is unconscious or otherwise nonautonomous) signifies an implied consent to the routine treatment. A variation on this theme is an explanatory claim about patients often heard in teaching hospitals: When a person decides (consents) to be a patient in such an institution, he or she has thereby given implied consent in that patient role to a range of standard practices common to such institutions (e.g., medical students and residents having defined roles pertaining to the care of patients).

How does this version of consent apply to human tissue research? The same kind of reasoning is used by some of the advocates of the general consent model discussed above. They claim that any time a person voluntarily becomes a patient in a hospital, especially a teaching hospital affiliated with a medical school, that person thereby gives implied consent to participate via his or her stored tissues in the various human tissue research studies carried out in that hospital and by that hospital's scientific investigators.

It does not seem to matter to advocates of this view whether this implied consent exists separately from a general consent to research that patients give during the admissions process or is an ongoing subset of general consent used as a rationale for specific research studies never mentioned to patients. What does matter is that the research-oriented hospital situation itself—combined with the previous actions of persons to be admitted as patients—creates the inference that such persons have given implied consent to research that may be done with tissues obtained from them. As noted earlier, the patients inferred to have given this implied consent to tissue-based research studies may not have understood or intended such an implication.

Presumed Consent. This model of consent also exists without oral expression or written documentation on the part of the person or persons said to have consented. When this kind of consent is claimed to have taken place, it exists apart from specific situations or other actions by individuals that might form the basis for an inference about implied consent. Presumed consent is therefore tantamount to *tacit consent:* Not only does an individual not have or exercise a chance to opt in to a new opportunity, policy, or program with which he or she agrees (e.g., by voting, sending money, or giving informed consent), he or she also fails to opt out by registering in a designated manner disagreement with the opportunity, policy, or program being promoted. Thus, individuals sometimes fail to vote against a referendum item they oppose, remain silent in the midst of a group discussion that seems to favor a course of action with which they disagree, or fail to return an opt-out card or letter to a company in a designated manner and time period to register official dissent with a new company policy they dislike. The result is that this silence or inaction is interpreted as representing agreement, there being insufficient evidence to the contrary, thereby permitting persons in positions of power to claim they are carrying out a new policy or program with the presumed consent of the persons involved.

This is the approach currently being used by Kari Stefansson and his supporters in Iceland to claim public support for DeCODE's monopolistic marketing of the Icelandic Healthcare Database. Since the concept of presumed consent was included as a political strategy in the 1998 Icelandic law, DeCODE has been able to claim substantial public support for the company's DNA banking practices because only a small percentage of adult Icelanders (approximately 10%, according to published figures) have chosen to carry out the one officially recognized way of expressing dissent, namely by completing opt-out cards, sending them to Iceland's director of public health, and requesting that their personal and medical information already contained in the IHD be removed.

Although not backed by similar monopolistic legislation, other investigators in other countries also use presumed consent as a political strategy for gaining public support for their research. In the United States, for example, this strategy is used in some state laws to enable investigators to obtain neonatal blood spots for research purposes without adequately informed parental consent. In Denmark and Norway, the geneticists directing the 100,000 Birth Cohort Study also use this strategy to claim that their work, perhaps correctly, is being done with the consent of parents.

The benefits of using presumed consent for biomedical research are similar to the benefits of using the model of general consent: it is an efficient way for investigators to gain authorization for their research, and, along the way, they and their research teams save time, cut down on administrative paperwork, and avoid hassles with research participants. Equally important to investigators, this methodology enables them to gain virtually unrestricted use of very large numbers of tissue samples, backed by the tacit consent of "the silent majority" that does not opt out from the planned way of gaining access to the samples. In contrast to the model of general consent, the methodology of presumed consent produces no explicit, written authorization (i.e., no signed consent document) from individual participants in the research. This approach, however, is also somewhat more restrictive on investigators because they must provide a few details to individuals and/or a community about their planned research as a necessary step toward getting the tacit consent they desire.

According to Gulcher and Steffanson, the benefits of using presumed consent for their DNA research with the coded samples and data in the IHD are clear and important. They are not constrained by any conventional approach to individualized informed consent that seeks consent for a particular "hypothesis-driven" research study. Rather, using the presumed consent (or as they say, "broad consent") of most Icelanders, they are able to carry out a new type of biomedical research in which they will be able to "mine large data sets" of health information about individuals, cross-reference phenotypic information with genotypic and genealogic data, study the interactions of genes with other genes and with the environment, possibly combine information from the IHD with information from other databases, and discover new methods of diagnosing and treating common diseases.[61] The use of presumed consent is justified by several claims: this kind of consent is necessary as an efficient way of gaining access to and using large amounts of genetic information; it (or more accurately, implied consent) is a standard methodology for claiming consensual authorization widely used by researchers working with medical records; it is acceptable to most "fully alert people of reasonable intelligence in Iceland"; and the research it authorizes will not likely lead to any subsequent discrimination against individuals or families in Iceland.[62] A benefit left unstated, of course, is considerable commercial gain for the DeCODE scientists and profits for the investors in this for-profit U.S. corporation.

Problems with the opt-out approach to consent are many, yet they are possibly manageable whenever there are convincing ethical reasons for investigators not to seek express, appropriately specific and adequately informed consent from individuals. The fundamental problem with presumed consent as a consent model for human tissue research is that it places more priority on the importance of gaining scientific knowledge in an efficient manner (another version of "What they don't know won't hurt them") than it does on gaining scientific knowledge with the trust and support of an informed population. Scientists who claim, as the DeCODE scientists do, that the population clearly supports their DNA banking and long-term research efforts are unable to back up that claim because the opt-out mechanism may show support for their work, or it may simply hide a combination of ignorance, apathy, forgetfulness, and procrastination on the part of a substantial percentage of the population. In Iceland, it is clear that the legally defined opt-out mechanism precluded the option of opting out for children and nonautonomous adults—and fueled the suspicions about the DeCODE research on the part of the Mannvernd group and many other critics in Iceland.[63]

In addition, the DeCODE scientists make a problematic claim when they assert that presumed consent is sufficient for DNA-based research because it has long been the ethical standard used for research on health-care data. This parallel simply does not work, for at least two reasons: the general content in a patient's medical record (unlike one's DNA information) is already known (or could be known) by the patient, and the results of the retrospective research that is typically done on health-care data are not usually linked to identified persons. Neither of these points is correct for the kind of DNA-based research on coded samples and data being done at DeCODE, Inc.[64]

Nevertheless, depending on the details in specific cases, the model of presumed consent can be ethically acceptable when scientists cannot seek the explicit, informed consent of individuals for large-scale DNA banking and research for reasonable reasons of impracticability. At the very least, the model of presumed consent can, depending on the details, be carried out in a manner that meets the three tests mentioned earlier: it can provide adequate disclosure to individuals, enable individuals and families to make voluntary choices about participation, and contain a procedure according to which an individual's banked DNA and data (or at least some of it) would be destroyed at that person's request. Childress suggests other requirements:

The potential consenter must be aware of what is going on and know that consent or refusal is appropriate, must have a reasonable period of time for objection . . . must understand that expressions of dissent will not be allowed after this period ends . . . must understand the accepted means for expressing dissent, and these means must be reasonable and relatively easy to perform.[65]

No Consent. The last option on the spectrum is the polar opposite of the express, appropriately specific, and adequately informed consent that has been discussed throughout this chapter. With this option, there is no question about whether a potential research participant has had the kind of information disclosed to him or her about a research study that a reasonable person in that situation would want to have. There has been *no disclosure* of any research-related information. Likewise, there is no point in raising questions about whether the individuals from whom tissue samples came were able to make deliberative and voluntary choices about participating in a given research project. They were not given the opportunity to make such choices.

Yet this option seems to be widely practiced by investigators doing human tissue research, with most of that research potentially important for a variety of scientific reasons. There are multiple justifications for scientists to do unconsented research on stored tissues, ranging from legal use of federal "waived consent" policies to claims about what nonscientists want or do not want to know about human tissue research using their tissues ("Most people wouldn't want to be bothered") to views about the ownership or abandonment of tissues ("Once it's in the lab, it's ours") to attempted rationales using other consent models (often, some version of general or implied consent). Added to these are other possible motivating reasons, including the need for research to be done as efficiently as possible, the belief that most people simply do not care what kinds of research may be done with their post-diagnostic or post-surgical "waste" tissue, and, perhaps for some scientists, the unstated desire for substantial personal financial gain from human tissue research that need not be shared in any way with the unknowing, unconsenting individuals from whom the tissues came.

We have a strong desire to see important human tissue research studies continue and increase in number, but we continue to advance the rationale for research done with banked tissues to be carried out in new and different ways, ways that strongly affirm the rights of individuals to be informed and to make voluntary choices about how their stored tissues will be used in long-term biomedical research. Yet we know that many responsible, ethically sensitive scientific investigators, along with some bioethicists and health-law attorneys, simply see no problems with at least some types of unconsented research (e.g., with anonymized tissues) continuing to be done.[66]

Thus the option of research done with no consent is not only practiced by many investigators in the United States and other countries, but it is sometimes defended as an option that has a legitimate place within the varieties of consent. In the next chapter, we discuss a number of types of research frequently done without informed consent to examine the claims for and criticisms against this option.

We conclude this chapter by reaffirming the need to update the informed consent process and the importance of using the reasonable person standard of disclosure in clinical and research settings, including research using DNA banking. The best way of updating the informed consent process for our time is not through the continued use of poor substitutes for informed consent (e.g., general consent, implied consent, presumed consent), but collectively working hard to develop new, practical ways of enabling potential research participants and patients to have *informed, appropriately specific choice* about the conditions under which their stored tissues will be used for research purposes. Not only is this the right course of action to take, but we also believe and hope that changing the interpersonal dynamics of human tissue research from limited or insufficient disclosure to openness and informed choices will lead to more public trust and support for biomedical research.

We are also convinced that improving the informed consent process can be done *without seriously impeding important scientific research*. Some attitudes will need to change about the importance of informed consent, and some logistical challenges will have to be managed, but it can be done. To support this claim, we point to a study done at the M.D. Anderson Cancer Center in Houston. Some investigators decided to find out if revised consent documents, expanded in 1997 to give patients more information and choice about banked tissues, would prove detrimental to the recruitment of participants for an ongoing genetic study on susceptibility to melanoma. The study's findings: 7% of potential participants refused participation when the earlier consent form was in use—and exactly the same 7% of potential participants (out of 257 consecutive persons over several months) refused participation when the revised forms were used. No one who declined participation indicated that the additional information and questions played a role in their decision. The investigators concluded: "the addition of these questions presented no obstacle to research participation."[67]

Cases and Vignettes

The search for disease-causing genes can be very effective in populations that have been geographically or culturally isolated for long periods of time because these populations have much more uniform genetic backgrounds than the general population does. Consequently, genetics investigators, biotechnology firms, pharmaceutical companies, and universities collaborate to make contact with indigenous populations and gather DNA samples for population-based genetics research. These "gene hunting" ventures are done in many places and funded by numerous companies. For example, Sequana (San Diego) funded a study on asthma done with DNA samples from Tristan de Cunha; AMRAD (Melbourne) has an agreement to get DNA samples from Tasmanians; and Genset (Paris) has a collection of DNA samples from North African populations. In one instance, a gene-hunting company used local physicians to collect blood samples, mapped a disease gene, and announced its discovery to the world—without ever telling the local people who participated in the study that it was being done as a commercial venture.[68]

The Samuel Lunenfeld Research Institute at the University of Toronto collaborated with Sequana in gathering DNA samples from the population of the tiny island of Tristan de Cunha in the Atlantic Ocean. They were trying to discover a gene that causes asthma.

The Institute's first research trip to the island was problematic. The investigators obtained blood samples without written consent from individuals in the English-speaking population (though they did have "community consent" from the island's ruling council), and the islanders were left feeling like "guinea pigs." Three years later, the investigators improved their procedures: They sent educational brochures to the islanders about the research study, gained both group and individuals' consents for additional blood draws, and agreed to provide free medications to the island if the study resulted in the development of new drugs.[69]

Jeff Murray, Ron Munger, and members of their research team have made trips for over a decade to the Philippines as part of Operation Smile, searching for scientific answers for the causes of cleft lip and palate. Murray, a pediatrician and geneticist, works on the genetic causes of cleft lip and palate. Munger, an epidemiologist with a focus on nutrition, seeks to discover the vitamin deficiencies that can trigger the condition. Both make trips to the Philippines looking for more blood samples because they are convinced that "the answers are buried, coiled and encrypted in the blood." The blood is collected in two ways: some of it ends up as dried blood spots on cards that are mailed back to Murray's lab in Iowa City, and some of it is put in vials that are carried back to Munger's lab in chests filled with dry ice. Getting the blood samples, however, involves many problems, one of which is informed consent. The research team uses a condensed form of a University of Iowa consent document, translated into Cebuano, the local language. The document mentions the minimal physical risks connected with blood draws, but does not mention any of the psychosocial risks, certainly not the U.S.-specific risk about the possible loss of health insurance after genetic testing. Do the individuals who sign the form do so because they voluntarily consent to provide a blood sample for DNA research, or for other reasons, such as the hope of getting surgery for their cleft lip and palate? The Americans cannot know for sure.[70]

A book reviewer commented about the common practice of doing human tissue studies without consent. In a review of an edited book on stored tissue samples, he remarked, "Many of these samples have been collected without the informed consent of the donor and may be useful to researchers for purposes other than the ones that justified the initial collection." For example, "British scientists recently examined stored human appendix and tonsil tissues dating back to the 1980s to gauge the rate of infection from variant Creutzfeldt-Jakob disease, the human form of 'mad cow' disease, a condition that was unknown when the samples were initially taken."[71]

David Snowdon, an epidemiologist at the University of Kentucky, has for 15 years been directing a remarkable study of the aging process and the onset of Alzeimer disease. Called the Nun Study, this longitudinal research study has focused on 678 nuns living in convents in seven states; 295 of the nuns are alive, and all of them are over 85 years old. The study is remarkable because it includes genetic analysis of blood and other tissues, repeated measurements of balance and strength, memory tests, personality tests, and a linguistic analysis of the autobiographical essays they wrote when they entered their order in their 20s. Among the things they have consented to do, sometimes with reluctance, is to donate their brains to the Nun Study after they die. (The brains are analyzed and stored in jars in a laboratory.) An administrator at one convent persuaded the nuns to donate their brains by reminding them that they had made "the difficult decision not to have children. This is another way of giving life."[72]

Notes

1. Jeffrey Gulcher and Kari Stefansson, "The Icelandic Healthcare Database and Informed Consent," *N Engl J Med* 342 (2000): 1827.
2. George Annas, "Rules for Research on Human Genetic Variation—Lessons from Iceland," *N Engl J Med* 342 (2000): 1831–32.
3. J. Krominga et al., "Shared Decision Making Using Interactive Programs," *FHP Journal of Clinical Research* 4 (1994): 27–32; and Marshall Kapp, "Managed Care and Mandatory Movies," *JAMA* 276 (1996): 1023.
4. T. Garry, "New Malpractice Armor Custom-Made for You," *OBG Management* (1995): 1–4.
5. For information about the Patient Education Institute's programs, see their Web site: www.patient-education.com.
6. For information about the Gene Trust DNA bank, go to their Web site: www.DNA.com.
7. Robert J. Levine, *Ethics and Regulation of Clinical Research,* 2nd ed. (New Haven: Yale University Press, 1988), pp. 95–153; and Ruth R. Faden and Tom L. Beauchamp, *A History and Theory of Informed Consent* (New York: Oxford University Press, 1986).
8. Robert F. Weir, *Abating Treatment with Critically Ill Patients* (New York: Oxford University Press, 1989), p. 350.
9. See, for example, Henry K. Beecher, "Ethics and Clinical Research," *N Engl J Med* 274 (1966): 1354–60; Henry K. Beecher, *Research and the Individual* (Boston: Little, Brown and Co., 1970); Jay Katz, *Experimentation with Human Beings* (New York: Russell Sage Foundation, 1972); and James H. Jones, *Bad Blood* (New York: Free Press, 1981).
10. Ellen Wright Clayton, "Informed Consent and Genetic Research," in Mark A. Rothstein, ed., *Genetic Secrets: Protecting Privacy and Confidentiality in the Genetic Era* (New Haven: Yale University Press, 1997), pp. 126–36.
11. Elisa Eiseman and Susanne B. Haga, *Handbook of Human Tissue Resources: A National Resource of Human Tissue Samples* (Santa Monica, Calif.: RAND, 1999).
12. Committee on Ethical and Legal Issues, Council of Regional Networks for Genetic Services (CORN), "Issues in the Use of Archived Specimens for Genetics Research: Points to Consider," unpublished manuscript, January, 1997, pp. 3–4.
13. Association of American Medical Colleges (AAMC), "Patient Privacy and the Use of Archival Patient Material and Information in Research," unpublished paper, April, 1997, p. 4.
14. Robert Weir and Robert Olick, "Pilot Study of Family Medicine Patients," part of an NIH grant proposal entitled "Informed Consent for Research on Stored Tissue Samples," Iowa City, Iowa, 1998, p. 34.
15. Robert Weir and Jay Horton, "DNA Banking and Informed Consent: Part 1," *IRB* 17/4 (1995): 1–3; and Weir and Horton, "DNA Banking and Informed Consent: Part 2," *IRB* 17/5 (1995): 1–8.
16. Anne McTiernan et al., "Informed Consent in the Women's Health Initiative Clinical Trial and Observational Study," *J Womens Health* 4 (1995): 519–29. We also had access to several of the consent documents used in the WHI.
17. See, for example, Norman L. Cantor, *Advance Directives and the Pursuit of Death with Dignity* (Bloomington: Indiana University Press, 1993).
18. See Robert S. Olick, *Taking Advance Directives Seriously: Prospective Autonomy and Decisions Near the End of Life* (Washington, D.C.: Georgetown University Press, 2001).

19. National Bioethics Advisory Commission, *Research Involving Persons with Mental Disorders That May Affect Decisionmaking Capacity*, 2 vols. (Rockville, Md.: USGPO, 1998); and NBAC, *Research Involving Human Biological Materials: Ethical Issues and Policy Guidance*, Vol. I (Rockville, Md.: National Bioethics Advisory Commission, 1999).

20. Medical Research Council of Canada, National Sciences and Engineering Research Council of Canada, and Social Sciences and Humanities Research Council of Canada, *Tri-Council Policy Statement: Ethical Conduct for Research Involving Humans* (Ottawa: Public Works and Government Services, 1998), p. 10.2.

21. Pallava Bagla, "New Guidelines Promise Stronger Bioethics," *Science* 290 (2000): 919. Also see Indian Council of Medical Research, *Ethical Guidelines for Biomedical Research on Human Subjects* (New Delhi: ICMR, 2000).

22. June Gibbs Brown, Inspector General, Department of Health and Human Services, *Institutional Review Boards: A Time for Reform*, June, 1998. The text of this report is on this Web site: http://www.researchroundtable.com/pdfiles/time_reform.pdf.

23. Dena Davis, "Legal Trends in Bioethics," *J Clin Ethics* 11 (2000), p. 189.

24. The NIH's Web-based tutorial is available on this Web site: http://cmc.nci.nih.gov/.

25. See the criticisms and suggestions made in Ellen Wright Clayton et al., "Informed Consent for Genetic Research on Stored Tissue Samples," *JAMA* 274 (1995); and the recommendations made in NBAC, *Research Involving Human Biological Materials*, Vol. I, pp. 55–76.

26. See the University of Iowa Ethical, Legal, and Social Implications Committee, "IRB Guidelines for Genetic Research," unpublished manuscript, 1994, pp. 1–27.

27. Sheryl Gay Stolberg, "Experts Call For New Rules On Research," *New York Times*, April 14, 2001, p. A14.

28. The IOM report, "Responsible Research: A Systems Approach to Protecting Research Participants," is available at http://www.iom.edu. For an overview of the report, see Brian Vastag, "New Focus on Research Participant Protection," *JAMA* (2002): 1973.

29. For more information about the new Federalwide Assurance (FWA) requirement for investigators and institutions, see this Web site: http://ohrp.osophs.dhhs.gov/irbasur.htm.

30. Compare these documents: American College of Medical Genetics (ACMG), "Statement on Storage and Use of Genetic Materials," *Am J Hum Genet* 57 (1995): 1499–1500; American Society of Human Genetics (ASHG), "Statement on Informed Consent for Genetic Research," *Am J Hum Genet* 59 (1996): 471–74; CORN, 1997; and AAMC, "Patient Privacy and the Use of Archival Patient Material and Information in Research," a paper later expanded and published as part of *Medical Records and Genetic Privacy, Health Data Security, Patient Privacy, and the Use of Archival Patient Materials in Research* (Washington, D.C.: AMA, 1997). The documents were discussed in Chapter 3.

31. Jon F. Merz, Pamela Sankar, Simon Yoo, "Hospital Consent for Disclosure of Medical Records," *J Law Med Ethics* 26 (1998): 241–48; and Jon F. Merz, Pamela Sankar, Sheila Taube, and Virginia Livoisi, "Use of Human Tissues in Research: Clarifying Clinician and Researcher Roles and Information Flows," *J Investig Med* 45 (1997): 252–57.

32. La. Stat. Ann. sec. 213.7F.

33. Faden and Beauchamp, pp. 32, 46.

34. *Ibid.*, p. 46.

35. Weir and Horton, "DNA Banking and Informed Consent," pp. 1–3.

36. See Weir and Horton, p. 2, for the original list of seven items, which we identified as seven categories of content needed in consent documents for genetics studies. For

investigators and their teams, the core of eight information items we now think that reasonable persons would want disclosed before consenting to participate in research studies should be considered as supplementary information to the eight required items of information listed in the Common Rule. For careful readers, we point out that the eight information items we list has no particular connection with the same number (8) of reasons we earlier gave for updating the informed consent process.

37. ACMG, pp. 1499–1500; and CORN, pp. 3–4.

38. College of American Pathologists, "Uses of Human Tissue," August 1996, pp. 7–8.

39. William Shakespeare, *Romeo and Juliet,* Act II, line 33.

40. James F. Childress, *Practical Reasoning in Bioethics* (Bloomington: Indiana University Press, 1997), p. 268.

41. *Ibid.,* p. 277.

42. *Ibid.* He gives a slightly different arrangement of these varieties of consent in another publication. See Tom Beauchamp and James F. Childress, *Principles of Biomedical Ethics,* 4th ed. (New York: Oxford University Press, 1994), pp. 128–30.

43. CORN, pp. 1–4.

44. See R. L. Gold et al., "Model Consent Forms for DNA Storage and Linkage Analysis," *Am J Med Genet* 47 (1993): 1223–24; and Bartha Maria Knoppers, Claude Laberge, Kathleen Cranley Glass, and Beatrice Godard, "Proposed Model Consent Form for DNA Sampling and Storage for Medical Research," *Legal Rights and Human Genetic Material* (Montreal: Emond Montgomery Publications Limited, 1996), 179–80.

45. *Tri-Council Policy Statement,* p. 8.7; and NBAC, *Research Involving Human Biological Materials,* p. 66.

46. See Prospect Associates, *National Action Plan on Breast Cancer* (Rockville, Md.: Prospect Associates, 1997).

47. CAP, pp. 1–2.

48. Sherman Elias and George Annas, "Generic Consent for Genetic Screening," *N Engl J Med* 333 (1994): 1611–13.

49. Committee on Bioethics, American Academy of Pediatrics, "Informed Consent, Parental Permission, and Assent in Pediatric Practice," *Pediatrics* 95 (1995): 315.

50. *Ibid.,* pp. 316–17.

51. *Ibid.,* pp. 315–16.

52. Robert Weir and Charles Peters, "Affirming the Decisions Adolescents Make about Life and Death," *Hastings Cent Rep* 27 (1997): 29–40. For a contrary view, see Lainie Friedman Ross, "Health Care Decisionmaking by Children: Is It in Their Best Interest?" *Hastings Cent Rep* 27 (1997): 41–45.

53. Loretta M. Kopelman, "Children as Research Subjects: A Dilemma," *J Med Philos* 25 (2000): 749.

54. Robert F. Weir and Jay Horton, "Genetic Research, Adolescents, and Informed Consent," *Theor Med* 16 (1995): 349–75.

55. Nuffield Council on Bioethics, *Human Tissue: Ethical and Legal Issues* (London: Nuffield Council on Bioethics, 1995), p. 47.

56. Henry Greely, "The Control of Genetic Research: Involving the Groups Between," *Houston Law Rev* 33 (1997): 1397–1430; and Henry Greely, "Informed Consent, Stored Tissue Samples, and the Human Genome Diversity Project: Protecting the Rights of Research Participants," in Robert F. Weir, ed., *Stored Tissue Samples: Ethical, Legal, and Public Policy Implications* (Iowa City: University of Iowa Press, 1998): pp. 89–108.

57. North American Regional Committee, Human Genome Diversity Project, "Proposed Model Ethical Protocol for Collecting DNA Samples," *Houston Law Rev* 33 (1997): 1431–73.

58. Committee on Human Genome Diversity, Commission on Life Sciences, National Research Council, *Evaluating Human Genetic Diversity* (Washington, D.C.: National Academy Press, 1997), pp. 62–63.
59. Eric Juengst, "Groups as Gatekeepers to Genomic Research: Conceptually Confusing, Morally Hazardous, and Practically Useless," *Kennedy Inst Ethics J* 8 (1998): 183–200; Eric Juengst, "Group Identity and Human Diversity: Keeping Biology Straight from Culture," *Am J Hum Genet* 63 (1998): 673–77; and Dena Davis, "Groups, Communities, and Contested Identities in Genetic Research," *Hastings Cent Rep* 30 (2000): 38–45.
60. William Freeman, "The Role of Community in Research with Stored Tissue Samples," in Robert Weir, ed., *Stored Tissue Samples,* pp. 267–301.
61. Gulcher and Steffanson, pp. 1827–28.
62. *Ibid.*, pp. 1828–29.
63. Hrobjartur Jonatansson, "Iceland's Health Sector Database: A Significant Head Start in the Search for the Biological Grail or an Irreversible Error," *Am J Law Med* 26 (2000): 31–67; David Winickoff, "The Icelandic Healthcare Database" (letter), *N Engl J Med* 343 (2000): 1734; and Einar Arnason, "The Icelandic Healthcare Database" (letter), *N Engl J Med* 343 (2000): 1734.
64. George Annas, pp. 1832–33.
65. Childress, p. 277.
66. See, for example, George Annas, Leonard Glantz, and Patricia Roche, "The Genetic Privacy Act," unpublished model law, February 1995; ASHG, pp. 471–74; and Bartha Koppers et al., "Control of DNA Samples and Information," *Genomics* 50 (1998): 387–92.
67. Rebecca Pentz et al., "Informed Consent for Tissue Research" (letter), *JAMA* 282 (1999): 1625.
68. Vicki Brower, "Mining the Genetic Riches of Human Populations," *Nat Biotechnol* 16 (1998): 337.
69. *Ibid.*, p. 338.
70. Lisa Belkin, "The Clues Are in the Blood," *New York Times Mag,* April 26, 1998, pp. 46–52, 54, 120–21.
71. Jack Wilson, review of Robert F. Weir, ed., *Stored Tissue Samples, Ethics* 111 (July 2001): 851.
72. Pam Belluck, "Nuns Offer Clues to Alzheimer's and Aging," *New York Times,* May 7, 2001, pp. A1, A14.

10

Beyond Informed Consent: Other Ethical Issues and Concerns

> Research using anonymous samples can have effects about which the sources may have grave concerns. To begin with a rather farfetched example, I, as a woman, would be very troubled were my DNA used to find a "dumb" gene to explain why women are not good at mathematics. However, more realistic examples illustrate my point. Native Americans may be quite concerned about efforts to find an "alcoholism" gene common to their population. Similar fears may be expressed by gays and lesbians about searches for a "homosexuality" gene.
>
> Ellen Wright Clayton, 1995
> Vanderbilt University Schools of Law and Medicine[1]

> 7. All people have the right to genetic privacy including the right to prevent the taking or storing of bodily samples for genetic information without their voluntary informed consent.
> 8. All people have the right to be free from genetic discrimination.
> 9. All people have the right to DNA tests to defend themselves in criminal proceedings.
>
> The Genetic Bill of Rights, 2000[2]

Much of the recent international debate about research practices with stored tissues has been characterized by differing views about the process of informed consent: what it is, when it is done in ethically appropriate ways, how much disclosure is needed in different research settings, when disclosure and informed consent are legally required, and so on. The debate is not limited, however, to questions about the necessity, appropriateness, or situational impracticability of informed consent. Rather, the debate goes beyond informed consent to include a number of other issues and concerns about human tissue research, some involving questions about law, most pertaining to research ethics, and all having to do with practices common to biomedical research in the era of genomic medicine.

We address many of these issues and concerns in this chapter. We do not discuss them to the same degree that we analyzed the concept of informed consent in the last chapter because these other matters, as important as they are, do not have the same prominence in the debate that informed consent does. But we try to be clear about why each issue and concern is important, why reasonable people sometimes disagree about them, and, when appropriate, what our views are concerning these other points of disagreement in the ongoing debate.

The Relevance of Ethical Principles to the Debate

Ethical principles have had a role in the framing and interpreting of research ethics for decades. Most notably, this country's first national ethics commission (the National Commission) organized its recommendations for improved research ethics around three central ethical principles: respect for persons, beneficence, and justice.[3] These ethical principles unquestionably influenced the development and wording of the federal regulations on research practices in the late 1970s. Moreover, at least to some degree, these ethical principles, often supplemented by the principle of nonmaleficence, continue to influence the thinking and conduct of many scientific investigators, if for no other reason than the mandated use of the federal regulations by national funding agencies and local IRBs.

Yet, the relevance of these ethical principles—or other ethical principles—to contemporary international research practices with stored tissues is debatable. The Health Council of the Netherlands emphasized only the principle of respect for persons in its report; England's Nuffield Council on Bioethics found traditional ethical principles to be impractical and used only two ethics "tests" for tissue-based research (honoring consent, avoiding "gratuitous" harm); and the NBAC only briefly discussed the importance of the earlier *Belmont Report* principles for guiding biomedical research, then used them cursorily in its recommendations. By contrast, the three research councils in Canada expanded the traditional list of three to four ethical principles applicable to biomedicine by issuing a policy statement based on eight revised ethical principles, including respect for human dignity and respect for vulnerable persons.[4]

Are ethical principles relevant to the current debate about research practices with stored tissues? More important, are they relevant as possible action-guides for investigators now doing human tissue research—research that depends as much on tissue samples collected from thousands of patients and research participants worldwide as it does on tissue samples obtained from individual patients, patients similar, perhaps, to John Moore?

In our view, the answer to both questions is affirmative, for three reasons. First, the ethical principle of beneficence helps to explain the views of many biomedical investigators, just as it often sheds light on the views of physicians and other health professionals in clinical settings. Thus the motivations, urgency, and energetic drive that investigators commonly express about continuing to pursue the scientific benefits available through human tissue research can correctly be understood as a lab-based formulation of this principle, an ethical principle in biomedicine that calls on biomedical scientists, as well as physicians and other health professionals, to try to promote the health and welfare of persons professionally entrusted to them. For investigators and research teams, however, the persons entrusted to them are not only individual patients who might be helped by their research findings, but all humans, worldwide, who potentially stand to benefit from the generalizable knowledge discovered through the research on banked tissues in their laboratories. To a lesser degree, perhaps, this ethical principle helps to explain the altruism of many persons who regularly contribute blood to blood banks, or who donate blood, skin tissue from buccal smears, or other tissue samples as participants in various research studies, even though they have been told they are unlikely to gain medical benefit from any particular research study themselves. The motivation for at least some of these research participants can correctly be attributed to a more general version of the principle of beneficence, which they would likely explain as simply their attempts to "make things better" for the next generation, "help others with the same genetic condition," or other words carrying a similar meaning.

Second, the other ethical principles also often used in contemporary biomedical ethics—respect for autonomy, nonmaleficence, and justice—help to explain the motivations and reasons behind some concerns expressed by many persons in recent years about some of the research done with stored tissues. These concerns are especially significant when voiced by individuals and groups normally supportive of biomedical research. Thus the questions and objections that have been raised about some current research practices—by patients, parents and other relatives of patients, bioethicists, attorneys, patient advocates, research scientists themselves, members of some identifiable groups (e.g., Ashkenazi Jews, Native Americans, breast cancer support groups), and members of indigenous communities—can frequently be understood, correctly, as expressions of these other ethical principles. These ethical principles call on all of us, investigators included, to respect (usually) the choices made by other people, to avoid harming others on balance, and to promote equity in the distribution of life's burdens and benefits, whether in research settings or elsewhere.

Third, these ethical principles can serve as action-guides, in a dual sense. They sometimes motivate individuals to question widely held views and common practices, especially when they conclude that common views and practices cause harm to others or violate their rights in fundamental ways. These ethical principles can occasionally also motivate individuals and groups actually to change their views or patterns of behavior, at least when they become convinced that these views and practices fail certain ethics "tests," such as those against causing, on balance, either significant harm or offense to others. One recent example in human tissue research is noteworthy. Although impossible to document on a global scale, a significant change seems to have taken place in recent years regarding previously common research practices with the tissues of indigenous people in various parts of the world. Based on our limited knowledge, we detect a gradual, but notable, change in the research practices of at least some investigators from the United States and other developed countries. Rather than continuing to ignore the traditions and values of specific indigenous groups, these investigators increasingly seem to be working with appropriate community representatives to design some of the details of their research studies—and thereby gain community approval—before they try to obtain tissue samples from any individuals in the groups. One of the significant causes of this change in research practices has been the cumulative efforts in recent years by multiple indigenous groups, advocates of the proposed but unfunded Human Genome Diversity Project, members of the National Research Council Committee on Human Genome Diversity (U.S.), and a number of individual scholars who have collectively emphasized that the previous scientific practices of collecting tissue samples without adequate community knowledge and approval were both harmful to the groups and violations of their rights.[5]

Some Special Issues Involving Research Without Adequate Consent

There are a number of clinical and research settings in which research is often done on stored tissues without express, appropriately specific consent from the sources of the tissues, their legal representatives, or their families. If consent is solicited for research, the consent is frequently (1) some version of general consent for undisclosed research purposes or (2) a version of presumed consent with an opt-out procedure. We will address some of the issues in seven research practices involving banked tissues. (Some of these practices have been briefly discussed in earlier chapters, while others appear for the first time.)

Neonatal Blood Spots in Government-Sponsored DNA Banks. There are an estimated 13.5 million dried blood spots currently being stored in newborn screening laboratories in the United States.[6] Hundreds of thousands of additional dried blood spots are stored each year in this country, with numerous other neonatal blood spots being stored in other countries and shared by genetics investigators and other scientists for a variety of national and international research studies. Yet the limited data available indicates that many, if not most, of the parents of these children have virtually no information disclosed to them about either (1) the screening tests or (2) the inclusion of their children's DNA in a government-sponsored DNA bank.[7] This absence of appropriate disclosure is unfortunate because dried blood spots from newborns are a constant and increasing source of banked DNA readily available for research and other secondary purposes that may be unrelated to the health of any individual newborn. Some research studies use dried blood spots that are linked to specific children; other population-based studies use anonymized spots.[8]

Our interest in neonatal blood spots at this point does not involve the widely variable practices among newborn screening programs, the important public health benefits produced through these programs, the presumed consent that most states use for the screening, or the significant contributions to newborn screening now possible with the analytic techniques of molecular genetics. Rather, our interest concerns the process of *informed* consent (not merely assent, general consent, or an unacceptable version of presumed consent) that could and should take place before research is done with the stored spots. In particular, at least some information should be disclosed to the parent(s) about post-screening research: plans for research with the dried blood spots stored in a specific neonatal DNA bank; plans regarding the identity status (coded or anonymized?) of their baby's blood spots after screening; time limits, if any, for the long-term storage of the spots on Guthrie cards or in genetics labs; information about future access by third parties to the dried samples and/or to the data about the samples stored in investigators' databases; and options parents have to communicate their consent (or refusal) to the post-screening research.

Such disclosures might be made in research consent documents given to prospective parents late in pregnancy. Or, at least some prospective parents could be encouraged to complete research advance directives designed for the possibility of post-screening research with their child's DNA.[9] Another alternative would be to use two pediatrician contact points with new parents to present them with consent documents for research with the dried blood spots, once in the hospital nursery and again at a baby's first check-up.

Secondary Research. DNA banks comprised of dried neonatal blood spots are but one example of the practices known as secondary research and secondary use. Other examples of secondary research abound (e.g., the data provided by the Health Council of the Netherlands), as do examples of other secondary uses of stored tissue samples (for education, commercial products, and forensic purposes).[10] The term *secondary research* refers to the use of a tissue sample or cell line by scientists other than the original investigator(s), or for scientific purposes unrelated to the original research study. More specifically, secondary research with stored tissues can take four forms: (*1*) use of the tissue samples by the principal investigator (PI) for a different research purpose (having a different overall goal, or pertaining to a different medical condition); (*2*) use of the tissues by other investigators in the PI's lab for different purposes than the original study; (*3*) use of the samples by other investigators outside the PI's lab for the same scientific purposes (e.g., to validate the results for publication); and (*4*) use of the materials by other investigators outside the PI's lab for different research purposes.[11]

Secondary research seems rarely to be mentioned in conversations between investigators and prospective research participants or in consent documents for research studies in which secondary research is either (*1*) planned in advance or (*2*) known at the time of recruitment to be a likely future possibility. Thus, to take one example, persons participating in a research study focusing on the genetic causes of a type of breast cancer would probably not be informed that their blood samples might subsequently also be used in a different research study, this one pertaining to the genetic causes of a particular trait studied in behavioral genetics (e.g., violence, drug use, sexual preference).

Yet secondary research is a common practice in research institutions, as is the practice of nondisclosure about it. For many persons, the result of these combined practices is nonproblematic, especially if the tissue samples used for secondary research purposes have been stripped of personal identifiers. Even anonymized samples, however, present some ethical problems. But the ethical problems connected with nondisclosure about secondary research practices using identified or linked samples are surely more significant, in part because the possibility of psychosocial harm to the identifiable sources is greater. A preferable practice would be for investigators routinely to disclose information about *planned (and even likely)* secondary research to prospective research participants so that these persons can factor that information into their thinking about possible participation in the original study via their tissue samples, regardless of what identity status their samples will have.

Post-Diagnostic Research. Nondisclosure by physician-investigators (and, sometimes, by other physicians) about planned or likely post-diagnostic research, a version of secondary use, is a related problem that occurs with some frequency in clinical settings, as previously discussed. To cite one example, only when asked by one of us (in a patient's role, prior to signing a vaguely worded consent document and having knee surgery) did an orthopaedic surgeon acknowledge with some apparent reluctance that, yes, after the diagnostic tests and surgical treatment were done, some of the excised knee cartilage would be turned over to a surgical colleague who does research studies on cartilage tissue. In nonsurgical clinical settings, the absence of disclosure about planned or likely post-diagnostic research can be even more problematic because, frequently, the physician/patient (or nurse/patient) conversation involves no consent document, especially when a tissue sample such as the "common" blood draw is obtained from a patient and sent to multiple research labs.

This problem can best be addressed by encouraging physicians and other health professionals to adopt a practice of regular disclosure about the possibility of post-diagnostic research (especially in research institutions), not only out of respect for patients but also as a way of contributing to the process of more adequately informed consent in specific clinical settings. This practice of disclosure should be supplemented, as noted earlier, with other disclosures about post-diagnostic research, namely by hospitals and clinical departments via the information they regularly provide to patients about hospital procedures.

These disclosures should also help reduce the times in which physician-investigators carry out research on clinically derived tissue samples without gaining IRB approval for the research. This unapproved research on biopsied tissues can become sufficiently problematic within a teaching hospital that all physicians are sent a written reminder about post-diagnostic research. These reminders tell them that research on biopsied tissues is acceptable only with IRB approval and compliance with institutional by-laws, such as the requirement that tissue specimens be sent to the hospital pathology laboratory for pathologic examination before any research is done with them.

Anonymized Tissues. Research studies with tissues that have been anonymized are widely regarded by many investigators as problem-free, at least in terms of ethical problems. Not only does anonymization remove the names and other identifiers of the sources of tissue samples, it also, according to a very common view, removes the ethical problems from human tissue research as well because the individual sources, whoever they were, do not retain any personal interests in any anonymized samples. Even if anonymization of tissue samples is frequently done without consent from patients (using their diagnostic samples) or research participants, it still presents no significant ethical problems when balanced against the beneficial value of research, at least according to the federal regulations, the American Society of Human Genetics, and NBAC.[12]

We disagree, as do some others.[13] The common practice of anonymizing tissue samples without consent does have some ethical problems, with one of the problems having significant clinical implications. That problem is the result of a trade-off made by investigators: in exchange for making selected tissue samples anonymous, thereby removing the possibility that the confidentiality and privacy of the sample sources might be breached, the investigators and their research teams produce samples for which *no clinical follow-up is possible* because the identity of each sample source is permanently deleted. Thus, even if investigators should find out some information from a particular anonymized sample and have good medical reasons for wanting to arrange for a clinical follow-up to be done with the person who provided the sample, the recommendation of this desirable clinical step would be impossible because the person could not be identified. If the samples had been truly anonymized (e.g., by pooling thousands of samples), the desirable clinical follow-up would be absolutely impossible. For some physician-investigators, this undesirable result of anonymizing tissue samples is a sufficient reason for keeping samples identifiable through some kind of linkage with the individuals from whom the samples came.[14]

Often there are, of course, good reasons for anonymizing samples, especially when thousands of samples are needed for population-based genetics studies. Yet the fact that removing all identifiers from samples is frequently done without consent compounds the ethical difficulty of this common practice. Other ethical problems are related to depriving research participants from having either (*1*) knowledge about or (*2*) any "say" in how the tissues obtained from their bodies may be used in research. Therefore, in addition to being deprived of a choice (much less an informed choice) about whether tissues obtained from them will remain identifiable, the sources of to-be-anonymized samples are usually not given the options of indicating that some kinds of research (even when done with anonymized samples) are *objectionable to them* (e.g., the attempts to find the "alcoholism," "homosexuality," and "violence" genes mentioned earlier). Individuals' reasons for finding even some kinds of anonymized research objectionable may be personal, familial, or group related, perhaps because they believe that even this type of research may cause psychosocial harm to themselves, their families, and/or members of their group or community.[15]

For instance, women who are opposed to abortion and regard prenatal diagnosis procedures as "search and destroy missions" might not want any of their tissues, even if anonymized, to be used for research that might lead to improved prenatal diagnostic techniques. Some African Americans likely would object to the use of their anonymized DNA samples in "research about the alleged genetic bases of intelligence."[16] In addition, many who are opposed to embryonic stem cell research (because the research involves the destruction of individual embryos) would not want their cryopreserved embryos in a fertility clinic's lab used for research, even if the embryonic stored tissues were anonymized. At least some parents, as illustrated by the Everett case at the conclusion of this chapter, do not want the DNA samples from one of their children used for research purposes that would be "irresponsible or disrespectful" of that child.[17]

For these reasons, the scientific practice of anonymizing samples needs to be changed in several ways. Even when there are good reasons for anonymizing samples, the practice can be improved, often, by providing the individual sources of samples with understandable information about this research practice (including its clinical implications), a choice about whether their currently identifiable samples may have the identifiers permanently removed, and a chance to indicate whether there are some types of research they would not want to participate in (even via anonymized samples) because they object to that research.[18] In addition, the common IRB practice of exempting all planned research studies with anonymized samples from serious committee review needs to be changed as well, thereby creating the possibility of IRB discussion about some of the ethical problems listed above.

Research on Tissues from the Now Dead. There are an estimated 160 million tissue specimens stored in pathology labs in this country, with more than 8 million additional specimens being added each year.[19] Pathologists, sometimes called the "custodians" or "stewards of the wax," carry out a variety of diagnostic procedures with these numerous tissue samples (solid tissues and body fluids), conduct retrospective research studies with these millions of archived specimens, and welcome new investigative methods for stored tissues, whether in molecular genetics, hematology, immunology, or other scientific fields. They take professional pride in the stewardship they exercise in handling stored specimens, emphasize the importance of protecting the confidentiality (and the anonymity, when needed) of the persons from whom the samples came, and are often open to the possibility of updating laboratory procedures in order to provide a "fire wall" of identity protection between diagnostic samples and samples being used for research.[20] We return to this last point in the next chapter.

By contrast, pathologists do not welcome suggestions from outside the field that some institutional and laboratory procedures governing the consent of patients and research participants need to be updated.[21] As a large professional group, the CAP publicly defends the traditional practice of giving patients only one option, namely that of general, or "simple," consent.[22] Any expansion of consent requirements in pathology will, they fear, severely restrict access to archival clinical specimens by pathologists, geneticists, and other investigators of human disease.[23]

The choice between defending the status quo or "being put out of business," as a leading pathologist put it to one of us, does not present the only options available. Rather, some significant changes can be made to the consent procedures in pathology that will greatly improve patient (and family) choice about research on stored samples without greatly damaging the important work that pathologists do. These suggested changes may well involve more time, effort, and expense on the part of some personnel in pathology labs, but it is past time to make these patient- and family-oriented changes, given the scientific possibilities now provided by molecular genetics.

In particular, two initiatives would be very helpful in improving the process of informed consent in pathology. First, all patients scheduled to have surgical procedures and all research participants who will have tissue samples stored in pathology labs need to be given more information, to the extent possible, about the type of research studies that may be done with their tissue samples. Surgical patients also should be informed about any research plans for the "extra" or "waste" tissue left over from surgery. In addition, patients and research participants need to be given adequate opportunity to communicate *express, informed consent* about the planned (or possible) research. Documents used to record this consent need not be very long, minutely detailed, or present more choices than most patients would want or could understand, but they do need to permit the sources of tissue samples that will be stored in the future (possibly for years, long after some of these persons die) to express some of their preferences and concerns about research that might be done with their tissues, including after their death, if they have preferences and concerns to communicate.

Second, the personal, familial, and predictive information now discoverable via molecular genetic techniques, as well as through the investigative methods of some other scientific fields, should persuade physicians, investigators, and administrators in pathology departments to rethink the issue of recontacting or reconsenting the living descendants of individuals whose cadaveric tissues are now stored in pathology labs, especially the families of individuals who died in recent years.

Of course, if those archived tissues have been truly anonymized, then making contact with any living descendants is impossible. Moreover, there certainly are circumstances (e.g., in some rural portions of most countries) when contacting any of the living descendants of deceased sample sources would be impracticable, if not impossible. Trying to recontact the immediate family members of all the cadaveric specimens in most pathology labs would also be impracticable, if not impossible. But that still leaves numerous identified or linked cadaveric specimens that have been in pathology labs for 10 years or less, with each specimen potentially containing personal, clinically significant, and familial information that may be important to one or more living family members.

Individuals who provided tissue samples to pathology labs in recent years—and the immediate family members who now survive them—will be better served and their interests given greater respect if some of the personnel in pathology labs are responsible for making at least a good-faith effort to contact one or more living family members before any new retrospective research studies are conducted with these identified or linkable cadaveric tissues. The purpose would be twofold: to give family members (or at least a representative) an opportunity to give informed consent (or refusal) for these new studies, and to enable them to carry out the decedent's previously expressed preferences, if any, thus protecting his or her interests that survive and remain important post-mortem (such as the meaning of genetics research for one's family or ethnic or religious group). If such future contact with survivors were to become a regular feature of pathology department practices, communication mechanisms could be established early (by phone and fax numbers, addresses, e-mail addresses, Web sites) that would make future contact with the survivors of stored cadaveric tissue sources less impracticable than it has been in the past.

Research with Cryopreserved Human Embryos. Some types of research that might be objectionable to the individual sources of stored DNA samples can, depending on details, take the form of post-diagnostic research or secondary research. Either way, the sources of the stored tissues probably never find out about the research and thus have no way of expressing their objections to the research. Similarly, investigators who direct most research studies currently done with (*1*) the anonymized tissues of living patients and research participants or (*2*) the identified, linked, or anonymized tissues from cadavers apparently never have to deal with the issue of objectionable research. The reason, it seems, is straightforward: persons participating in the studies via their anonymized tissues (and family members surviving the cadavers) seldom have either knowledge or choice about the types of research that may be done with these tissues.

By contrast, research studies currently being done with cryopreserved embryos are highly visible because of news coverage in recent years about human embryonic stem (ES) cell research and the possible federal funding of that research. These studies are very controversial because of the types of tissue involved. They are objectionable to many people, even if not to many couples who have donated their "extra" embryos to reproductive medicine clinics for research purposes.[24] The limited data indicates that 10% of couples with cryopreserved embryos stored for two years choose, with general consent, to donate their frozen embryos for undisclosed research purposes (34% opt to have their frozen embryos discarded).[25]

As discussed in Chapter 4, cryopreserved human embryos are a special type of stored tissue precisely because these tissues have the capacity—if removed from cylinders of liquid nitrogen, successfully implanted into women's bodies, and nourished there throughout gestation—of becoming *persons*. According to some religious beliefs and philosophical views, frozen human embryos, even though produced with technological assistance and with only eight cells, are genetically unique tissues, already have the moral status of persons, and have been persons since fertilization occurred. Therefore, these stored tissues should never be used for research, especially any research that would destroy these embryos, such as research on ES cells and the production of ES cell lines. Some individuals and groups, therefore, advocate a federal ban on this type of research. By contrast, many scientists and others hope that ES cell research may provide medical benefits to numerous patients, particularly those with heart disease, diabetes, Parkinson disease, Alzheimer disease, and spinal cord injuries.[26]

A thorough analysis of the ethical issues in ES cell research is beyond the scope of this book and has been done by other authors.[27] Rather, we limit our discussion of ES cell research to the context of this book, namely the use of these special stored tissues for research purposes. We focus on cryopreserved embryos as a source for ES cells because the thousands of often unnecessary, frequently unwanted, and largely unregulated frozen embryos in this and other developed countries represent either a wonderful source of banked human DNA research material or a multitude of absolutely vulnerable, nonconsenting participants in biomedical research, depending on one's views.

There are three important questions about this research. What are the ethical positions now being staked out on ES cell research? What are the major ethical arguments about doing stem cell research with this specific type of stored human tissue? If some stem cell research with cryopreserved embryos is ethically justifiable, as we think it is, how can the process of informed consent by the biological parents of frozen embryos be improved?

There are at least five ethical positions currently being advocated by individuals and groups participating in a national and international debate about ES cell research. Some of these positions have been enacted as national policy in a few countries.[28] Like many other ethical issues in biomedicine, this issue has prompted a variety of responses, ranging across a philosophical spectrum from the most conservative position to the most liberal.[29] For the advocates of each position, the task of articulating a particular view on the spectrum often involves ethical line-drawing, a standard move in ethics whereby the proponents of a position give reasons why they are willing to go "this far, but no further" in defending or justifying a specific practice.

Position 1 is straightforward: research with human embryonic stem cells is never justifiable. This view is held by persons and groups who have a conservative "pro-life" position, usually grounded in specific religious beliefs about God's creative action and the sanctity of human life. Advocates of this perspective maintain that each individual human life is created by God, morally protectable human life begins at fertilization, the only morally justifiable abortions are therapeutic abortions done in genuine conflict-of-life situations, and *any* intentional destruction of a human embryo is tantamount to murder. The implications of this view for any proposed ES cell research are clear: such research simply cannot be justified, even given the possibilities of substantial medical benefit to numerous adults that might occur through this research. Proponents include Pope John Paul II, who regards this kind of research as inherently wrong and on a par with infanticide and euthanasia.[30] In the United States, those holding this position are the strongest advocates for a federal ban of this research, but they often voice no opposition to research with adult stem cells.

Position 2 is a more nuanced "pro-life" position: research with embryonic stem cells is justifiable only with existing stem cell lines. This view, of course, is the widely publicized "compromise" position taken by President George W. Bush on August 9, 2001.[31] President Bush announced that the federal government would soon begin funding ES cell research, but in a very limited way. For members of his conservative constituency, he affirmed his belief in the sanctity of life, the intrinsic value of each human embryo, and the inherent wrongness of intentionally killing human embryos for scientific gain. For scientists projecting unprecedented therapeutic options achievable through stem cell research, he announced that the NIH had located 64 embryonic stem cell lines from embryos already destroyed, that the federal government would limit funding for stem cell research to these cell lines (if Congress agreed), and that federal funding would not be available for the destruction or creation of additional embryos for research purposes. The key point of the president's announced compromise is a clear example of the "this far, and no further" type of ethical line-drawing. His position does not depend on the accuracy of the announced number of 64 cell lines, but on drawing a line between any intentional destruction of human embryos in the future/and any type of ES cell research that might qualify for federal funding.

Position 3 moves beyond the Bush line: research with embryonic stem cells is justifiable with cryopreserved embryos, within appropriate limits. Advocates of this position maintain that early human embryos *are* acceptable to use for ES cell research, given the combination of (*1*) the promise of substantial benefit from this research for many suffering patients and (*2*) the fact that these *ex utero* embryos will be destroyed at some point anyway. Three ways of deriving such cells exist: from aborted fetuses, from frozen embryos stored in connection with fertility programs, and by creating embryos technologically for the purpose of ES cell research. Of these alternatives, proponents of Position 3 are convinced that the second option is better than the other two: using cryopreserved embryos is morally and politically preferable to using cadaveric fetal tissue, and, likewise, it is morally preferable to use "extra" embryos for ES cell research that are currently frozen in cylinders of liquid nitrogen than to create additional embryos for that same scientific purpose. Advocates of this view include NBAC and the American Academy of Pediatrics, both of which have called for a change in federal law to permit funding of ES cell research with frozen embryos donated for that purpose.[32]

Position 4 goes further: creating human embryos for stem cell research is justifiable, even if the embryos will later be destroyed. This position, known variously as *research cloning, nonreproductive cloning,* or *nuclear transfer research,* involves an attempt to apply laboratory cloning techniques to ES cell research, but with no intention of ever trying to implant the embryos in female uteri. Some advocates of this position maintain that the electrically stimulated genetic material is not actually an "embryo," because the ova are never fertilized with sperm.[33] All advocates of this view are convinced that the potential medical benefits to be gained from using cloning techniques, or somatic cell nuclear transfer, in ES cell research are sufficiently great for large numbers of patients that they justify the technological creation of human embryos for this specific research purpose, *even if* all the embryos (or nonfertilized, dividing human cells) will be destroyed. Proponents maintain the fundamental advantage of this approach, also called *therapeutic cloning,* is that the resulting cells are genetically matched to the person who provided the somatic cell, thus avoiding the problem of immune rejection by the body. Advocates of this position, which include the National Academy of Sciences, therefore believe that this nonreproductive use of cloning technology has substantial benefits in ES cell research compared with the use of frozen embryos.[34]

Position 5 stands at the far end of the spectrum: creating human embryos for implantation and birth is justifiable as a logical extension of cloning technology. This position, known as *reproductive cloning,* seems to have few outspoken advocates other than a small religious group of Raelians, but persons who hold this view are convinced that the successful use of somatic cell nuclear transfer by scientists to produce a variety of cloned nonhuman animals can be repeated as a scientific form of reproduction for humans as well. More than that, they are convinced that reproductive cloning *should* be done using human cells, especially when this extended use of cloning technology might be beneficial in a number of ways: the replacement of a dead child with a delayed genetic "twin," the creation of a one-generation-younger version of a dead spouse using stored DNA from that person, or the fulfillment of a basic desire for a child by an infertile couple. Not deterred by the numerous problems in nonhuman reproductive cloning efforts, the ethical arguments against this type of cloning, or its illegal status in this and many other countries, at least a few scientists have announced plans actually to try to clone a human baby. The Clonaid organization made unsubstantiated claims in 2002 of having done so.[35]

As suggested by these brief descriptions, advocates for each of these positions use a variety of ethical arguments to define their views and distinguish their positions from alternative views regarding ES cell research. Nevertheless, the advocates of the first four positions all agree about the goal being sought: unprecedented medical benefits for millions of patients now suffering from a variety of medical conditions, with a shared hope that those medical benefits will include curative treatments not presently available. The disagreement is over the morally acceptable means of achieving that goal. And this fundamental disagreement produces multiple ethical arguments about ES cell research, with the central ethical points consisting of drawing lines beyond which it is not morally acceptable to move.

At the time of writing, it is impossible for us to know which of these ethical arguments will carry the day in the United States and, therefore, which of the five ethical options will become the dominant, mainstream position in this country. Likewise, it is impossible to know how public policy regarding ES cell research will develop. At the present time legislators at the federal and state levels are embroiled in an important debate about banning human cloning. More specifically, they are trying to decide whether to pass legislation that will ban both research cloning and reproductive cloning, or only to ban reproductive cloning and thereby permit scientists to do research cloning as one form of ES cell research.

When the dust settles, we anticipate that ES cell research will continue in some form as an ongoing scientific endeavor. Some of that research will probably be done with cryopreserved embryos currently in storage at numerous fertility clinics. Given that expectation, we recommend that fertility clinics move beyond the kind of general, simple consent they commonly request from couples who are willing to donate their stored embryos for undisclosed research purposes. A better option would be to provide parents with pertinent information about ES cell research and any other research studies that might be done (and research that would not be done) with their frozen embryos, permitting them to make a more informed choice about donation. Alternatively, such information would enable parents to give an informed refusal if they find some of the planned research morally objectionable or if they prefer another option (continued storage at parental expense, donation to one or more other couples, or destruction by thawing). A disclosure policy along these lines would also be consistent with NBAC recommendations.[36]

Vulnerable Research Participants. Many, if not most, persons who participate in human tissue research via their banked DNA samples can be regarded as vulnerable in that they are insufficiently informed about research that will be done with their tissues to give adequately informed consent. To stop with that point, however, is to paint with too broad a brush. A better way of calling attention to the unusual consent problems presented by especially vulnerable research participants can be seen in the approaches taken by two national bioethics committees. The Nuffield Council on Bioethics rightly points out that some individuals, because of advanced age, young age, or neurological disability, lack the decision-making capacity to give voluntary, informed consent to tissue-based research with their stored tissues.[37] NBAC recommends that the federal regulations be revised to contain alternative consent requirements when prospective research participants "either do not have or have lost the capacity to provide consent."[38]

We select adolescents as an example of the consent problems that some vulnerable individuals have when placed in the situation of being prospective participants in human tissue research studies, specifically a variety of genetics studies. The Iowa Study of consent documents, discussed in earlier chapters, contained as one of its parts an analysis of 70 consent documents provided by genetics investigators who conduct research with children and adolescents on 44 medical conditions. The analysts in this study found that (1) most of the documents were unclear about the decision-making capacity of neurologically normal adolescents; (2) most of them failed to given adolescents a "voice" independent of parents; (3) none of the documents addressed adolescents as capable decision makers in clinical or research settings; and (4) none of them provided any information about the psychosocial risks connected with participation in genetics research.[39] As a result, adolescents may be especially vulnerable and inadequately informed when a physician-investigator seeks their consent to participate in a research study (e.g., cystic fibrosis, leukemia), particularly if they are already personally, perhaps desperately, interested in wanting to help find a cure for that disease.

The Risks of Other Kinds of Psychosocial Harm

Much conventional thinking by physicians, nurses, and investigators regarding risks of harm to patients and research participants focuses almost exclusively on the risks of physical harm. This is the sort of harm that can be observed, measured, documented in a medical chart or research record, and reviewed by others. A pervasive example of this view is the warning about physical risks that nurses or phlebotomists typically give patients prior to a blood draw: some brief pain from a needle stick, perhaps some bruising of the skin, and a remote chance of infection. Although other kinds of harm in biomedical settings are discussed in the literature, most biomedical professionals, it seems, continue to think about risks of harm as being primarily risks of physical injury and the physiological effects of such injury.[40]

One consequence of this view is that many biomedical professionals are skeptical about some of the claims advanced in recent years concerning the nonphysical harms that may occur to patients and research participants who participate, via their tissue samples, in research studies, especially when those studies involve molecular genetics. When ethicists, attorneys, members of patient advocacy groups, and leaders of genetic support groups point to the potential psychosocial harm to participants in research studies using banked DNA samples, scientific investigators often respond with critical questions, rebuttals about self-reported cases and possible self-deception in personal claims about discrimination, and requests for information about actually documented cases, not just "anecdotal" cases. Giving limited credence to claims about possible psychosocial harm (such as loss of privacy, stigmatization, or unconsented participation in objectionable research), investigators frequently insist on actual, documented instances of breaches of confidentiality or genetic discrimination and assert that these risks are both uncommon and usually precluded with anonymized samples.

Nevertheless, beyond the risks of genetic discrimination through loss of health insurance or in the workplace, there are other, even less quantifiable risks of psychosocial harm that should be considered—and should remain as part of the debate about the benefits and risks involved in research with banked DNA samples. Table 10.1 lists several types of risks of psychosocial harm to participants in some

Table 10.1 The risks of psychosocial harm in some genetics studies

WITH IDENTIFIED OR CODED SAMPLES	WITH ANONYMOUS OR ANONYMIZED SAMPLES
1. Risks regarding loss of privacy	1. Risks of having one's samples anonymized and used for research without one's knowledge or consent
2. Risks regarding breaches of confidential genetic information	2. Risks of missing a possible opportunity for future treatment and improved health because no clinical follow-up can be done
3. Risks concerning loss of health insurance	
4. Employment risks	3. Risks of one's samples being used for objectionable research because the type of research is offensive to the sample source
5. Psychological risks in gaining new self-knowledge (about one's genetic heritage, genetic makeup, genetic propensity toward unwanted medical problems, or presymptomatic status for a late-onset genetic condition)	4. Additional risks of one's samples being used for objectionable research because the type of research may be harmful to the sample source, that person's family, or the group with which that individual is personally identified
6. Additional psychological risks based on disclosure policies or actions of some investigators (risks related to new family knowledge about each other, risks to interpersonal relationships, and risks of being stigmatized)	5. Risks to investigators and research teams of becoming "ethically blind" to some of the possible problems with anonymizing samples without the sample source's consent

genetics studies, with the possible harms being grouped according to the identity status of tissue samples in various studies. The two descriptive lists build on the earlier work of a multidisciplinary committee at the University of Iowa College of Medicine, comprised of several physician-investigators, research nurses in genetics, IRB members, ethicists, and attorneys, with one of us (RFW) as a member.[41] In updating the work of that committee, we include anonymized samples as one of the descriptive categories.

Like the Iowa committee, we are convinced that some of these risks are more real than others and that some risks remain theoretical in nature (or are not yet suitably documented) and thus represent only potential problems about which participants in some genetics studies should be aware. Pertinent information about some of these psychosocial risks needs to be included in all consent documents for genetics studies with adolescents and adults. Moreover, IRBs need to require that relevant information about psychosocial risks be put in all consent documents before committee approval, as many IRBs are already doing. How much information should be included and how specific that information needs to be are matters that will depend on the views of various IRBs and the differing disclosure policies of investigators directing the studies.

The Ownership of Body Parts

Putting aside the legal doctrines, did John Moore have a legitimate claim that his bodily tissues were *his* property? We believe that most people would agree that he did, that the concept of property and ownership captures something important about the intrinsic connection between a person and his or her body. As William F. May writes, for centuries people have been identified with their bodies "in such a way as to render the dignity of the two inseparable. A man not only *has* a body, he *is* his body."[42] Susan Lawrence argues that "beliefs about the location of humanness and personal identity—in the body, the brain, the soul, or combinations of these places—shape the meaning and value that humans ascribe to body parts."[43] These comments also illuminate why many of our laws and practices legitimate and protect autonomy over one's own body, and why many persons experience deep offense, as did John Moore, at the idea of a person's body parts being used by another without permission.

The difficulty and the controversy come from the fact that much of current biomedical research—and its enormous promise for advancement of medicine, health, and other societal goods—rests on using human tissue and genetic information as the "raw materials" of research. Thus the concept of ownership of one's tissues raises fundamental questions about the relationship of individuals to their communities, and whether, for example, the greater good should permit society through its institutions, such as hospitals and academic health centers, to lay claim to human tissue in some circumstances. Attempts to balance the sometimes competing interests of research participants, investigators, research institutions, and the public present controversial questions about what rights of transfer and control a research participant ought to have and how those rights should be recognized in the conduct of human tissue research. Parallel questions concern what rights researchers should have to acquire and *own* human tissues without consent and how these tissues and the genetic information derived from them may be used, including the nature, dissemination, and possible commercialization of the research.

Borrowing again from James Childress's work on organ procurement (see Chapter 9), we can posit at least six ways of thinking about the acquisition (transfer) of human tissues. Taken together, these concepts portray a spectrum of approaches to allocating dispositional authority and control between the individual (or a legal representative) and the community (through its institutions). Childress argues that human body parts may be acquired or transferred by (*1*) express donation, (*2*) presumed donation, (*3*) routine removal, (*4*) expropriation, (*5*) abandonment, or (*6*) sale/purchase.[44] Each of these approaches finds expression in the debate over stored tissue research.

Federal policy strongly embraces express donation through the mechanism of informed consent. Exceptions for anonymous research seemingly rely on some form of implied or presumed consent, such as when a hospital consent form includes permission to use tissues removed for clinical purposes for unspecified, future research stripped of identifying information, putting the onus on the patient to opt out. Secondary research, such as with pathology samples "on the shelf" obtained originally by other physicians in the course of clinical care, might be justified on grounds of implied consent, presumed consent, or abandonment, depending on the circumstances. A strong statement on abandonment comes from the Nuffield Council's position that consent to clinical use constitutes abandonment of removed tissues to which researchers may lay claim. Research practices with anonymized and anonymous samples and the arguments as to why consent is unnecessary typically focus on the minimal risk involved for participants—the central concept of federal policy—but sometimes also appeal to communitarian values to assert the importance and priority of societal claims to the pursuit of biomedical research.

In addition, appeal to a societal obligation to contribute to research for the benefit of all, placing the good of society above that of the individual, justifies, so the argument goes, routine use (but not routine removal). Though rarely expressed in the stark terms of a societal right to expropriate (mine) human biological materials, a weaker version of this view can be found among those who believe that post-mortem research with previously collected samples is exempt from federal oversight and does not require consent. In effect, this means that any rights and interests the sample source may have had are extinguished with death. The claim that biomedical progress takes precedence over the (possible) objections of ethnic or religious groups to particular research studies also suggests a form of societal ownership and entitlement in the name of the greater good.

Finally, there is a lively debate about whether we should cast aside the gift model of the federal policy in favor of commercial rights in the body. Proposals for recognition of commercial rights for research participants advance the merits of full-fledged property rights, including the right to sue successfully for compensation,[45] and argue for various ways to share in the profits,[46] such as through creation of a government-regulated royalty clearinghouse,[47] government-standardized and regulated licensing agreements,[48] or a hybrid. Legally structured, a hybrid system would favor donation with remuneration to be provided in unusual cases where tissues proved to be especially valuable.[49]

As should be evident, we maintain that many of our property-like interests in exercising control over what happens with our bodily tissues and the information derived from them can be recognized, respected, and protected by commitment to a more robust informed consent process. Meaningful movement in this direction would include more forthright and routine disclosures to research participants about the nature of a research study, plans and possibilities of future research studies, the prospects of financial gain for investigators and institutions, and the realistic possibilities for commercialization from the fruits of completing especially valuable research studies. Whenever reasonable, consent should be express, not presumed or implied. We reject any systematic reliance on the doctrine of abandonment or other models (routine use, expropriation) that would deny individuals even the opportunity to say no to the use of their tissues in genetics and other biomedical research.

This position goes only part way in addressing research participants' interests in and claims to compensation, the question taken up in the next section. Without assessing the merits of the various proposals for allowing research participants to share in the profits, we call for at least modest change in this direction, leaving open whether future approaches, with advances in biotechnology and biomedicine, might balance competing interests differently.

Concerns About Commercialism

Just as molecular genetics has transformed the practice of clinical medicine, so the laboratory techniques of molecular biology and genetics have transformed the basic biological sciences and the culture of biomedical research, including the ways academic scientists think about their work beyond the confines of the laboratory. Years ago (at least before the recombinant DNA research of the 1970s), the "old scientific method" consisted of formulating a hypothesis, accumulating data, doing extensive experimentation (sometimes with human participants), and publishing the results, thereby sharing them with the scientific community. Scientists directing these studies seem to have hoped that research results would be verified by other scientists, regarded as significant contributions to science, and rewarded in salary increases, promotions, and awards.

The "new scientific method," especially in the biological sciences, sometimes seems to consist of formulating a hypothesis, accumulating data, doing limited experimentation up front, often refraining from sharing this research information with other scientists, seeking funding to support the research, later applying for a patent based on the preliminary research findings, and then seeking a lucrative agreement with a biotechnology firm, a pharmaceutical company, venture capitalists, or the federal government to continue the research. The new scientific method occasionally consists of seeking a patent on an innovative, useful product (often some kind of diagnostic test) and then charging hospitals, physicians, and patients every time the product is used. A small number of scientists seem motivated to use their scientific skills, expensive laboratory equipment, and large research teams to achieve enormous personal wealth, perhaps allowing their own scientific standing, contributions to science, and production of benefits to others to be secondary. Examples of scientist-entrepreneurs abound, including Herbert Boyer's founding of Genentech in the 1970s; Kari Stefansson's establishment of DeCODE Inc., in Iceland; Craig Venter's move from the NIH to the private Institute for Genomic Research, then (giving up a reported $38 million) to Celera Genomics, and then to his own genomics company; and the annual publication of a list of "molecular millionaires," most of whom are scientists working with or for biotechnology companies.[50]

The many facets of the commercialization of biomedical research are well chronicled by Lori Andrews, Dorothy Nelkin, Bartha Knoppers, and others.[51] Our concerns build on their work but focus primarily on the problematic implications of this process of commercialization for human tissue research, the rights of research participants, and public support for this research. There are, in our view, at least six current problems.

First, the increasing commercialization of biomedical research influences the way we commonly think about human tissues. Rather than regarding our solid organs and bodily fluids as important biological components of who we are as individual human beings, many of us are, perhaps imperceptibly, beginning to think of many of our tissues (blood, sperm, ova, umbilical cord blood, an "extra" kidney) as disposable, potential income-producing parts of our bodies, depending on the circumstances and price. The result is a move away from altruistic acts, from donations of organs and tissues to others in need, and from the ethic of beneficence toward the ethic of the market place. Tissues are thus beginning to be viewed as commodities to be bought and sold, as illustrated by the advertised offers for ova from idealized women possessing specified physical features and mental abilities (e.g., the offer of $80,000 for ova from a "special egg donor" recently published in a university student newspaper).[52]

Second, the commodification of tissues reflects some of the current business aspects of much human tissue research, with companies selling all kinds of human tissues to scientific investigators, commercial catalogs listing specific types of tissues available for set prices (sometimes linkable to specific persons as sources), and some physicians becoming modern versions of bounty hunters. For example, the catalog from the American Type Culture Collection lists thousands of tissues and cell lines for sale to investigators, with entries providing some minimal descriptive information (age, medical condition, racial/ethnic background) about the persons from whom these samples came.[53] As to the bounty hunter description, some academic oncologists get paid "per head" for recruiting specific types of patients for funded cancer studies; other physicians occasionally contact geneticists and offer to "sell you my families," meaning that they will, for a fee, give investigators their patients' blood samples.[54]

Third, the increasing commercialization of biomedical research creates unprecedented conflicts of interest for academic scientists doing biomedical research. These conflicts, while not new in kind, are unprecedented in degree and scope because biomedical investigators working in academia have never before had the opportunity to get rich "on the side" while remaining on a university payroll, nor have they had the recurring opportunity to get rich by quitting their university job, joining (or founding) a biotechnology company down the street, and entering into direct competition with their previous employer. These conflicts of interest can take many forms, with some of the conflicts involving scientists' personal financial interests and others involving conflicts of commitment (in terms of time, effort, interest, or obligation) between working for a university employer and also working for private industry. Whenever such conflicts for academic scientists (or other professionals) are suspected or documented, they raise questions about the objectivity of research findings, validity of data, and compromises in science and/or ethics that may have been made along the way.[55]

The fourth problem is that this commercialization influences the way biological scientists work with each other. There are now conflicts among geneticists, other biological scientists, and multidisciplinary scientific groups working on the same scientific problems that, while not new in kind, are unprecedented in degree and scope because of the huge amounts of money involved. For decades, of course, scientists and scientific teams have engaged in competitive races to be first in making major scientific discoveries. Now, some of the characteristic features of this normal scientific competition have changed, partially because the rewards have changed from winning major scientific awards to accumulating staggering amounts of money, often by getting patents and then establishing business monopolies. The unfortunate results are several, ranging from some geneticists reluctantly seeking patents out of commercial self-defense (to preserve the right to work with genes discovered in their labs), to many scientists being increasingly reticent to share or even publish scientific data before getting patent protection, to notable groups of geneticists who worked on the Human Genome Project (the international consortium and Celera Genomics) refusing to share data cooperatively or insisting on payment for the use of generated data.[56]

Fifth, the commercialization of human tissue research sometimes has a negative impact on research participants who provide the tissues, in several different ways. Some individuals feel cheated because, like John Moore, they provide identified or linkable tissue samples that subsequently become scientifically important (e.g., by helping to identify a test for a specific type of cancer or a test for the HIV-resistant gene) and lead to patents and wealth for the investigators, while the patients and research participants get left out. Some groups of parents with genetically abnormal children feel cheated when they locate a qualified investigator to search for the specific disease-causing gene affecting their families, provide many tissue samples (blood, urine, skin) "to be used for the public good," raise funding to help the research study continue, and then experience disappointment, anger, and betrayal when, as in the Canavan disease case, the hospital employing the scientist gets a gene patent for a diagnostic test and now charges a royalty fee every time the test is used (see Chapter 7).[57] Some indigenous groups feel cheated when they provide tissue samples to a visiting scientist, receive no subsequent monetary benefit for individuals or the group itself, and conclude that they have been victims of "biopiracy." The latter example has occurred often enough that the Genetic Bill of Rights, partially quoted at the beginning of the chapter, includes this statement: "All indigenous peoples have the right to manage their own biological resources ... and to protect these from expropriation and biopiracy by scientific, corporate or government interests."[58]

The final problem is a consequence of all these factors, namely, that the increasing commercialization of human tissue research may, if current trends continue, *have a negative impact on public support for biomedical research.* Even with the recent increases in federal funding for biomedical research (in the United States and England), storm clouds are gathering. Those clouds hanging over national programs of biomedical research have to do with a fundamental issue: public trust in the research enterprise either leads to or away from expanded public support for research studies. Our concern is that publicity about academic scientists' financial relationships with industry, the money-driven conflicts within science over shared or patent-protected data, and the reluctance of scientists to disclose the commercial aspects of their work or to share their profits with research participants may collectively lead to diminished public trust and public funding. Catherine DeAngelis, the editor of *JAMA,* expresses the concern this way: "Our decision to publish this study [on conflicts of interest among scientists] is based on the belief that the integrity of the research process must be protected and preserved."[59]

We are not suggesting that these problems are currently widespread. Nor do we propose workable solutions for each of them. We do think, however, that there are ways of addressing the last two problems that are consistent with the themes developed in this book: *more disclosure* by investigators, *more information and choice* for research participants, and *greater collaboration* between investigators and participants as they work for beneficial research goals that will benefit us all.

There are, of course, multiple ways of dealing with some of the commercial aspects of human tissue research, and in particular, the reluctance of investigators to offer participants reasonable alternatives regarding any commercially valuable products that may result from a study. Some participants in research, perhaps having read about the John Moore case or other problematic cases, occasionally demand money up front before providing tissue samples. Other participants, who have reason to think that their DNA samples will be particularly valuable to a study, occasionally produce contracts that spell out their entitlements in advance and then provide tissue samples only if the investigator(s) have signed the agreement. For example, prior to signing a consent document to participate in a study of pseudoxanthoma elasticum (PXE), a rare genetic disease, two parents having children with the disease persuaded researchers to sign a contract giving them and all other participating families rights to share in the profits that might come from the discovery of the disease gene.[60] (We return to this case in Chapter 11.)

Investigators should begin to take the initiative in addressing concerns about personal commercial benefits from studies of stored DNA, rather than merely responding to the demands or proffered legal contracts of research participants. Directors of human tissue research studies, as well as directors of clinical programs in which post-diagnostic/post-therapeutic research is a distinct possibility (e.g., reproductive medicine programs), can contribute to the development of a more collaborative research climate with participants by making as many as three changes in all their consent documents:

1. Disclose that commercial use of the stored tissue samples is (*a*) possible, but very unlikely because that result is neither intended nor anticipated or (*b*) one of the goals of the study for the investigator and/or other scientists who will be able to use the stored tissues for secondary research purposes.
2. Inform research participants that if commercial use of stored, *identified, or linked* samples does occur, the investigator(s) agrees to contribute a percentage of the profits (10%?) to one or more identified charitable organizations.
3. Inform research participants that if commercial use of stored, *anonymized* samples occurs, the investigator(s) also agrees to contribute a percentage of the profits (5%?) to one or more identified charitable organizations.[61]

By increasing the amount of disclosure to research participants in this manner, investigators will meet the reasonable person standard of disclosure. They will also, we hope, help raise the level of trust necessary for collaborative research studies. (We elaborate on these recommendations in the next chapter.)

Research Using Databases

The use of databases—many of them constantly evolving—is an integral feature of human tissue research and DNA banking, or "biobanking." Yet as indicated earlier, most of the controversy and debate about research with stored tissues has focused primarily on the first kind of storage used in DNA banking: storing human biological materials for long periods of time in research labs, followed by variable practices of analyzing, replicating, and sometimes sharing portions of tissue samples, extracted DNA, or cell lines with other investigators. The second kind of storage, the *storing of genetic data* derived from the banked samples, has received less attention in the debate, at least in this country, even though many of the same ethical and legal concerns in DNA banking continue as the focal point of scientific interest moves from the genetic and predictive information contained in a DNA sample to the visual and analytic portrayal of that genetic information electronically in one or more databases. In both cases a central concern is access to and use of genetic information. Only persons in countries that have established, or are considering establishing, a national database using DNA samples—Iceland, of course, but also Denmark, Estonia, England, and others—seem to have had sufficient experiential reasons to include this second part of DNA banking as a topic of public concern and debate.

Yet, there can be little doubt that the use of research databases, apart from DNA banking practices, has transformed all the biological sciences over the past 10 to 15 years, as well as virtually all other professional fields worldwide. Rapid changes, with always faster and more powerful computers, the Internet, dramatically improved search engines, the genomics revolution, and online information databases, have dramatically altered the way that geneticists, other biologists, and, for that matter, many of the rest of us do research. For biological scientists, the explosion in numbers and types of publicly accessible information databases has led to efforts to organize them in terms of somewhat arbitrary categories, such as popularity (GenBank, SWISS-PROT, Pfam, SMART),[62] size and sophistication of Web sites providing DNA sequence data (Web sites of NCBI, Ensembl, UCSC),[63] and specialized types of databases within the Molecular Biology Database Collection (major public sequence repositories, comparative genomics, gene expression, genetic and physical maps, genomics, mutations, RNA sequences, transgenics).[64]

No similar effort has been made, to our knowledge, to formulate descriptive categories for the various human tissue databases that are used nationally and internationally, often developed locally by geneticists and other biomedical investigators who engage in DNA banking studies. We thus suggest that these databases (international, national, and local) used in connection with human tissue studies can be grouped along the following category lines:

- *Publicly accessible databases.* Hundreds of human tissue databases (GenBank and some others also contain some model nonhuman DNA sequences) are accessible, without charge or required password, to qualified scientists, with portions of the databases accessible to anyone in the world using a computer with an Internet connection.

- *National DNA databases.* Already existing or planned in several countries, these databases are often comprehensive, with links to numerous medical databases, multiple demographic databases, banked DNA samples, and, sometimes, personal identification numbers.

- *Commercial, password-protected databases.* Many other human tissue databases (e.g., Celera and other biotech companies) are restricted to scientists willing to pay to have access to the DNA sequences, SNPs, patented genes, and other protected information contained in these specialized genetics databases.

- *State-based or national epidemiological databases.* These databases provide personal, familial, and demographic data about individuals from whom tissue samples were obtained (e.g., state neonatal screening programs, NHANES and other CDC studies, the SEER tumor registries administered by the National Cancer Institute), with access to the databases being restricted to authorized professionals.

- *Clinical research databases.* Developed by and restricted to authorized clinical investigators (e.g., in oncology, pathology, psychiatry) in several academic medical centers, these databases contain genetics and other biomedical information about consenting individual patients derived from their clinically collected tissues, with the electronic data sometimes being transmitted to a central database at NIH or elsewhere.

- *Clinical department databases.* In academic medical centers, these databases are developed by some departments to store clinical and research information, with access restricted by password to authorized departmental personnel and any data pertaining to funded human tissue studies available only by links to other, more specialized, databases managed by research investigators in the department.

- *Databases for future clinical research studies.* These databases, developed by an investigator with no current research hypothesis, are authorized by a funding source, protected by password, and approved by a local IRB for the scientific purpose of gathering, storing, and organizing multiple items of information (names, ages, diagnoses) about numerous patients in particular clinical areas (neonatology, ophthalmology, oncology, etc.), with informed consent or parental permission, and with the expectation that this coded data will later be used in specific human tissue studies.

- *Study-specific, genetics databases.* The prototype for organized data storage in DNA banking studies, these research databases are typically developed by investigators in a federally or commercially funded human tissue study, authorized by the funding source and a local IRB, used according to an approved research protocol (including informed consent), administered by a database manager, protected by physical and electronic security measures, and restricted to grant-funded personnel (whether in local labs or labs elsewhere).

- *Non-study-specific, genetics databases.* These DNA databases, which can be national in scope (Iceland), are developed without a specific research hypothesis or informed consent from sample sources, possibly owned by a commercial biotech company (DeCODE), and protected by various in-house security measures, with investigators systematically juxtaposing large data sets in the database in a search for unusual if not unique DNA "finds" or "hits."[65]

Our interest in these research databases is twofold, and limited to those that store and organize DNA-derived information as part of human tissue research. First, the long-term storage of genetic information in DNA banking needs to meet an abbreviated version of the same standard of disclosure as the long-term storage of tissue samples for research purposes, namely *the reasonable person standard of disclosure.* This standard of disclosure, when used in the context of obtaining informed consent for the storage of tissues in DNA banking, requires that investigators and other key members of a research team use the process of informed consent (including informed consent documents) to address the interests and concerns of a reasonable person in the situation of a potential research participant.

When applied to the projected, long-term storage of *tissue samples,* this standard of disclosure focuses on the interests and concerns of a reasonable person that were identified earlier: (*1*) the identity status of the samples, (*2*) the privacy and confidentiality of personal information, (*3*) the control and ownership of samples, (*4*) the right of withdrawal from a study, (*5*) the length of tissue storage, (*6*) personal access to clinically relevant information derived from the samples, (*7*) possible third-party access to the samples, and (*8*) possible use of the samples for secondary research purposes. When applied to the projected, long-term storage of *genetic information*—with its personal, familial, predictive, and possibly group implications—in one or more databases, disclosures to a potential research participant required by the reasonable person standard are slightly condensed, but equally important:

- The identity status of the information in the database (Will it be identified by name or other descriptors, or coded in a sufficiently protected manner?)
- The security measures (locked rooms, limited keys, computer passwords, protected files) that will be used to protect the privacy and confidentiality of this intimately personal information
- The control and ownership of this computerized, yet personal data
- The limitations placed on the right to withdraw this data from a database with information about many other research participants
- The protection of the data from unwarranted third-party access
- The protection of the personal data (by being anonymized) if shared with other investigators doing secondary research studies.[66]

Second, research institutions, possibly through their IRBs, need to do a better job of monitoring and regulating the research databases used in connection with DNA banking. Given the reality that directors of large research labs engaged in human tissue studies often have multiple databases storing, tracking, and organizing DNA-derived information from thousands of persons in several countries, and the fact that large research institutions now have hundreds of investigators doing long-term human tissue studies, the task of keeping track of these thousands of research information databases is daunting. Doing so will require that research institutions develop one or more *institutional databases* that will enable IRB administrators to be able—at least—to document how many research databases in the institution are involved in DNA banking and which labs or individual investigators have them.

More oversight of research databases would be even better. No one wants a research administration to take on a "big brother" role or to micromanage the use of research databases. Yet it would be very helpful if administrators of in-stitutional research programs, possibly working with a committee mandated to develop institution-wide standards, would begin to enforce some core standards for databases used in human tissue studies. For starters, those standards could pertain to institutional ownership of research databases, expected disclosures to research par-ticipants, requirements regarding limited access to databases, and required security measures for equipment.

Some Special Issues in Forensic Settings

As indicated earlier, some DNA tissues are special and raise special issues because they are stored and analyzed for nonbiomedical purposes. Perhaps the best known of the special DNA tissues used for nonbiomedical purposes are those used for identification of human remains from destructive scenes of death, whether the deaths occur through warfare, explosion, fire, plane crash, or terrorist action. A notable example is the Department of Defense's DNA Repository, established in 1991 during Operation Desert Storm as a technological leap beyond the use of "dog tags," dental remains, and fingerprints for identification purposes. This tissue repository now has over 2 million DNA specimens (from mandatory blood-stain cards and cheek swab samples from all military personnel), along with a database that matches each DNA sample with the Social Security Number and abbreviated last name of the individual from whom it came.[67]

A more recent example of human remains identification after tragic deaths is the work of numerous pathologists in New York and other states as they have tried to identify the thousands of persons killed by terrorists on September 11, 2001. Using the analytical methods of molecular genetics (e.g., analyzing 13 biological markers in DNA samples), these pathologists have painstakingly identified the remains of many persons killed that day, working to match some of the deteriorated remains with amplifiable DNA removed from the victims' belongings collected from victims' families.[68]

A more publicized and controversial use of stored tissues—and DNA databanks—for nonbiomedical purposes is the practice of using DNA evidence in court to convict (or sometimes exonerate) individuals facing criminal charges. This widely used practice of DNA forensics has been carried out in a number of countries since it began in England in 1985, with the British legal system providing substantial support over the years for the ever-widening use of this law enforcement technology, including the controversial practice of "sweeps" (the collection of large numbers of DNA samples from persons living in an area where a terrible crime occurred). Now, laws for forensic DNA databanks have been enacted in Australia, Canada, China, France, Germany, and several other countries.[69]

Likewise, all 50 states enacted laws for forensic DNA databases in the 1990s. These laws have many purposes. They encourage and sometimes fund state crime labs to use the state-of-the-art analytic technologies of molecular genetics with items of evidence from crime scenes, and enable state forensic databases to be connected with the FBI's CODIS (Combined DNA Index System) databases. In addition, they provide law enforcement officials with the legal option of using DNA evidence to connect an alleged perpetrator with a crime (rape, burglary, murder, etc.) lacking witnesses, and give prosecutors the possibility of using a piece of circumstantial evidence that has extraordinary mathematical probabilities of being correct.

By using DNA evidence, prosecutors gain two advantages. First, DNA (blood, hair, semen, saliva residue, skin particles, fingerprints, hand smudges, etc.) is often more abundant at crime scenes than other pieces of evidence. Second, the comparative genetics analysis of DNA samples from a crime scene and from one or more suspects–amplifying very small amounts of DNA by PCR, separating the amplified products by electrophoresis, using fluorescent tags with the samples, and analyzing 13 short tandem repeats (STRs) of repetitive DNA in the samples—sometimes results in a DNA match that is difficult to refute in court.[70] Barring countervailing evidence of inadvertent or malicious handling of the DNA samples by police or forensic scientists, this DNA evidence often proves to be decisive.

Equally important, especially in societies that are supposed to presume the innocence of suspects until solid evidence proves otherwise, DNA evidence is also being used to exonerate persons who have been wrongly accused of crimes and, increasingly, to free prisoners who have spent years incarcerated for crimes they did not commit. As documented by the Innocence Project at the Cardozo School of Law in New York, more than 130 prisoners in the United States have been exonerated in recent years through the post-conviction use of DNA evidence that was not used in their trials.[71] At this writing, every few weeks the media carries yet another story about a prisoner released because DNA evidence established his or her innocence.[72]

The use of DNA evidence for both of these purposes—criminal convictions and exonerations of the innocent—is likely to increase in the future, especially as the field of molecular genetics changes with the development of new analytic technologies that can be used in the pursuit of justice. Equally predictable, the forensic DNA database laws in the United States and other countries are likely to undergo many changes in the future as crime rates, imprisonment numbers, government budgets, public opinion polls, and civil libertarian concerns rise or fall.

Many aspects of the topic of forensic DNA samples, including a discussion about research that may be done with these collected tissues, go beyond the scope of this book. Still, we can identify some of the concerns and questions that should be part of the ongoing public debate about using stored DNA samples and DNA databases in the context of the criminal justice system. We thus conclude this chapter with a suggested list of 10 substantive issues that seem imperative for legislators (and other citizens) to consider regarding existing DNA database laws, possible revisions of those laws, or any new laws authorizing the collection of DNA samples and use of DNA databases for forensic purposes:

- *Crimes targeted by the laws.* Only sexual felonies? Also property crimes? Various non-violent crimes? "White-collar" crimes? All felonies? Specific misdemeanors as well?
- *Inclusion of juvenile offenders.* Included in the databank along with adult criminals, or personal/familial DNA data placed in a separate database for legal minors?
- *Timing of collection of DNA samples.* Blood sample and/or cheek swab sample to be obtained after conviction of a specified crime? After arrest? Before parole from prison?
- *Length of sample and data storage.* Retain the sample after the DNA profile has been put in the forensic database? Retain the sample and/or data for 50 years? For the lifetimes of the convicted criminals?
- *Procedures for destruction/deletion.* What is to happen to the stored samples and data pertaining to individuals who are *exonerated?*
- *Use(s) of stored samples and data.* Restricted to "law enforcement"? To "identification purposes"? Or also to be used for research on forensic techniques? What about use in *non-forensic DNA research?*
- *Identity status and forensic research use.* If samples and/or data are to be used for forensic research purposes, will they still be identified or coded, or will they be anonymized for this use?
- *Security provisions and third-party access.* What security measures are needed for forensic DNA databases? How are employers, insurance companies, private detectives, and others to be prevented from unwarranted access?
- *Provisions for unauthorized disclosures.* Is there a criminal penalty for unauthorized disclosures of private/familial DNA information from stored samples or a databank? Is there a financial penalty?
- *Population-wide DNA profiling.* What is to be done about recurring proposals, in Britain and the United States, regarding establishing an all-inclusive, national

DNA databank for forensic and identification purposes, perhaps connecting DNA profiling at birth with currently mandated neonatal screening programs?[73]

Cases and Vignettes

Margaret Everett asks, "What would happen if we lost the ability to make decisions about how our DNA is used?" Her question is raised out of personal experience, not philosophical reflection. When her son Jack was born with a rare genetic disorder, she "found out first hand what it was like to become the subject of DNA research." After Jack's death, researchers requested the parents' consent to analyze and transform the blood samples obtained earlier from Jack's body. Consent was easily given "because we believe the research is important and because we trusted the geneticists, who treated our child with respect and sensitivity." But Everett says it is strange "to think that our son is dead and yet his cells are growing in at least three labs in three different countries." Are those cells Jack? No, she says. "Jack was the baby I held in my arms ... not some disembodied lab samples." Then she emphasizes, "But I also know those are more than 'just cells.' It bothers me to think that his DNA might be handled in a way that is irresponsible or disrespectful of my son. By retaining some control over how his cells are used, I feel that I am continuing to act as a responsible parent." For her, it comes down "to not wanting researchers to ever be able to forget that there is a human being connected to those cells."[74]

Boston University (BU), which administers the Framingham Heart Study under a contract with the NIH, had to give up a grand plan because of concerns about public data, ethics, and commercial interests. BU's plan, announced in 2000, was to provide data from the study's 160 different databases (plus pre-computer-era data stored in boxes and file cabinets) to a private company that intended to provide, for a profit, genomic analysis of the vast data. The benefits to be gained from this genomic analysis would be unmatched, since this longest epidemiologic study in medicine has collected an enormous amount of coded data from the original participants, dating from 1948. It has added more coded data from their children since 1971 and is now beginning to collect coded data from their grandchildren (see Chapters 1 and 2 for descriptions of this study). If the plan had worked, a BU-generated private company, Framingham Genomic Medicine, would have created an unparalleled database from the extensive and diverse Framingham data, a database that, as initially proposed, would have been freely available to investigators who requested specific data. The plan for this public-private collaboration collapsed, however, over concerns at NIH that this deal would give too much control to a for-profit company, especially when the company wanted exclusive rights to some of the data for a period of time.[75]

The Mayo Clinic, in Rochester, Minnesota, is creating a database that will ultimately contain medical and genetic information about all of its patients. Collaborating with computer experts from IBM, some physicians, scientific investigators, and systems-information administrators at Mayo are working on plans for a comprehensive database that will include not only the six million patient records at Mayo, but eventually also contain detailed genetic information about these persons. As one of the database experts declared, "We are basically planning for the ability to have everyone's complete genome in there." According to the plan, Mayo physicians in the future will be able to provide "personalized medicine" for patients. At the present time there are no plans to make the database available to non-Mayo medical professionals. But for Mayo physicians, the computerized future of medicine is promising. An oncologist, for example, anticipates the time when he will be able to assemble a group of colon-cancer patients from similar geographic areas whose cancer developed earlier in life, retrieve their tissue samples from storage, and then analyze their differing DNA from a portion of each sample for clues about their common medical condition.[76]

Matt Myers, a junior at the University of Iowa, is willing to participate for money in virtually any scientific study. For the past three years, he has checked the university's list of current research studies each morning, trekked from one study site to another, and made additional money by referring other persons to the study sites. He has provided blood samples, offered his sperm and urine (for a price) to investigators, and endured bimonthly bronchoscopies to extract cells from his lungs. He has made over $4,000 for being "numbed, shaved, pricked, infected, and rammed." Matt's perspective on his entrepreneurship is simple: "I've always been money-conscious and trying to find new ways of making money, but I [had] never thought about experimenting with my own body."[77]

Rosie Gordon, an 11-year-old girl living in a Washington, D.C., suburb, was abducted from the street in front of her home. Her body was found two days later about five miles away. Based on the circumstances of her disappearance and death, behavioral specialists from the National Center for the Analysis of Violent Crime in Quantico, Virginia, developed a criminal profile of the perpetrator. They also studied reports of similar incidents in area suburbs over the three years before the Gordon case. They turned up four cases with common features: daylight abductions, female victims, residential neighborhoods, possible sexual molestation. Moreover, they studied DNA samples from the cases and discovered that they came from the same man, a fact that had not been known until the DNA testing was done. A suspect was identified, arrested, and subsequently convicted of abduction and rape in the four cases; he is now in prison. Although criminal investigators could not produce sufficient evidence to convict him of killing Rosie Gordon, they are reasonably sure of one thing: If DNA technology and the FBI's CODIS system had been in place earlier, some of these girls would not have been victimized and Rosie Gordon would not have been killed.[78]

Notes

1. Ellen Wright Clayton, "Panel Comment: Why the Use of Anonymous Samples for Research Matters," *J Law Med Ethics* 23 (1995): 375–77.
2. Board of Directors, Council for Responsible Genetics, "The Genetic Bill of Rights," Cambridge, Mass., 2000.
3. National Commission for the Protection of Human Subjects of Biomedical and Behavioral Research, *The Belmont Report: Ethical Principles and Guidelines for the Protection of Human Subjects of Research* (Washington, D.C.: DHEW Publication 78-0012, 1978); and Robert Levine, *Ethics and Regulation of Clinical Research,* 2nd ed. (New Haven: Yale University Press, 1988), pp. 1–18.
4. See Chapter 5 and Chapter 8 for more details.
5. Commission on Life Sciences, National Research Council, *Evaluating Human Genetic Diversity* (Washington, D.C.: National Academy Press, 1997).
6. Elisa Eiseman and Suzanne Haga, *Handbook of Human Tissue Sources* (Rockville, Md.: RAND, 1999), p. 141.

7. Therese Lysaught et al., "A Pilot Test of DNA-based Analysis Using Anonymized Newborn Screening Cards in Iowa," in Robert Weir, ed., *Stored Tissue Samples* (Iowa City: University of Iowa Press, 1998), pp. 3–31; Philip Reilly, "Panel Comment: The Impact of the Genetic Privacy Act on Medicine," *J Law Med Ethics* 23 (1995): 379; Ellen Wright Clayton, "Issues in State Newborn Screening Programs," *Pediatrics* 90 (1992): 641–46; Jean McEwen and Philip Reilly, "Stored Guthrie Cards as DNA 'Banks,'" *Am J Hum Genet* 55 (1994): 196–200; and Ellen Wright Clayton, "Informed Consent and Genetic Research," in Mark Rothstein, ed., *Genetic Secrets: Protecting Privacy and Confidentiality in the Genetic Era* (New Haven: Yale University Press, 1997), pp. 134–35.

8. Lysaught et al., pp. 5–8.

9. Robert F. Weir, "Advance Directives for the Use of Stored Tissue Samples," in Weir, *Stored Tissue Samples,* pp. 236–66.

10. Health Council of the Netherlands, *Proper Use of Human Tissue* (The Hague: Health Council, 1994).

11. Multidisciplinary committee at the University of Iowa, "IRB Guidelines for Genetic Research," 1995, pp. 21–22 of an unpublished document.

12. 45 C.F.R. 46 (Subpart A); American Society of Human Genetics, "Statement on Informed Consent for Genetic Research," *Am J Hum Genet* 59 (1996): 471–74; and National Bioethics Advisory Commission, *Research Involving Human Biological Materials* (Rockville, Md.: NBAC, 1999).

13. Anita L. Allen, "Genetic Privacy: Emerging Concepts and Values," in Rothstein, pp. 44–45; and Clayton, "Panel Comment," pp. 375–77.

14. Jon F. Merz and Pamela Sankar, "DNA Banking: An Empirical Study of a Proposed Consent Form," in Weir, *Stored Tissue Samples,* pp. 198–225.

15. Clayton, "Panel Comment," p. 376.

16. Allen, p. 45.

17. Margaret Everett, "Commentary," *The Oregonian,* June 2, 1999. This commentary is also available through the Web site of Geneforum, an Oregon educational organization: http://www.geneforum.org.

18. Council of Regional Networks for Genetic Services, "Issues in the Use of Archived Specimens for Genetics Research," unpublished manuscript, 1997, pp. 3–5.

19. Eiseman and Haga, p. 141.

20. See Jon Merz, Pamela Sankar, Sheila Taube, and Virginia Livolsi, "Use of Human Tissues in Research: Clarifying Clinician and Researcher Roles and Information Flows," *J Investig Med* 45 (1997): 252–57.

21. Ellen Wright Clayton et al., "Informed Consent for Genetic Research on Stored Tissue Samples," *JAMA* 247 (1995): 1786–92.

22. College of American Pathologists, "Uses of Human Tissue," unpublished policy statement, 1996; and William Grizzle et al., "Recommended Policies for Uses of Human Tissue in Research, Education, and Quality Control," *Arch Pathol Lab Med* 123 (1999): 296–300.

23. Wayne Grody, "Molecular Pathology, Informed Consent, and the Paraffin Block," *Diagn Mol Pathol* 4 (1995): 156.

24. See several articles in a thematic section on ethical aspects of human embryonic stem cell research in the *Kennedy Inst Ethics J* 9 (1999): 109–88; a number of articles in a thematic section on stem cell research and ethics in *Science* 287 (2000): 1417–46; Sharon Begley, "Cellular Divide," *Newsweek,* July 9, 2001, pp. 22–27; and Evan Thomas and Eleanor Clift, "Battle for Bush's Soul," *Newsweek,* July 9, 2001, pp. 28–30.

25. Bradley Van Voorhis, Dan Grinstead, Amy Sparks, and Robert Weir, "Establishment of a Successful Donor Embryo Program: Medical, Ethical, and Policy Issues," *Fertil Steril* 71 (1999): 604–08.

26. Gilbert Meilaender, "The Point of a Ban: Or, How to Think about Stem Cell Research," *Hastings Cent Rep* 31 (2001): 9–16; and the university professors who supported a federal ban on this research in a letter to President Bush, which is available at this Web site: http://pewforum.org/projects/stemcell/antiletter.pdf. For a contrasting view, see Michael J. Meyer and Lawrence J. Nelson, "Respecting What We Destroy: Reflections on Human Embryo Research," *Hastings Cent Rep* 31 (2001): 16–23.

27. See Ronald M. Green, *The Human Embryo Research Debates* (New York: Oxford University Press, 2001); Shirley J. Wright, "Human Embryonic Stem-Cell Research: Science and Ethics," *Am Sci* 87 (1999): 352–61; Geron Ethics Advisory Board, "Research with Human Embryonic Stem Cells: Ethical Considerations," *Hastings Cent Rep* 29 (1999): 31–36; American Association for the Advancement of Science, *Stem Cell Research and Applications: Monitoring the Frontiers of Biomedical Research* (Washington, D.C.: AAAS, 1999); National Bioethics Advisory Commission, *Ethical Issues in Human Stem Cell Research,* 2 vols. (Rockville, Md.: NBAC, 1999); and Eliot Marshall, "The Business of Stem Cells," *Science* 287 (2000): 1419–21.

28. For the official views of several countries, see Gretchen Vogel, "Bush Squeezes Between the Lines on Stem Cells," *Science* 292 (2001): 1242–45; Vogel, "In the Mideast, Pushing Back the Stem Cell Frontier," *Science* 295 (2002): 1818–20; and Vogel, "Regulations Constrain Stem Cell Research Across the Globe," *Science* 297 (2002): 924.

29. For examples of positions on some other ethical issues in biomedicine, see Robert F. Weir, *Selective Nontreatment of Handicapped Newborns* (New York: Oxford University Press, 1984); and Weir, *Abating Treatment with Critically Ill Patients* (New York: Oxford, 1989).

30. Alessandra Stanley, "Bush Hears Pope Condemn Research in Human Embryos," *New York Times,* July 24, 2001. Some of the description of some of these ethical views is gleaned from earlier discussions in these sources: Eric Juengst and Michael Fossel, "The Ethics of Embryonic Stem Cells—Now and Forever, Cells Without End," *JAMA* 284 (2000): 3180–84; and Nicholas Wade, "Grappling With the Ethics of Stem Cell Research," *New York Times,* July 24, 2001, p. D3.

31. Katharine Seelye, "Bush Gives His Backing For Limited Research On Existing Stem Cells," *New York Times,* August 10, 2001, p. A1, A16; and Frank Bruni, "Bush Says He Will Veto Any Bill Broadening His Stem Cell Policy," *New York Times,* August 14, 2001, p. A1, A14.

32. NBAC, *Ethical Issues in Human Stem Cell Research,* Vol. I, pp. 3–6; and the American Academy of Pediatrics, "Human Embryo Research," published online July 13, 2001, at this Web site: http://www.aap.org/policy/s0104.html.

33. Editorial, "The Pro-Life Case for Cloning," *New York Times,* May 2, 2002, p. A26.

34. Commission on Life Sciences, National Academy of Sciences, *Stem Cells and the Future of Regenerative Medicine* (Washington, D.C.: National Academy Press, 2001).

35. Brian Vastag, "At the Cloning Circus Sideshows Abound, While Scientists Seek a Wider Audience," *JAMA* 286 (2001): 1437–38; and Gregory Pence, *Who's Afraid of Human Cloning?* (Lanham, Md.: Rowman and Littlefield, 1998). Also see Jeremy Manier, "Cloning of Baby Doubted, Damned," *Chicago Tribune,* December 28, 2002, pp. 1, 8; and Linda Greenhouse, "F.D.A. Exploring Human Cloning Claim," *New York Times,* December 30, 2002, p. A9.

36. NBAC, *Ethical Issues in Human Stem Cell Research,* Vol. I, pp. 6–7.
37. Nuffield Council on Bioethics, *Human Tissue: Ethical and Legal Issues* (London: Nuffield Council, 1995), p. 47.
38. National Bioethics Advisory Commission, *Ethical and Policy Issues in Research Involving Human Participants* (Rockville, Md.: NBAC, 2001), p. 67.
39. Robert F. Weir and Jay R. Horton, "Genetic Research, Adolescents, and Informed Consent," *Theor Med* 16 (1995): 347–73.
40. For a discussion of other types of harm in biomedicine, see Weir, *Abating Treatment with Critically Ill Patients,* pp. 350–54.
41. See note 10 above.
42. William F. May, "Attitudes toward the newly dead," *Hastings Cent Stud* 1: (1973): 3.
43. Susan C. Lawrence, "Beyond the Grave—The Use and Meaning of Human Body Parts: A Historical Introduction," in Weir, *Stored Tissue Samples,* p. 112.
44. James F. Childress, *Practical Reasoning in Bioethics* (Bloomington: Indiana University Press, 1997), p. 268.
45. Catherine Caturano Horan, "Your Spleen is Not Worth What it Used to Be: Moore v. Regents of UCLA," *Creighton Law Review* 24 (1991): 1423–48.
46. William Boulier, "Sperm, Spleens, and Other Valuables: The Need to Recognize Property Rights in Human Body Parts," *Hofstra Law Review* 23 (1995): 693–731.
47. Michael M.J. Lin, "Conferring a Federal Property Right in Genetic Material: Stepping into the Future With the Genetic Privacy Act," *Am J Law Med* 22 (1996): 109–34.
48. Mary Taylor Danforth, "Cells, Sales, and Royalties: The Patient's Right to a Portion of the Profits," *Yale Law and Policy Review* 6 (1988): 179–202.
49. Charlotte H. Harrison, "Neither Moore nor the Market: Alternative Models for Compensating Contributors of Human Tissue," *Am J Law Med* 28 (2002): 77–105.
50. Dorothy Nelkin and Lori Andrews, "Homo Economicus: The Commercialization of Body Tissue in the Age of Biotechnology," *Hastings Cent Rep* 28 (1998): 33, 37; and Lori Andrews and Dorothy Nelkin, *Body Bazaar: The Market for Human Tissue in the Biotechnology Age* (New York: Crown Publishers, 2001), pp. 45–46.
51. See the article and book cited immediately above. Also see Bartha Knoppers, Marie Hirtle, and Kathleen Glass, "Commercialization of Genetic Research and Public Policy," *Science* 286 (1999): 2277–78; and Bartha Knoppers, Claude Laberge, and Marie Hirtle, eds., *Human DNA: Law and Policy* (The Hague: Kluwer Law International, 1997), pp. 341–83.
52. See *The Daily Iowan,* July 27, 2001, p. 4. Also see Rebecca Mead, "Eggs for Sale," *The New Yorker,* August 9, 1999, pp. 56–65.
53. Andrews and Nelkin, *Body Bazaar,* pp. 25, 31.
54. Nelkin and Andrews, "Homo Economicus," p. 31.
55. See Elizabeth A. Boyd and Lisa A. Bero, "Assessing Faculty Financial Relationships With Industry," *JAMA* 284 (2000): 2209–14; Mildred K. Cho et al., "Policies on Faculty Conflicts of Interest at US Universities," *JAMA* 284 (2000): 2203–08; David Korn, "Conflicts of Interest in Biomedical Research," *JAMA* 284 (2000): 2234–37; and Colin Macilwain, "Scientists defy their ethics codes and take gifts from industry," *Nature* 392 (1998): 427.
56. Eliot Marshall, "NIH Considers Paying to Use Private Database," *Science* 291 (2001): 223–24; Eric Campbell et al., "Data Withholding in Academic Genetics: Evidence From a National Survey," *JAMA* 287 (2002): 473–80; and Van McCrary et al., "A National Survey of Policies on Disclosure of Conflicts of Interest in Biomedical Research," *N Engl J Med* 343 (2000): 1621–26.

57. Gina Kolata, "Sharing of Profits Is Debated As the Value of Tissue Rises," *New York Times,* May 15, 2000, pp. A1, A15; *Greenberg v. Miami Children's Hosp. Research Institute,* 264 F. Supp. 2d 1064.

58. Board of Directors, Council for Responsible Genetics, "The Genetic Bill of Rights," statement #4. Also see Quirin Schiermeier, "Traditional Owners 'Should Be Paid,' " *Nature* 419 (2002): 423.

59. Catherine D. DeAngelis, "Conflict of Interest and the Public Trust," *JAMA* 284 (2000): 2237–38; and Robert P. Kelch, "Maintaining the Public Trust in Clinical Research," *N Engl J Med* 346 (2002): 285–87. Also see the Task Force on Financial Conflicts of Interest in Clinical Research, Association of American Medical Colleges, "Protecting Subjects, Preserving Trust, Promoting Progress—Policy and Guidelines for the Oversight of Individual Financial Interests in Human Subjects Research," available online at Task Force Web site (http://www.aamc.org/members/coitf/). The same concern exists in other countries. See, for example, Dennis Normile, "Japan Readies Rules That Allow Research," *Science* 293 (2001): 775, where a leading developmental biologist says, "Strict regulation [of embryonic stem cell research] is necessary to obtain public support."

60. Kolata, "Sharing of Profits," p. A15; and Paul Smaglik, "Tissue donors use their influence in deal over gene patent terms," *Nature* 407 (2000): 821.

61. See note 10 above, "IRB Guidelines," pp. 22–23; and Mary Taylor Danforth, "Cells, Sales, and Royalties: The Patient's Right to a Portion of the Profits," *Yale Law and Policy Review* 6 (1988): 179–202. Also see NBAC, *Ethical Issues in Human Stem Cell Research,* Vol. I, p. 7, where Recommendation 5 calls for the disclosure of "the *source of funding and expected commercial benefits* of the research with the embryos, if known" (emphasis added).

62. Jennifer Fisher Wilson, "The Rise of Biological Databases," *The Scientist* 16 (2002): 34–35; and Isabelle Hirtzlin et al., "An Empirical Survey of Biobanking of Human Genetic Material and Data in Six EU Countries," *Euro J Hum Genet* 11 (2003): 475–88.

63. Andreas Baxevanis, "The Molecular Biology Database Collection: 2002 Update," *Nucleic Acids Research* 30 (2002): 1–2.

64. *Ibid.,* pp. 3–12.

65. For other assessments of genetics databases and ethics, see Bartha Knoppers and Claude Laberge, "Ethical Guideposts for Allelic Variation Databases," *Hum Mutat* 15 (2000): 30–35; and Ruth Chadwick and Kare Berg, "Solidarity and Equity: New Ethical Frameworks for Genetic Databases," *Nat Genet* 2 (2001): 318–21. The latter is available at this Web site: www.nature.com/reviews/genetics.

66. For two discussions of ethical and legal issues with research databases, see Beverly Woodward, "Medical Record Confidentiality and Data Collection: Current Dilemmas," *J Law Med Ethics* 25 (1997): 88–97; and Latanya Sweeney, "Weaving Technology and Policy Together to Maintain Confidentiality," *J Law Med Ethics* 25 (1997): 98–110.

67. Victor Weedn, "Stored Biologic Specimens for Military Identification: The Department of Defense DNA Registry," in Weir, *Stored Tissue Samples,* pp. 345–57.

68. See Lawrence Altman, "Forensics Lab Is Prepared For 20,000 DNA Tests," *New York Times,* September 14, 2001; and Eric Lipton and James Glanz, "Limits of DNA Research Pressed To Identify the Dead of Sept. 11," *New York Times,* April 22, 2002, pp. A1, A14.

69. Phil Reilly, "Legal and Public Policy Issues in DNA Forensics," *Nat Rev Genet* 2 (2001): 313.

70. Reilly, p. 314. Also see Ian Evett and Bruce S. Weir, *Interpreting DNA Evidence: Statistical Genetics for Forensic Scientists* (Sunderland, Mass.: Sinauer Associates, 1998).

71. Jodi Wilgoren, "Confession Had His Signature; DNA Did Not," *New York Times,* August 26, 2002, p. A1. For the best compilation of cases in which DNA evidence has been used to exonerate persons wrongly imprisoned, see Barry Scheck, Peter Neufeld, and Jim Dwyer, *Actual Innocence: When Justice Goes Wrong and How to Make It Right* (New York: Signet, 2001).

72. See, as examples, Jim Yardley, "In Rape Case Gone Awry, New Suspect," *New York Times,* August 29, 2001, p. A12; and William Glaberson, "6 Years After Conviction, DNA Clears Man in Murder," *New York Times,* April 25, 2002, p. A30.

73. For helpful discussions of these substantive matters, see Reilly, "Legal and Public Policy Issues," pp. 313–17; Jonathan Kimmelman, "Risking Ethical Insolvency: A Survey of Trends in Criminal DNA Databanking," *J Law Med Ethics* 28 (2000): 209–21; and Jean McEwen, "Storing Genes to Solve Crimes," in Weir, *Stored Tissue Samples,* pp. 311–28.

74. Everett, "Commentary," see note 17 above.

75. Gina Kolata, "Boston U. Founds Company to Sift Leading Heart Data," *New York Times,* June 17, 2000; and Andrew Lawler, "NIH Kills Deal to Upgrade Heart Data," *Science* 291 (2001): 27–28.

76. David Hamilton, "Mayo to Build Patient Database; It Will Include Genetic Profiles," online version of *The Wall Street Journal,* March 25, 2002 (http://online.wsj.com).

77. Lauren Smiley, "Donating His Life to Science, 1 Cell at a Time," *The Daily Iowan,* May 9, 2003, pp. 1A, 4A.

78. John W. Hicks, "The Use and Development of DNA Databanks in Law Enforcement," in Weir, *Stored Tissue Samples,* pp. 309–10.

11

An Agenda for the *Near* Future

Throughout this book we have made the case for greater disclosure and more appropriately informed consent concerning the collection, storage, and scientific uses of human tissue samples. Our clarion call for policy and practice reforms that will better empower research participants in the exercises of choice in no way diminishes our steadfast support for biomedical research. We know how essential the use of human tissues is to that research and have great hope that biomedical investigators doing research with stored DNA samples will continue to lead the way toward patient-specific treatments and the promise of better health for all of us in the era of genomic medicine.

We also know that the scientific achievement of better medicines and treatments is dependent in a fundamentally important way on public support and federal funding for the research that investigators do in their labs. That support and funding, in turn, depends on public perceptions and attitudes about the types of research being done, the ways in which the research is carried out, the victories being achieved in the name of scientific progress, and the costs of those victories, both financial and moral. These public perceptions and attitudes about biomedical research are often difficult to gauge accurately. In general, they reflect the degree to which the public believes that biomedical scientists, especially those employed in academia, are through their research studies both "doing the right thing" and doing it the right way. In democracies, that's roughly how nonscientists assess the work that scientists do. This general assessment is one of the important factors that motivates many individuals to help science progress by participating in human studies, frequently with their tissues. Others do not to want to participate in such studies, if they know about them, possibly because they are insufficiently informed, simply uninterested in participating, concerned about genetic discrimination and other possible psychosocial harms, or, for some other reasons, distrustful of scientists and scientific research.

As documented earlier (see Chapter 2), a significant portion of the American public has vaguely described concerns about some biomedical research being done, especially in genetics. Moreover, a significant number of persons are troubled by what they know or hear about common research practices, chiefly human tissue research with stored samples here and elsewhere. At least five surveys published in this country indicate that much of this public concern focuses on the lack of disclosure about the types of research being done, the lack of appropriate informed consent to the use of one's tissues, and the possibility that the personal, familial, and predictive information in one's DNA samples might end up being used for discriminatory purposes by employers, health insurance companies, or governments.

Whether these concerns are experientially based is open to debate. What does not seem debatable, however, is that a significant portion of American society *perceives* the loss of genetic privacy and the possibility of genetic discrimination to be sufficiently real and important threats that they have serious reservations about the use of their DNA samples in biomedical research. How much concern the public has about other possible psychosocial harms, such as psychological risks in gaining new self-knowledge or the risks of one's tissues being used for objectionable research, connected with some types of research studies is not as clear, but it cannot simply be dismissed.

We *stand at a crossroads* for human tissue research. Beyond surveys of public opinion, organized opposition groups in Iceland have tried for years to stop the DNA banking and research database of DeCODE, a coalition of churches and human rights groups in the Kingdom of Tonga successfully blocked the government's business deal with Autogen, an Australian biotech company, and at least two groups are trying to stop UK BioBank from being established.[1] In each instance, the groups opposing DNA banking and research databases have been motivated by concerns over inadequate informed consent, possible loss of genetic privacy, commercialism in research, and other issues.

We hope that these concerns will be addressed satisfactorily by advocates of biomedical research worldwide. We also hope that the general public's support of research with stored tissue samples can be strengthened and federal funding for this research significantly increased. Further, and equally important, we hope that citizens in the United States and other countries will be empowered in an unprecedented way in their individual roles as informed, collaborative participants in human tissue research.

To these ends, we conclude with a series of recommendations. We do so for three reasons. First, a "business as usual" approach in human tissue research, based in part on a traditional system of minimal disclosure about the collection, storage, and long-term research uses of human tissues, does not and will not address the concerns increasingly expressed by nonscientists when they think about their DNA samples being used for unknown research purposes. Second, our recommendations, if implemented, will demonstrate greater respect for the autonomy of potential and actual research participants, help promote their interests in genetic privacy, and provide them, perhaps, with greater protection against the real-life possibilities of genetic discrimination and other psychosocial harms. Third, the long-term consequence of these changes will be beneficial for all of us. We envision a revised understanding of human tissue research as a *collaborative process* in which skilled investigators and appropriately informed participants jointly contribute to new scientific achievements and help produce a better, more healthful future for children and adults worldwide.

Recommendations

In earlier chapters we discussed an assortment of suggestions, proposals, and recommendations for improving some practices used in human tissue research and made a number of suggestions and proposals ourselves. The formal recommendations discussed in Chapters 5 and 8 came from multidisciplinary committees in the Netherlands, England, Canada, the Human Genome Organization, the Council of Europe, and the United States. Now we advocate a set of recommendations that are intended to be reasonable, realistic, and productive of significant change. We hope that the changes produced, if our recommendations are followed, will have an impact on the major players in the human tissue research enterprise: the individuals and families who give of themselves, literally, to participate in human tissue research studies; the investigators who devote their time, talent, and technological skills to the successful completion of much-needed research; and the administrative leaders in hospitals, clinics, and organizations that sponsor biomedical research.

Recommendations for Individuals and Families

As Regular, Ordinary People. We live in a fast-paced, constantly changing world. Part of the change that influences an increasing number of persons comes from the unprecedented achievements now occurring through molecular genetics and other fields of biomedical research. Whether reading about the discovery of the latest "gene-of-the-week," watching the depiction of a genetically programmed and stratified future society in the movie "Gattaca," hearing about Dolly the sheep and other reproductive cloning events, or worrying about a relative diagnosed with a genetically associated form of breast cancer or Alzheimer disease, most of us are both amazed and concerned about recent, all but inescapable developments in genetics.

We hope that individuals and families neither ignore the latest publicized discoveries in genetics nor spend a lot of time worrying vaguely about genetics, biomedical investigators, the possibility of being victimized through genetic discrimination, or, like John Moore, about participation in a human tissue research study. Instead, we hope that individuals and families will talk, when opportunities arise, about some of their research-related concerns, such as the risk to personal and familial privacy, and try to become more informed, educated citizens.

1. To acknowledge the concerns that many persons have about participating in genetics research, individuals and families should be open, candid, and realistic. They should try to think, talk, and learn together to try to determine if their concerns are based in reality, especially those about research done with tissue samples that have been (or might be) obtained from family members, alive or dead.

American families do not typically discuss these matters at the dinner table (though many high school students now discuss genetics and bioethics in biology and social science classes), much less talk about the latest gene-of-the-week, multifactorial inheritance patterns, mitochrondrial DNA, polymerase chain reaction, or other facts about genetics. But more common, family-related factors relating to genetics and other biomedical research could well be occasional topics of conversation. For example, why not try to find out if other family members have concerns about possibly losing some personal and familial privacy, becoming victims of genetic discrimination, or discovering that the wrong third party (e.g., employer, health insurance company, government) has gained access to important personal information contained in one's stored DNA sample? Just as many American families have begun in recent years to have serious, family-centered conversations about matters pertaining to death, dying, and life-prolonging medical treatments (without, perhaps, much clinical or technical knowledge), so too, should we engage in family dialogue about the possible benefits and risks of participating in genetics or other research studies.

2. To address the limited knowledge that many persons have about genetics and other biomedical research, we recommend that families begin to have conversations, being as specific as possible, about some of the possible benefits and risks of living in the time when one's DNA has become a valued commodity to biomedical researchers, research institutions, and biotechnology companies. Should these conversations become frustrating or produce more questions than answers, we should look for help from primary

care physicians, knowledgeable nurses, or appropriate organizations (e.g., Genetic Alliance in Washington, D.C.; GeneForum in Portland, Oregon; other well-informed organizations and their Web sites; the federal government's Web site that provides information about the health aspects of genetics research).[2]

As Patients in Hospitals and Clinics. Most persons, at least in technologically developed countries, are patients from time to time in hospitals and clinics. We run at least some risk that we will be asked for a blood, urine, or skin sample for diagnostic purposes—and that this tissue sample will subsequently be used for one or more post-diagnostic research studies. Whether we are informed about this research possibility, whether the tissue sample will actually be used in biomedical research, whether we are given an opportunity to give express, informed consent for this research, whether the sample will remain identified/ be coded/ or be anonymized in a lab, and whether the tissue-based research will be done in-house or external to the institution all depend on a number of variables. However these variables play out, some of us will, either with appropriately disclosed information or in ignorance, provide tissues that will later end up being used for research.

We hope that patients will increasingly be both aware of and informed about the possibility of post-diagnostic research and other secondary forms of research. For that to happen, several changes need to take place, among them a change in patients' perspectives about the possibility of human tissue research being done with tissues obtained from their bodies. If nonscientists are to become more knowledgeable about common research practices, and if they are to move from vague, worrisome concerns about genetics research to greater awareness about what physician-investigators, genetics investigators, and other biomedical researchers can do with stored tissues, questions need to be asked of surgeons, other physicians, nurses, genetic counselors, and other knowledgeable medical professionals. In addition, we should make our preferences and wishes known, perhaps in writing, about research studies that might be done with our tissue samples.

Of course, not everyone will formulate and express their preferences, much less put them in writing. Sometimes this is due to the huge knowledge gap between patients/participants and professionals. Historical experience with end-of-life decisions is instructive. For years many adults were reluctant to talk about critical or terminal illness with their families and physicians, complete an advance directive, or write down their own preferences about life-sustaining treatments in some clinical circumstances. Yet over the past two or three decades, millions of adult Americans have begun to talk about these important matters with their physicians, to fill out advance directives to communicate preferences for treatments wanted or not wanted, and to give, in writing, a trusted relative or friend the authorization to make surrogate health-care decisions should the need arise. (By most estimates, only 15%–20% of us have put our preferences regarding decisions near the end of life in writing, but knowledge and dialogue about these matters are far more pervasive in our society than they were just a quarter century ago.)

It is time—past time—openly and vigorously to address common concerns about research with stored tissues, whether that research takes place with clinically derived tissues or with tissues obtained from participants in standard research studies. Thoughtful patients and research participants should have the option of completing an advance directive for human tissue research studies, to make plain their desired role in this collaborative enterprise.

3. To provide adults with an alternative way of communicating choice about the use of personal tissues in research, we recommend that research advance directives become an acceptable option for use by patients and research participants who want to use these documents as a way of indicating their preferences for research studies done with their tissues.[3]

As Participants in Research Studies. As noted earlier, public opinion surveys regarding biomedical research indicate that many adults have concerns about the prospect of sometime participating in a genetics study via their stored tissues. *The concerns expressed are several:* loss of privacy, loss of control, inadequate confidentiality with tissue samples and derivative databases, the profit motive of some biomedical investigators, absent or inadequate disclosure about research plans, lack of opt-in or specific informed consent, and inadequate compensation for personal tissue samples used in successful, potentially lucrative research studies. The bottom-line implication of these concerns, so to speak, is both simple and stark: Should the limited findings of these surveys be substantiated by other surveys using different scientific methods and larger numbers of persons surveyed (including surveys in other countries), the results would certainly be cause for concern, not only for investigators at research institutions, but for all of us who support and value biomedical research.

We project two potentially beneficial options for dealing with these concerns in the near future, with both options already beginning to take place in a limited fashion. First, we call upon investigators, administrators of research institutions, and makers of public policy to speed up the public recognition that human tissue research is a collaborative process that needs to have the active, willing participation of both partners in the process if it is to proceed toward the completion of innumerable, fundamentally important research studies. Without more participants willing to provide tissues for research purposes, and without more and better funded investigators willing to dream the dreams, write the grants, and do the work in laboratories, the collective "we" simply will not realize some of the benefits we hope to see in the era of genomic medicine.

As just noted, patients (especially those in research-related hospitals) and potential research participants need to ask more questions, seek better information about tissue-based research studies, and become more involved in making informed decisions about their own participation in such studies with their tissue samples. Equally important, to make collaborative research studies more widely accepted by the general public, investigators need to be more forthright and informative in disclosures to potential research participants, administrators of research institutions need to increase public trust by making more information about research practices regularly available and by establishing greater institutional protections for stored tissues and research databases, and lawmakers need to make some long-overdue changes in the federal policy for research with human participants.

Second, we anticipate that an increasing number of interested, willing, and informed individuals and families will begin to take action themselves to try to ensure that human tissue research, especially research studies done on some specific medical conditions, is more collaborative in the future than it has been in the past. There are good reasons for such collaboration for both sets of partners in the research process. For example, some individuals and families are vitally interested in a specific genetic condition because it has had a profound, tragic role in their family history. They want, perhaps desperately, to help geneticists identify the gene or genes that cause the condition (or contribute to, or predispose toward the inheritance of the condition), be definitive about the inheritance pattern and penetrance of the gene(s), provide helpful information related to future procreation efforts, and move more rapidly toward effective treatment possibilities. Because they have familial experience with the heightened morbidity and mortality rates connected with the condition, they also have a heightened interest in helping investigators by providing tissues—and also, possibly, by eliciting tissues from other families with the same condition, so that, together, they can solve this particular medical mystery.

Some investigators also have reasons to pursue more explicitly collaborative arrangements than in the past. If, for instance, linked or coded samples are more scientifically and medically valuable, and/or more commercially valuable than anonymized samples in work on a particular genetic condition, there are good reasons to collaborate and maintain contact with the persons who have provided or may provide needed samples and information. In contrast to research with anonymized samples, where one blood sample is indistinguishable from hundreds or thousands of others in terms of individual origination, blood samples or other tissues that are linked with identifiable sample sources can often provide very important demographic and medical information. This additional information can, in turn, add to the possible commercial value of specific, coded samples that are scientifically unusual. Investigators and research teams working with coded samples also have two other options not possible with anonymous or anonymized samples: follow-ups for some individuals and families with helpful, periodically updated research information and clinically related information; and, if commercial profits are to be realized from particularly important research studies, the possibility of sharing this commercial gain in a way that is meaningful to the individual participants and, possibly, to their communities.

Two cases in recent years provide contrasting evidence that a more explicitly collaborative approach to human tissue research is sometimes possible, necessary, and mutually beneficial. Both cases began approximately the same way: Two American families with young children who have inherited different, rare, devastating genetic conditions. The parents in both cases were determined to help solve these medical mysteries and were not content to wait and hope for a scientific breakthrough. The parents' efforts in both cases involved, initially, contacting a few geneticists whose work seemed promising. They offered to contribute to cooperative geneticists' research studies by providing tissues for research, recruiting additional research participants from other families having the same genetic conditions, and, should more help become necessary, raising research funds and helping to manage databanks for the studies. The parents thus initiated several steps that were "revolutionary" in nature, in the sense of causing a paradigm shift to occur.[4] Rather than waiting to be recruited by one or more investigators working on these specific genetic conditions, the parents themselves initiated action with investigators and, thereby, clearly had collaborative roles in the subsequent scientific achievements.

Unfortunately, both cases have not, to date, had equally successful outcomes. In the Canavan disease case, briefly discussed in Chapter 7, the children's parents collaborated with a geneticist at Miami Children's Hospital to aid his successful efforts to isolate the gene associated with the disease. Subsequently, the geneticist went to another institution, the hospital got a patent and received exclusive licensing on a diagnostic test for Canavan disease, and the parents were sufficiently upset that they joined the Canavan Foundation and other plaintiffs in partially successful legal action against the hospital.[5]

By contrast, in a case briefly mentioned in Chapter 10, the parents of two children with PXE, a genetic disorder that causes calcification of connective tissues, have been more successful in meeting some of their important parental goals through collaboration with genetics investigators. Rather than waiting for geneticists to isolate the gene associated with PXE, and concerned, if the PXE gene should be found, that a scientist or a research institution might gain exclusive rights to the gene, Sharon and Patrick Terry decided to become activists in the pursuit of an effective medical treatment for their children's PXE. They established an advocacy group, PXE International, and found some cooperative geneticists at the University of Hawaii. The resulting collaboration was extraordinary. The Terrys provided the geneticists with blood and other tissue samples, solicited other families with PXE for tissue samples, set up their own tissue bank and registry (to protect the interests of patients and research participants), and had numerous conversations with other families and the Hawaii scientists about the symptoms of PXE. The geneticists succeeded in isolating the PXE gene in 1999, and the University of Hawaii joined

PXE International in taking the novel step of jointly applying for a patent on the diagnostic test for the gene. When both organizations received a provisional patent, they began negotiating the details for the final patent application that would enable them to keep the costs of genetic tests low and also to split any profits between the collaborators.[6]

4. To affirm that collaborative human tissue studies can take many forms, we recommend that potential research participants consider, depending on their situations, becoming more active in seeking new ways to strengthen and expand their roles in research studies.

Recommendations for Physician-Investigators and Other Biomedical Investigators

Most of our reasoned arguments, suggestions, and proposals in earlier chapters were intended for investigators, as well as IRBs, primarily, but not solely, those in academic institutions. Most investigators are aware of many of the ethical and regulatory aspects of their professional work. With this in mind, the following 10 recommendations are presented without further elaboration of their collective rationale and without attaching significance to their order. Each stands alone, all are interrelated, and all should lead to more collaborative human tissue studies in the future than in the past.

1. To affirm and protect the basic right of privacy, specifically *informational privacy,* investigators should make written information available to all potential research participants about the security measures that will be used (in the lab, with computer systems, and external to the lab) to protect (*a*) stored tissues and (*b*) the privacy and confidentiality of any personal and familial information contained in the tissues or in the databases that will be used in a research study.

2. To affirm and protect the important interest that many persons have in giving express, appropriately informed consent regarding what happens to tissues removed from their bodies for *long-term research studies,* investigators should disclose, in writing, several items of information to potential research participants about their policies and practices related to DNA banking (see Chapter 9):
   - the identity status of the DNA samples (identified, linked, anonymized) and the stored DNA data
   - the security measures for protecting samples and databases
   - the ownership of identified or linked samples in the lab
   - the procedures for withdrawing identified/linked samples and computerized data from the study
   - the planned length of storage of samples and data

- the policies for handling clinically relevant information discovered in identified or linked samples
- the policies regarding third-party access to identified/linked samples and data
- the research team's policies regarding re-use of identified/linked samples and data for secondary research purposes

3. To affirm and protect the important interest that many persons have in giving express, appropriately informed consent regarding what happens to tissues removed from their bodies (or their children's bodies) for diagnostic, therapeutic, and research reasons, physician-investigators and other researchers should go beyond the language of standard consent documents to *disclose additional items of information* to potential research participants, including appropriate patients, or parents/guardians of appropriate pediatric patients (see Chapters 9–10):

- the possibility of post-diagnostic research with the tissues
- the possibility of secondary research for other research purposes
- plans regarding anonymization of tissue samples, and what that means for persons from whom the samples were obtained
- plans regarding obtaining and using "extra tissue" for research
- relevant information about the investigator's financial interests in the planned research study
- possible, identifiable psychosocial harms to individuals (or group members) participating in the planned tissue study
- any options research participants have to indicate choices about acceptable or objectionable uses of their tissues (whether the samples remain identified, or will be coded or anonymized)

Implementation of HIPAA's privacy and security rules has already moved the research enterprise in some of these directions. Investigators and IRBs should assume responsibility for going still further. These recommendations are not intended to propose unnecessary impediments to timely research studies or to advocate impracticable, time-consuming, and seemingly endless lists of information to be included in consent documents. Rather, investigators (or members of their research teams) might handle these disclosures by formulating a multistudy template for items that can be used, with some specific-study tailoring, with multiple research studies.

The CDC sponsored a multidisciplinary task force a few years ago that produced a very helpful template for consent documents for population-based research involving genetics.[7] This model, appropriately modified, could well offer a useful foundation.

4. To address the general concern about ownership of tissues after they have been obtained from research participants, investigators should communicate to potential study participants, in writing, that after tissues have been

obtained from their bodies, the tissues (and derivative information from them stored in databases) are *owned, with limited property rights,* by the university or company employing the principal investigator. (This statement of ownership may have already been disclosed, but it will need to be revised to reflect joint ownership of tissue samples in unusual cases where such an arrangement has been negotiated in advance.)

5. To address the right of research participants to withdraw from research studies, investigators should affirm this right of participants in human tissue studies by describing, in writing, (*a*) the procedures that will need to be followed if a research participant requests the destruction of identified/linked tissue samples or database information, (*b*) any time limits on such requests, and (*c*) the practical limits on such requests whenever tissues and computerized data have been anonymized. (This statement may also have been previously covered.)

These two recommendations address one of the most contentious issues in the debate about human tissue research with banked DNA samples, whether the tissues are from living patients and research participants or from cadaveric bodies in pathology labs. We argued in earlier chapters that individuals—John Moore and the rest of us—are on sound moral and legal ground when we claim property-like interests in our bodily tissues, certainly while these tissues are part of our bodies but also, and more importantly, after these tissues have been removed from our bodies for diagnostic, therapeutic, or research purposes. As human beings, we have the moral right to exercise control over our bodies; the extent and scope of our legal right to do so depends on the laws of the country (or state) in which we live.

Under normal conditions of life (outside wars, prisons, and hospitals), we can legitimately claim to "own" our bodies in the sense of having *limited* property rights in our bodies, including tissues and organs. This moral and legal right is limited because we cannot do everything with our body parts that we can do with other things we own, and in which we have *full* property rights. For example, we cannot, with a few exceptions (e.g., blood, plasma, sperm, and occasionally ova), sell the tissues and organs in our bodies, but we can sell other items of property to which we have full property rights.[8]

The key question is whether, and to what extent, these limited property rights to our tissues and organs (and the personal information contained in those tissues) are retained once the tissues have been removed from our bodies. We maintain that, as a general matter, these limited property rights are grounded in the common moral and legal requirements of obtaining informed consent (or at least having implied or presumed consent) before anyone removes bodily tissues in a clinical or research setting. Consequently, we reject theories of abandonment, routine removal, expropriation, and social contract obligations, as these might be applied to the collection and use of tissues, to the extent each of these concepts asserts the rights of others, in particular investigators or society, to make claims in differing ways of complete ownership and use of our tissues without prior individual consent.

At the same time, in the context of human tissue research, the hospital, clinic, or company that employs the principal investigator and holds the stored tissues and any derivative information (usually in a lab), *also has limited property rights* to the same samples and related database information. If our description of human tissue research as a collaborative research process is correct, this *sequential sharing* of limited property rights to banked tissues, DNA, and data seems to follow. This means that both partners in this research endeavor either (*1*) retain or (*2*) come to have property-like interests in the tissues and information stored in the lab, but that both partners' property rights are limited, unless the research participant expressly transfers all rights to someone else. Thus participants retain the traditional right to withdraw from a research study at any time, and they may request that identified/linked tissue samples or database information be destroyed (correctly expecting this destruction and deletion to be done), but not if the samples and information have been anonymized.

The other partner's property rights are also limited. An investigator (and that person's employer or collaborator) obtain property rights in stored tissues and database information, but in a limited way. The investigator and/or employer have the options of selling anonymized samples, cell lines, and data, seeking a patent, or pursuing other commercial benefit from the stored tissues and data in a specific study, but they do not have the moral and legal right to sell identified tissues and data, nor should they, in our view, have the right to keep all the commercial gain from an unusual human tissue research study. Rather, as partners in a possibly lucrative research study, they should plan to share a portion of the profits in some way with the research participants who also contributed to the study.

6. To address the dual concerns about the profit motive of some investigators and the absence of standards regarding *any sharing of profits* in unusual, commercially gainful tissue studies with identified, linked, or anonymized samples, investigators should (*a*) make a disclosure about the role of personal profits in the research study (e.g., an investigator's financial interests in a for-profit company connected with the study) and also (*b*) make a written commitment to share a reasonable percentage (5%–10%) of any commercial profits from the study, if that should happen later, with one or more identified charitable organizations (see Chapter 10).

We know this recommendation is controversial. But we think that both disclosures are needed, for three reasons: to allay nonscientists' concerns about profit motives and conflicts of interest in biomedical research, to provide appropriate information for potential research participants as part of the process of informed consent, and to move human tissue studies toward a more genuinely collaborative model in which research participants have more of a personal stake in a research study even if, as is usually the case, they will not receive any medical benefits from their participation.

This recommendation is neither intended to contribute to the increasing commodification of the human body, nor to encourage the notion that human tissues should be bought and sold. Rather, as noted by the HUGO ethics committee, it is a realistic recognition of the large role that money plays in biomedical research and a call for a partial sharing of the financial rewards that, in rare cases, sometimes come to the investigators in unusually successful research studies. The reason for the range in the recommended percentage to be given to charity is simple. Because studies using anonymized samples are generally not dependent on specific individuals, it seems reasonable that the sharing of commercial profits from these studies be set at a lower rate than in other studies using identified tissues or samples linked to specific individuals.

7. To address the dual problems of possibly *objectionable research studies done with anonymized tissues* and the absence of clinical or informational follow-ups with anonymized tissues, we recommend that the frequent practice of anonymizing tissues for prospective research studies, often done for reasons of informational privacy protection and investigator convenience, be done only with the express, informed consent of the sample sources.

Tissue samples are often anonymized for good reasons. Yet an unknown number of thoughtful individuals and vulnerable groups find (or might find, if they knew about the studies) some types of research studies objectionable for personal reasons. Some, perhaps many, people neither want their tissues, even when anonymized, used for research purposes with which they do not agree, nor do they want their tissues, even when anonymized, used for research that might result in the stigmatization of a group or community to which they belong. Either way, an appropriate process of informed consent needs to make plain, in writing, a plan-to-anonymize-samples disclosure, thus giving potential research participants the option of making an informed choice.

8. To respond to the general concern about the lack of helpful follow-ups for research participants, investigators should develop a newsletter or some other mechanism for subsequent communications with identifiable participants in order to provide them, on a regular schedule or periodically, with updated information about relevant research studies and relevant clinical information.

9. To affirm that the human genome has been inherited from many individuals in earlier generations by all the world's peoples, investigators from technologically developed countries who collect DNA samples around the globe should agree to adhere to research practices that require (*a*) community

consultation and (*b*) a reasonable, site-specific combination of community approval and individual consent before tissue samples are obtained from indigenous groups for research studies (see Chapter 9).

10. To address the dual concerns that poorly educated individuals and groups in remote parts of the world are being coerced to give their DNA samples to Western scientists and that the DNA of indigenous peoples is being stolen from them, investigators should give appropriate community representatives a written commitment, in the dominant native language, pledging (*a*) to promote voluntary, informed participation in a research study and (*b*) to negotiate a percentage (5%–10%?) of any later profit from the study to be returned to the community for humanitarian purposes and community benefit.

The two previous recommendations affirm the developing trend of combining community consultation, community approval, and the individual consent of community members in research studies done with indigenous peoples. For reasons given in Chapter 9, the concept of "community consent" is unrealistic. At the same time, the elitist, paternalistic methods used in the past by some investigators from technologically advanced countries need to be changed. A specific way of carrying out a more collaborative model of research in any isolated location worldwide is for investigators to negotiate a contingent profit-sharing plan for tissue samples with community leaders if the unlikely should occur, namely that this specific research study should later end up making money.

Recommendations for Administrators of Research Institutions

All research-affiliated hospitals have policies that apply to the clinicians on staff, scientific investigators, patients, research participants, contractual agreements with external companies, institutional obligations to the federal government and accreditation bodies, and so forth. Included in this assortment of policies are codes of ethics, a patients' privacy notice and policies related to HIPAA requirements, a rights of patients statement, and similar documents. Also included in this panoply of policies are institutional statements pertaining to human tissues obtained by staff members for diagnostic, therapeutic, educational, and research purposes. Many other biomedical research institutions also have human-tissue-related documents that describe their policies on obtaining, storing, and using tissues for research.

If for some important reason (say, an upcoming accreditation visit), the central administrators of a research hospital needed to provide all human-tissue-related policies currently in effect, they could produce a variety of statements, guidelines, and policies: general consent documents for surgery, policy documents related to the pathology department, materials transfer agreements, and so on. Some of the policies would probably have been written decades ago, while others might have been developed in recent years. Three questions should be asked about these documents. How many were written with the interests of patients in mind? How many identify the rights and concerns that patients and research participants have related to their bodily tissues? How many commit the institution to an informative, collaborative, and appropriately consensual arrangement with patients and research participants?

Most administrators of research institutions are also quite aware of most of the ethical, legal, and regulatory aspects of their professional work. Still, the administrators of research-affiliated hospitals (and, when applicable, other research institutions)—central administrators, chairs of IRBs and other research committees, attorneys, department heads, chairs of tissue use committees, and chairs of institutional ethics committees—should consider the following recommendations.

1. To emphasize that adult patients have the right to make voluntary, informed choices about the future use of their tissues prior to letting a nurse, phlebotomist, or physician have one or more tissue samples, these administrators should initiate three changes in hospital policy and practice:

   (*a*) Make informed consent about the possible uses of human tissue (diagnostic, therapeutic, educational, and research) part of the *admissions process* by including a clear statement about these possible uses in an admissions document for all patients.

   (*b*) Produce two institution-wide lists: points of tissue collection that require the use of *written consent documents* (all surgeries, all skin biopsies, all tissues in assisted reproduction programs, all research with neonatal blood samples) and points of tissue collection that can function with less vigorous, sometimes *implied consent* (emergency rooms, critical care units, the treatment of patients lacking DMC, some diagnostic blood draws).

   (*c*) Make informed consent about the possible storage and long-term research use of personal tissue samples part of the *discharge planning process* by disclosing some information about research with stored DNA samples in a discharge document for all potentially affected patients, accompanied by a written opportunity for each patient or appropriate surrogate to consent to (or refuse) ongoing participation in this research option with stored tissues.

These recommendations emphasize the importance of institutional disclosure about research and other aspects of the informed consent process actually becoming a regular, multistep process in research institutions. Like many changes within complex institutions, implementation would take some time, patience, additional funding, and general acceptance before becoming a part of the institutional routine. But the benefits would be several: an affirmation that biomedical research is an essential feature of the institution, an increase in the disclosure about research practices (including post-diagnostic research) at several points of contact with patients, and a way of bringing substantially better informed patients into the loop of awareness about their participatory roles in that research process.

2. To address some of the general concerns that patients may have about biomedical research with their tissues and to increase their knowledge about and support for biomedical research, administrators should encourage physicians and physician-investigators in appropriate clinical areas to develop department-specific and clinic-specific informational brochures for patients (and family members in waiting rooms) to read about types of research studies currently being done or being planned for the near future, as well as appropriate Web sites for these educational purposes.

3. To clarify the matter of ownership of tissues, administrators should communicate in writing to all patients, as part of the admissions process, that after any tissues have been obtained from their bodies, the tissues are owned, with limited property rights, by the hospital (or university/company owning the hospital) and can be used, with a patient's written or implied consent, for diagnostic, therapeutic, and clinically related research purposes pertaining to the provision of medical care, as in much of the research done in a pathology department.

Disagreement about the ownership and control of tissue samples is compounded by the fact, discussed in earlier chapters, that tissues are sometimes obtained from patients' bodies in hospitals for one set of acknowledged purposes (improved diagnosis, more effective medical care), yet occasionally end up being used for another, secondary purpose (biomedical research). Human tissues are not "abandoned" when they are being used for either the primary purposes or the secondary purpose. Rather, when they are obtained from a patient's body in a hospital, they are then owned by that hospital, but in a limited way. This *sequential, limited ownership* means that if and when this tissue is to become part of a research study, an identifiable source of that sample takes on the rights of a research participant, including the right to consent to participation in the study and also the right to withdraw from the study by requesting that the research tissue sample and any derivative database information be destroyed.

It is equally true that a research hospital, having acquired tissue samples with consent, gains limited ownership of those samples. Thus investigators working in a research lab can take some of those tissue samples and use them in multiple ways for various research purposes, including possibly anonymizing some of them, transforming some of them into cell lines, and, in rare cases, seeking to use some of them for commercially gainful ends.

4. To respond to the concerns, expressed both by patients and investigators, about the comingling of clinical and research roles by physician-investigators

and the resulting difficulty of protecting the privacy and confidentiality of identifiable patients' tissue samples in research labs, institutional administrators should work with department heads to establish either (*a*) *a single institutional tissue bank* (providing an institutional "firewall" between the identifiable tissues collected by clinicians in all departments, and all biomedical investigators) or (*b*) a system of similarly organized departmental tissue banks.

Led by some pathologists, bioethicists, and health-law attorneys around the country, there has been an increasing effort in recent years to address these related problems in human tissue research, problems that are especially difficult to handle in the many, very complex biomedical research institutions that exist here. Separated from the institutional politics that make research-related practice changes difficult in any research institution, the position that has gained some backing is the one we summarized above.

With more details added, but still in summary form, this recommendation calls for research institutions to establish a single institutional tissue bank directed by a tissue bank "trustee." The tissue bank trustee (and other employees) would be given the fiduciary duty of protecting, on the institution's behalf and with IRB authorization, the anonymity of patients whose tissues are used for research by pathologists and investigators in other departments. To that end, the trustee and tissue-bank colleagues would function as a tissue-code-installing firewall between clinicians who collect and sometimes store *identified tissues* from patients (for reasons pertaining to the provision of medical care), and all investigators who would henceforth do research on tissues originally obtained from patients only with *coded* tissues distributed by the bank, as well as, of course, other tissues obtained from research participants and other tissue sources.[9]

5. To enable IRBs to do a more responsible job with the continually increasing demands placed on them, administrators should strengthen and update these review committees in several ways: add members with expertise in the research techniques of molecular genetics; compensate members more appropriately for the considerable committee work they do; give them a mandate to keep track of the numbers and types of tissues and related databases used for research purposes in the institution; encourage them to make more use of Web-based educational resources for IRB members and investigators; and provide them with opportunities to learn more about the traditions and values of indigenous research participants in other parts of the world.

IRBs can and should have a more significant role in human tissue research than they do. Beyond fine-tuning the language in consent documents, IRBs should be given an institutional mandate with an expanded oversight role for documenting, tracking, and managing certain parts of research studies using stored tissues. One specific way of doing this would be for institutions to require that IRBs review all protocols involving genetics studies with tissue samples from deceased individuals. Whenever that review determined that the proposed research would generate information that might be relevant to living family members, the investigators would be required to gain the informed consent of one or more family members.[10] As mentioned earlier, this approach involving IRB review and, possibly, subsequent family consent could be used as an alternative to the routine seeking of consent from the surviving family for all retrospective research with archived samples in pathology labs.

Producing significant change in institutions is never easy. Yet changing the ways that human tissue studies are done in research-oriented hospitals is important and long overdue. Equally important, *changing the ways that this biomedical research is portrayed* to patients and the general public is necessary. Our hope is that administrators will promote—not hide—the indispensably important research done with tissues collected from patients, as well as with tissues obtained from volunteer participants in research studies. By not continuing the "what they don't know won't hurt them" traditional approach, characterized by vague, uninformative general consent documents, administrators may bring about some needed changes in their institutions: disclosing more information about the human tissue research done there, doing a better job in protecting the interests of sample sources, and giving patients the public gratitude that is rightfully due them for their collaborative role in biomedical research.

Recommendations for Makers of Public Policy Related to Human Participants Research

We conclude with some general recommendations for the persons in the federal government who draft and interpret the regulations on research with human participants, the Common Rule.[11] Other persons and groups, notably the earlier NIH/CDC workshop group and, importantly, NBAC, have recommended multiple changes regarding the language of the regulations and their interpretation by the Office of Human Research Protections, local IRBs, and editors of research journals.

Taking a different path, we highlight five thematic changes that need to be made to the federal regulations, leaving to the appropriate policymakers the formidable task of crafting specific policy and regulatory changes consistent with the themes developed earlier. We hope that changes made in U.S. policies for research with DNA samples will be consistent with some of the better research policies in other technologically advanced countries.

The five themes for change are these:

1. Required, informative disclosure to potential research participants by scientific investigators, including disclosure of financial conflicts of interest and the prospects of commercial gain from a research study

2. Required, authentic expressions of informed consent, appropriate to specific clinical and research settings, including written consent (not implied, presumed, or general "consent") for secondary research with identified or coded samples and for permission to anonymize personal samples

3. Recognition of the right of self-determination, including the right not to participate, via one's stored tissue samples, in research studies that are objectionable to the sample source

4. Recognition of the traditions, values, and interests of identifiable groups being recruited for research purposes, whether in the United States or elsewhere in the world, with the requirement of community consultation and a combination of community approval and individual consent before any DNA samples are collected

5. Recognition of the psychosocial harms that can occur to participants (both individuals and groups) in genetics research studies, with an attendant raising of the bar in interpreting the regulatory "minimal risk of harm" so that nonphysical harms and harms to groups are included.

We do not expect that these proposed changes in the federal regulations, if implemented, will end the debate about research with stored tissues. That debate will and should continue, as illustrated by its inclusion in a recent "Controversies in Internal Medicine" issue of *Archives of Internal Medicine*.[12] One surgeon's emphatic description of the issue is telling: "There should be no doubt about what is at stake in developing policy for the use of stored samples: the fundamental right to decide whether and how one's body and its parts will be used in research."[13] The issues are indeed fundamental—and the stakes are high. We are convinced that greater public support for biomedical research, and more success in recruiting individuals and groups for important research studies, may depend, in part, on bringing about greater collaboration between investigators in human tissue studies and the persons from whom those tissues come.

Notes

1. Melissa Austin, Sarah Harding, and Courtney McElroy, "Genebanks: A Comparison of Eight Proposed International Genetic Databases," *Community Genet* 6 (2003): 37–45.

2. For more information, check these helpful Web sites. For information about groups in the Genetic Alliance, see http://www.geneticalliance.org/. For information provided by GeneForum about genetics, education, and public policy issues, see http://www.geneforum.org/. For information from the National Human Genome Research Institute about the health aspects of genetics research, see http://www.genome.gov.

3. For three model research advance directives, see Robert F. Weir, "Advance Directives for the Use of Stored Tissue Samples," in Robert Weir, ed., *Stored Tissue Samples* (Iowa City: University of Iowa, 1998): 236–66.

4. Thomas Kuhn, *The Structure of Scientific Revolutions* (Chicago: University of Chicago Press, 1970).

5. Gina Kolata, "Sharing of Profits Is Debated As the Value of Tissue Rises," *New York Times,* May 15, 2000, pp. A1, A15; Eliot Marshall, "Families Sue Hospital, Scientist For Control of Canavan Gene," *Science* 290 (2000): 1062; and *Greenberg v. Miami Children's Hosp. Research Institute,* 264 F. Supp. 2d 1064.

6. Paul Smaglik, "Tissue donors use their influence in deal over gene patent terms," *Nature* 407 (2000): 821. For additional information about PXE International, see their Web site: http://www.pxe.org.

7. Laura Beskow et al., "Informed Consent for Population-Based Research Involving Genetics," *JAMA* 286 (2001): 2315–21. The informed consent template is summarized in the article and printed on the CDC Web site: http://www.cdc.gov/genomics/info/reports/consent.htm.

8. James F. Childress, *Practical Reasoning in Bioethics* (Bloomington: Indiana University Press, 1997), pp. 282–300.

9. Jon Merz, Pamela Sankar, Sheila Taube, and Virginia Livolsi, "Use of Human Tissues in Research: Clarifying Clinician and Researcher Roles and Information Flows," *J Investig Med* 45 (1997): 252–57.

10. An anonymous reviewer of this manuscript indicated that the IRB at his or her institution is mandated to review protocols for some retrospective genetics studies in this manner.

11. 45 C.F.R. 46.

12. Farrell Lloyd and Adriane Budavari, "Controversies in Internal Medicine: A New Feature in the *Archives,*" *Arch Intern Med* 162 (2002): 1441.

13. Robert Sade, "Research on Stored Biological Samples Is Still Research," *Arch Intern Med* 162 (2002): 1440.

Appendix

Index of Acronyms

Index

Abandonment of tissues, 103, 106–9, 165, 169–71, 286–88
Abbott, Alison, 21*n*
Access to genetic information, 215, 309–10
Advisory Committee on Human Radiation Experiments, 202
Affymetrix, 64, 84
African Americans, 42, 277
Agilent Technologies, 84
AIDS, 18
Alder Hey Royal Liverpool Children's Hospital (England), 41
Allen, Anita, 194*n*, 198*n*, 301*n*
Altman, Lawrence, 304*n*
Alzheimer disease, 24, 31, 192, 227, 265, 309
American Academy of Pediatrics, 253–54, 268*n*, 282, 302*n*
American Association of Blood Banks, 4, 76
American Association of Medical Colleges (AAMC), 3, 20*n*, 57–63, 67*n*, 230, 251, 266*n*, 267*n*, 304*n*
American Association of Tissue Banks, 26
American College of Medical Genetics (ACMG), 51, 54, 59–62, 66*n*, 246, 249, 267*n*

American College of Obstetrics and Gynecology, 227
American Health Consultants, 219
American Healthstyles Survey, 30–31
American Journal of Human Genetics, 55
American Red Cross, 25
American Society for Reproductive Medicine, 77
American Society of Human Genetics, 54–55, 59–62, 66*n*, 267*n*, 276
American Type Culture Collection, 25, 290
Americans with Disabilities Act, 35, 186–91
AMRAD, 264
Anderson, Ross, 20*n*
Andrews, Edmund, 127*n*
Andrews, Lori, 66*n*, 171, 192*n*, 195*n*, 289, 303*n*
Annas, George, 21*n*, 50, 64, 66*n*, 67*n*, 194*n*, 198n, 223, 266*n*, 268*n*, 269*n*
Appelbaum, Paul, 152*n*
Arabian, Justice, 160
Arap, Wadih, 150
Armed Forces Institute of Pathology, 24, 205
Arnason, Einar, 269*n*
Ashburn, Ted, 22
Ashkenazi Jews, 17, 29–30, 145, 191, 272